Patient-Reported Outcomes

Measurement, Implementation and Interpretation

Chapman & Hall/CRC Biostatistics Series

Editor-in-Chief

Shein-Chung Chow, Ph.D., Professor, Department of Biostatistics and Bioinformatics,
Duke University School of Medicine, Durham, North Carolina

Series Editors

Byron Jones, Biometrical Fellow, Statistical Methodology, Integrated Information Sciences,
Novartis Pharma AG, Basel, Switzerland

Jen-pei Liu, Professor, Division of Biometry, Department of Agronomy,
National Taiwan University, Taipei, Taiwan

Karl E. Peace, Georgia Cancer Coalition, Distinguished Cancer Scholar, Senior Research Scientist
and Professor of Biostatistics, Jiann-Ping Hsu College of Public Health,
Georgia Southern University, Statesboro, Georgia

Bruce W. Turnbull, Professor, School of Operations Research and Industrial Engineering,
Cornell University, Ithaca, New York

Published Titles

Chapman & Hall/CRC Biostatistics Series

Patient-Reported Outcomes

Measurement, Implementation and Interpretation

Joseph C. Cappelleri
Kelly H. Zou
Andrew G. Bushmakin
Jose Ma. J. Alvir
Demissie Alemayehu
Tara Symonds

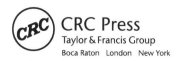

CRC Press
Taylor & Francis Group
Boca Raton London New York

CRC Press is an imprint of the
Taylor & Francis Group, an **informa** business

A CHAPMAN & HALL BOOK

CRC Press
Taylor & Francis Group
6000 Broken Sound Parkway NW, Suite 300
Boca Raton, FL 33487-2742

First issued in paperback 2016

© 2014 by Taylor & Francis Group, LLC
CRC Press is an imprint of Taylor & Francis Group, an Informa business

No claim to original U.S. Government works

Version Date: 20140331

ISBN 13: 978-1-138-19959-0 (pbk)
ISBN 13: 978-1-4398-7367-0 (hbk)

Library of Congress Cataloging-in-Publication Data

Cappelleri, Joseph C., author.
    Patient-reported outcomes : measurement, implementation and interpretation / Joseph C. Cappelleri [and 5 others].
        p. ; cm. -- (Chapman & Hall/CRC biostatistics series)
    Includes bibliographical references and index.
    Summary: "Covering conceptual and statistical methods, this book discusses the issues related to measuring and interpreting patient reported outcomes (PROs). It begins with a review and background information and then covers measurement scales, validity and reliability, item response theory, and missing data. The book also describes various statistical analysis techniques, including exploratory, cross-sectional, and longitudinal data analysis, and highlights the practical interpretation and application of the techniques in clinical and pharmaceutical settings. SAS code for all methods is available in an appendix and online"--Provided by publisher.
        ISBN 978-1-4398-7367-0 (hardback)
    I. Title. II. Series: Chapman & Hall/CRC biostatistics series (Unnumbered)
    [DNLM: 1. Data Interpretation, Statistical. 2. Outcome Assessment (Health Care) 3. Health Care Evaluation Mechanisms.
    4. Patient Participation. W 84.41]

    R853.S7
    610.72'7--dc23   2013034194

Visit the Taylor & Francis Web site at
http://www.taylorandfrancis.com

and the CRC Press Web site at
http://www.crcpress.com

Contents

Preface

A patient-reported outcome (PRO) is any report on the status of a patient's health condition that comes directly from the patient, without interpretation of the patient's response by a clinician or anyone else. This monograph serves as an up-to-date treatise on central and analytical issues of PRO measures. The monograph covers both introductory and advanced psychometric methods, with applications and illustrations given throughout as examples, infused with the current state of the science.

The purpose of this volume is to provide a current assessment of several key elements of PRO measures for the benefit of graduate students in a health discipline and especially to biopharmaceutical researchers and others in the health sciences community who wish to develop or enrich their understanding of PRO methodology, particularly from a quantitative perspective. Key concepts, infused with psychometric and biostatistical methods for constructing and analyzing PRO measures, are highlighted, illustrated, and advanced to inform and educate readers about the measurement, implementation, and interpretation of PRO measures. Real-life examples from the literature and simulated examples using SAS® are used to illustrate the concepts and the methodology.

The biopharmaceutical industry is the major sponsor of PRO measures. Our book is intended to cater to the needs of the biopharmaceutical industry, as well as to research enterprises collaborating with it, in order to advance the development, validation, and use of PRO measures.

All simulated datasets in this monograph are grounded in or motivated by real-life phenomena and placed in the context of the concepts and illustrations embodied in their corresponding chapters. As such, all simulated datasets are not artificially or randomly produced without direction; instead, they are targeted to practical scenarios. The simulations are intended as teaching tools to further grasp, more deeply, concepts and illustrations explained beforehand. Therefore, the simulations provide the opportunity to learn by doing and by example. In addition to serving as a primer, this volume also serves to document, align, and summarize the state of the science on several key aspects of PRO development and methodology.

We are all employees of Pfizer Inc, a research-based pharmaceutical company that manufactures and markets pregabalin, sildenafil, sunitinib, varenicline, and other medicines. Empirical examples are generally drawn from applications of Pfizer medicines and come from published and peer-reviewed sources based on research and scholarship that we were intimately involved in and are in the best position to communicate. These examples, chosen to highlight real-life applications based on our first-hand experience, are intended solely and strictly for educational and pedagogical purposes.

The content of new PRO measures should be developed rigorously and often iteratively. Chapter 1 introduces health measurement scales and follows with some key elements in the development of a PRO measure. Chapter 2 expands on the conceptual framework that should be an intrinsic part of the development of a PRO instrument, a framework used to depict the relationship between items in a PRO instrument and the concepts measured by it.

Validity, the evidence and extent that the PRO taps into the concept that it is purported to measure in a particular setting, is assessed in a number of ways: content validity and the various forms of construct validity. The reliability of a PRO instrument, the consistency or reproducibility of the measure, is assessed by internal consistency and test–retest reliability. Validity and reliability are discussed in Chapters 3 and 4, respectively.

Chapter 5 covers, in detail, exploratory and confirmatory factor analysis. Exploratory factor analysis can be used to find the number of concepts (also called factors or domains) and to determine which items go with which concepts. In doing so, it lends structure and validity to a PRO instrument. Confirmatory factor analysis of a PRO instrument is used when the concepts within the measure are known. Confirmatory factor analysis tests whether the observed pattern of correlations conforms to a prespecified number of factors and to a theoretical framework of which observed items are related and not related to which factors.

Chapter 6 covers item response theory (IRT), which has become more prominent in the validation of a measure, and complements the chapters on psychometrics that tend to focus generally on classical test theory (CTT), which assumes that the observed score for a subject is equal to the subject's true score plus some random error. Rather than replacing the CTT methodology, the IRT methodology can be more constructively viewed as a potentially important complement to CTT for scale development, evaluation, and refinement in certain circumstances.

Cross-sectional analysis of PRO items or domain scores is the analysis of data at a single time point. Chapter 7 highlights cross-sectional comparisons of two or more groups and testing of PRO endpoints. Chapter 8 covers longitudinal analysis of scores from a PRO measure based on an analysis of data over multiple time points, with each subject expected to have a series of repeated measurements on the PRO, and is an essential topic for determining the responsiveness of a PRO measure, a key attribute for any such measure.

Chapter 9 discusses mediation modeling as a way to identify and explain the mechanism that underlies an observed relationship between an independent variable (e.g., treatment) and a dependent variable (e.g., sleep disturbance) via the inclusion of a third explanatory variable (e.g., pain), known as a mediator variable. The independent variable, dependent variable, or the mediator variable, or all, can be a PRO measure.

Chapter 10 covers the subject of missing data on PRO measures. Missing data can take three forms: (1) missing data in the entire domain (i.e., subscale or concept of interest), (2) missing data in the entire questionnaire (all domains), and (3) missing items in a part of a multi-item domain. The chapter covers how to deal with missing data.

Finally, interpretation of PRO results extends beyond statistical significance to emphasize the meaning of results, and its clinical importance, especially as it relates to treatment benefit. Being intrinsically subjective, a PRO measure needs to have its scores interpreted, and this interpretation has become central to its usefulness as a measure of treatment outcome. Chapter 11 focuses on techniques to address this very important issue, along with the topic of multiple testing.

Of course, more topics related to PROs, such as sample size estimation, meta-analysis and generalizability theory, to name just a few, could have been included. The topics chosen reflect what we consider to be among the most relevant, given the book's objectives and space restrictions.

Numerous references are provided for a more detailed and comprehensive examination of the material. For readers who are interested in conducting statistical analyses of PRO measures and delving more into intricacies, most chapters contain SAS code and output that illustrate the methodology. Also being referenced is the final guidance from the US Food and Drug Administration (FDA) and a reflection paper from the European Medicines Agency on PRO measures in medical product development, which outline necessary steps required for regulatory purposes.

Joseph C. Cappelleri
Kelly H. Zou
Andrew G. Bushmakin
Jose Ma. J. Alvir
Demissie Alemayehu
Tara Symonds

Disclosure and Acknowledgment

All of us are current employees of Pfizer Inc. Additional editorial support was not provided. However, this monograph is intended strictly as a scientific and not commercial treatise for educational and instructional purposes, with emphasis on the methodology of patient-reported outcomes.

We are particularly grateful to a number of colleagues for reviewing this document and providing constructive comments as the work proceeded. Special thanks go to Lucy Abraham, Helen Bhattacharyya, Claire Burbridge, Friedhelm Leverkus, Natasa Rajicic, and Katja Rudell.

Authors

Joseph C. Cappelleri earned his MS in statistics from the City University of New York, his PhD in psychometrics from Cornell University, and his MPH in epidemiology from Harvard University. He is a senior director of statistics at Pfizer Inc. He is also an adjunct professor of medicine at Tufts Medical Center and an adjunct professor of statistics at the University of Connecticut. He has delivered numerous conference presentations and has published extensively on clinical and methodological topics. He has also been instrumental in developing and validating a number of patient-reported outcomes for different diseases and conditions. He is a fellow of the American Statistical Association.

Kelly H. Zou earned her MA and PhD in statistics from the University of Rochester. She completed her postdoctoral training in health-care policy and radiology at Harvard Medical School. She is a director of statistics at Pfizer Inc. She has served as an associate or deputy editor for *Statistics in Medicine*, *Radiology*, and *Academic Radiology*. She was an associate professor in radiology and director of biostatistics at Harvard Medical School. She is the lead author of *Statistical Evaluation of Diagnostic Performance: Topics in ROC Analysis* published by Chapman & Hall/CRC Press. She is a fellow of the American Statistical Association and an accredited professional statistician.

Andrew G. Bushmakin earned his MS in applied mathematics and physics from the National Research Nuclear University (former Moscow Engineering Physics Institute, Moscow, Russia). He has more than 20 years of experience in mathematical modeling and data analysis. He is an associate director of statistics at Pfizer Inc. He has coauthored numerous articles and presentations on topics ranging from mathematical modeling of neutron physics processes to patient-reported outcomes.

Jose Ma. J. Alvir earned his DrPH in epidemiology from Columbia University. He is a senior director of statistics at Pfizer Inc. He was an associate professor at the Albert Einstein College of Medicine of Yeshiva University and later at New York University School of Medicine. He has published extensively on clinical and methodological topics. He has served as the industry representative on the Medicare Evidence Development and Coverage Advisory Committee and is editor of the *Biopharmaceutical Report* of the American Statistical Association.

Demissie Alemayehu earned his PhD in statistics from the University of California, Berkeley. He is a vice president of statistics at Pfizer Inc. He has been on the faculties of Columbia University and Western Michigan University.

He is a fellow of the American Statistical Association. He has published widely and has served on the editorial boards of major journals, including the *Journal of the American Statistical Association* and the *Journal of Nonparametric Statistics*.

Tara Symonds earned her BSc in behavioral sciences and PhD in health psychology from Huddersfield University. She is a senior director of outcomes research at Pfizer Ltd. She is also a chartered health psychologist. She has more than 18 years of experience in developing and implementing patient-reported outcome (PRO) measures for use in clinical research. She has presented at numerous conferences and published widely covering various topics related to PRO measures.

1

Introduction

1.1 Patient-Reported Outcomes in Perspective

The US Food and Drug Administration (FDA, 2009) defines a patient-reported outcome (PRO) measure as follows:

> Any report of the status of a patient's health condition that comes directly from the patient, without interpretation of the patient's response by a clinician or anyone else. The outcome can be measured in absolute terms (e.g., severity of a symptom, sign, or state of a disease) or as a change from a previous measure. In clinical trials, a PRO instrument can be used to measure the effect of a medical intervention on one or more concepts (i.e., the thing being measured, such as a symptom or group of symptoms, effects on a particular function or group of functions, or a group of symptoms or functions shown to measure the severity of a health condition).

Thus, PRO is an umbrella term that includes a whole host of subjective outcomes such as pain, fatigue, depression, aspects of well-being (e.g., physical, functional, psychological), treatment satisfaction, health-related quality of life, and physical symptoms such as nausea and vomiting. While the term *health-related quality of life* (HRQL) has been frequently used instead of PRO, HRQL has a broad and encompassing definition that consumes a whole array of health attributes collectively, including general health, physical functioning, physical symptoms and toxicity, emotional functioning, cognitive functioning, role functioning, social well-being and functioning, and sexual functioning, among others. As a more suitable term than HRQL, PRO measures accommodate health questionnaires whose objective is to measure a patient's health, be it HRQL, symptom, satisfaction with treatment, functioning, well-being—whatever the purpose—from the patient's perspective rather than from a physician, caretaker, or biological measure.

PROs are often relevant in studying a variety of conditions—including pain, erectile dysfunction, fatigue, migraine, mental functioning, physical functioning, and depression—that cannot be assessed adequately without a patient's evaluation and whose key questions require patient's input on the impact of a disease or a treatment. After all the patient knows best. To be useful to patients and other decision makers (e.g., clinicians, researchers, regulatory agencies, reimbursement authorities), who are stakeholders in medical care, a PRO must undergo a validation process to confirm that it measures what it is intended to measure reliably and accurately.

The term *patient* in *patient-reported outcome* is apt because in this book interest centers mainly on individuals whose health is compromised enough to seek medical treatment. Although not all subjects as *patients* are ill or have a condition, and therefore do not seek medical treatment, the term *patient-reported outcome* as used here is broad enough to also include *healthy* subjects or persons who may also take part in an overall health survey, typically as part of a nontreatment intervention study. Self-report scores from healthy subjects can be useful for the purpose of better understanding the properties of a PRO and also to help enrich the meaning and interpretation of PRO scores.

Some PROs are intended for generic use, irrespective of the illness or condition of the patient, and may often be applicable to healthy people as well. Healthy people may complete a health questionnaire as part of a population or sample survey or as part of a method study to evaluate the PRO. Examples of generic PRO questionnaires that capture various aspects of health status include the EuroQoL (Brooks et al., 1996), Medical Outcomes Study 36-Item Short Form (Ware et al., 1993), Nottingham Health Profile (Hunt et al., 1981), and Sickness Impact Profile (Bergner et al., 1981), to name just a few.

There are many other PRO instruments that are useful for measuring the impact of a specific disease, PRO measures that are considered condition or disease specific. These types of PRO measures may capture certain aspects of health status found in the generic PROs, depending on their purpose, but are usually specifically tailored to measure the special characteristics found in particular conditions or diseases. Examples include the following (among others): The European Organisation for Research and Treatment of Cancer QLQ-C30 (Aaronson et al., 1993), Functional Assessment of Cancer Therapy–General (Cella et al., 1993), International Index of Erectile Function (Rosen et al., 1997), National Eye Institute Visual Functioning Questionnaire (Mangione et al., 2001), Paediatric Asthma Quality of Life Questionnaire (Juniper et al., 1996), Quality of Life in Epilepsy (Devinsky et al., 1995), and Rotterdam Symptom Checklist (de Haes et al., 1996). Hospital Anxiety and Depression Scale for measurement of anxiety and depression (Zigmond and Snaith, 1983), McGill Pain Questionnaire for measurement of pain (Melzack, 1975), Multidimensional Fatigue Inventory for measurement of fatigue (Smets et al., 1995), and Barthel Index of Disability for measurement of functional dependency (Shah et al., 1989).

1.2 Patient-Reported Outcomes in Clinical Research

In general, the same clinical trial design principles that apply to directly assessable clinical endpoint measures (be they clinician based or biologically based), such as blood pressure, also apply to PROs. Although not necessarily unique to PROs, at least five characteristics tend to be associated with PROs (Fairclough, 2004). One characteristic is that, by definition, PROs require the patient's active participation, resulting in the potential for missing data from not only missed assessments on an entire PRO but also nonresponse of some items on a PRO used in a clinical study. A second characteristic is that, being subjective and not an objective endpoint like death, PROs require their measurement properties to be assessed, leading to additional steps of validation (reliability and validity) prior to their analysis on treatment effect. A third characteristic, related to the second one of subjectivity, is that special steps and methods may be needed to enhance the interpretation of PROs. A fourth characteristic is that most PROs are multidimensional and hence produce multiple scores on various aspects of what is being measured, engendering multiple comparisons and testing of outcomes that need to be at least methodologically considered and possibly statistically addressed. The fifth characteristic is that the outcomes are generally repeated over time, calling for methods that effectively handle longitudinal data in the context of the research question.

Identifying which components of a PRO are relevant to measuring the impact of a disease or effect of a treatment is essential to good study design and subsequent scientific scrutiny. Successful measurement of PROs begins with the development of a protocol to provide a guide for the conduct of the study. The protocol provides not only key elements of the study design but also the scientific rationale and planned analysis for the study, which are inextricably linked to the study design.

Because the validation of PROs is an ongoing process, multiple protocols, each having its specific purpose, may often be necessary. A protocol for a study, be it a clinical trial or a method study, should contain several essential elements: the rationale for the specific aspect of PRO being measured, explicit research objectives and endpoints, rationale for timing of assessments, rationale for instrument selection, details for administration of PRO assessments to minimize bias and missing data, sample size estimation, and analytic plan (Fairclough, 2004, 2010).

A method study protocol involves, by definition, methodological considerations, such as which measurement properties of a PRO will be tested, and these considerations will define the design of the study. For example, if an objective is to obtain test–retest reliability data, data should be collected on at least two occasions. Contrary to a clinical trial design, which includes a preselected diseased population at baseline, method studies may not involve any treatment and may include a variety of subjects from healthy to severely ill for whom a PRO is designed to assess.

The CONSORT (Consolidated Standards of Reporting Trials) Statement, first published in 1996 and most recently revised in 2010 (Moher et al., 2010; Schulz et al., 2010), aims to improve the reporting of randomized controlled trials. The CONSORT PRO extension has been developed for use in conjunction with the CONSORT 2010 Statement and other explanation and elaboration articles (appropriate for the trial design, intervention, and outcomes) (Moher et al., 2010; Schulz et al., 2010). As the central part of the CONSORT PRO extension, five checklist items are recommended for randomized controlled trials in which PROs are primary or secondary endpoints: (1) that the PROs be identified as a primary or secondary outcome in the abstract, (2) that a description of the hypotheses of the PROs and its relevant domains be provided if applicable (i.e., if a multidimensional PRO tool has been used), (3) that evidence of the PRO instrument's validity and reliability be provided or cited, (4) that the statistical approaches for dealing with missing data be explicitly stated, and (5) that PRO-specific limitation of study findings and generalizability of result to other populations and clinical practice be discussed (Calvert et al., 2013). And we would argue for a sixth criterion of explicitly stating the responder definition or clinical important difference definition for each endpoint to aid in the interpretation of results.

1.2.1 Label Claims

Data generated by a PRO can provide a statement of a treatment benefit from the patient perspective. For a treatment benefit to be meaningful, though, there should be evidence that the PRO under consideration effectively measures the particular concept (or construct or attribute) that is studied. Generally, findings measured by PROs may be used to support claims in approved medical product labeling when the claims are derived from adequate and well-controlled investigations in which PROs measure specific concepts accurately and as intended. Such PROs can be developed and assessed in accordance with regulatory guidance documents from the FDA (2009) and the EMA (2005). Other published sources can be consulted (Chassany et al., 2002; Patrick et al., 2007; Revicki et al., 2007; Luo and Cappelleri, 2008; Bottomley et al., 2009; Coons et al., 2011; Fehnel et al., 2011; Hareendran et al., 2012). Even if the intent is not to seek a label claim, at least some elements (as part of good scientific practice) from these guidance documents will be helpful for questionnaire development and assessment.

A review of PRO labels granted from 1997 to 2002 in the United States showed that PRO evidence was cited in the clinical studies section of the label for 30% of the new medical product approvals and that 11% of the new products were approved on the basis of PROs alone (Willke et al., 2004). Since then, from 2006 to 2010 (the 5-year period since the release of the 2006 draft FDA guidance on PROs for a label claim), 116 medical products were identified (Gnanasakthy et al., 2012) with 28 (24%) being granted PRO claims; 24 of these 28 (86%) were symptoms and, of these, 9 (38%) were pain-related products. Of the 28 products with PRO claims, a PRO was a primary endpoint for 20 (71%), all symptom-related. During this 5-year period (2006–2010), the majority of accepted claims were supported by simple one-item scales or on the basis of measures traditionally accepted by reviewing divisions of the FDA. A purpose of this book is to provide the methodological rigor and scientific basis to expand the reach of potential PRO label claims into multi-item scales that are not necessarily symptom based.

Research has indicated that the EMA was more likely than the FDA to grant PRO claims and to do so for higher-order concepts such as functioning and health-related quality of life (DeMuro et al., in press). Despite this discordance, a general degree of concordance was found when label types (e.g., symptoms and functioning) were analyzed for products with PRO label claims granted by both the FDA and the EMA. It was concluded that further research that creates strategic alignment between agencies would be beneficial. In a related investigation, it was found that the primary reasons for FDA denial of a PRO label claim included issues of fit for purpose; issues of study design, data quality, interpretation; statistical issues; administrative issues; and lack of demonstrated treatment benefit (DeMuro et al., 2012).

Both the EMA and the FDA have provided guidance on the qualification process for drug development tools (DDTs) (EMA, 2009; FDA, 2010). These guidance documents on DDTs can serve as a complementary adjunct to the guidance on PROs for label claims to ensure expeditious review of the new measure for use in clinical trials and potential product labeling. All too frequently, innovative and improved DDTs are delayed, which results in missed opportunities for ensuring DDTs are adequate for allowing product labeling; hopefully, these new DDT processes will help with this situation.

If a DDT is qualified, analytically valid measurement on it can be relied upon to have a specific use and interpretable meaning in drug development. The objective is to develop innovative and improved DDTs that can help streamline the drug development process, improve the chances for clinical trial success, and yield more and better information about treatment or disease or both. Once a DDT is qualified for specific use, industry can use the DDT for the qualified purpose during drug development, and FDA/EMA reviewers can be confident in applying the DDT for the qualified use without the need to reconfirm the DDT's utility.

Therefore, the intent of the DDT qualification process is for FDA/EMA reviewers to work with industry sponsors of these tools in order to guide sponsors as they refine their tools and rigorously evaluate them for use in the regulatory landscape. Overall goals of the qualification process for PROs are to obtain PRO qualification and to provide concept identification, context of use, an overview of current PRO development status, development of PRO context and document of content validity (i.e., documentation that the PRO covers what patients consider most important), documentation of measurement properties, language translation and cultural adaptation (if applicable), data collection, copy of all existing final versions of the PRO measure, user manual, and list of relevant references.

1.2.2 Beyond Label Claims

While the FDA guidance is useful for regulatory and labeling purposes in the United States, this monograph is intended to be broad enough to serve as a reference whether or not the intention is to seek a label claim (a statement of treatment benefit) on a PRO in support of a medical product. PROs have merit that go beyond satisfying regulatory requirements for a US label claim (Doward et al., 2010). Payers both in the United States and Europe, clinicians, and patients themselves all have an interest in PROs that transcend a label claim for patient-reported symptoms or any other PRO. These key stakeholders help determine the availability, pricing, and value of medicinal products. And PROs can provide complementary and supplementary evidence distinct from other clinical outcomes in shaping the overall profile of a medical intervention. The publication of results from a well-developed PRO scale based on a well-conducted clinical study can identify distinguishing clinical aspects, favorable and not favorable, about the treatment or disease (or both) relevant to stakeholders.

1.2.3 Clinical Practice

The International Society for Quality of Life Research (ISOQOL) has developed a *User's Guide for Implementing Patient-Reported Outcomes Assessment in Clinical Practice* and has published a report summarizing the key issues from the *User's Guide* (Snyder et al., 2012). Using the literature, the ISOQOL team outlined considerations for using PROs in clinical practice; options for designing the interventions; and strengths, weaknesses, and resource requirements associated with each option. A number of methodological and practical decisions are involved for implementing routine PRO assessment in clinical practice: (1) identifying the goals for collecting PROs; (2) selecting the patients, settings, and timing of assessments; (3) determining which questionnaires to use; (4) choosing a mode of administering and scoring the questionnaire; (5) designing processes for reporting results; (6) identifying aids to facilitate score interpretation; (7) developing strategies for responding to issues identified by the questionnaires; and (8) evaluating the impact of the PRO intervention on clinical practice. Several measures such as the SF-36, Dartmouth COOP Charts, Sexual Health Inventory for Men, and Chronic Respiratory Questionnaire have been shown to identify key issues, improve patient–clinician communications, and improve and enhance patient care (Frost et al., 2007).

1.2.4 Comparative Effectiveness Research

The goal of comparative effectiveness research (CER) is to explain the differential benefits and harms of alternate methods to prevent, diagnose, treat, and monitor a clinical condition or to improve the delivery of care. CER encompasses all forms of data from controlled clinical trials to outside of them (so-called real-world data), including clinical practice, and PROs play a central role in CER (Alemayehu et al., 2011). Recommendations have been made for incorporating PROs in CER as a guide for researchers, clinicians, and policymakers in general (Ahmed et al., 2012) and in adult oncology in particular (Basch et al., 2012). Emerging changes that may facilitate CER using PROs include implementation of electronic and personal health records, implementation of hospital and population-based registries, and the use of PROs in national monitoring initiatives.

1.3 Terms and Definitions

Table 1.1, taken from the glossary in the FDA Final Guidance on PROs for label claims (FDA, 2009), contains a list of specialized vocabulary useful when reading and applying PROs. Most of these terms, which are applicable even when a label claim is not being sought, are also instructive and pertinent for understanding and learning some of the nomenclature used in this book. These terms, along with others, are explicated upon in subsequent chapters. Another useful source for terminology, not restricted to PROs, comes from the International Society of Pharmacoeconomic and Outcomes Research (Berger et al., 2007).

1.4 Measurement Scales

1.4.1 Properties and Types of Scales

A PRO is a measurement scale. Each scale of measurement satisfies one or more of the following properties of measurement:

- *Identity*: Each value on the measurement scale has a unique meaning.
- *Direction*: Values on the measurement scale have an ordered relationship to one another; that is, some values are larger and some are smaller.
- *Equal intervals*: Scale units along the scale are equal to one another; therefore, the difference between 1 and 2 would be equal to the difference between 19 and 20.
- *Absolute zero*: The scale has a true zero point, below which no values exist.

The *nominal scale of measurement* only satisfies the identity property of measurement. Values assigned to variables represent a descriptive category, but have no inherent numerical value with respect to direction. Gender is such an example. Individuals may be classified as *male* or *female*, but neither value represents more or less *gender* than the other. Religion and ethnicity are other examples of variables that are typically measured on a nominal scale. This type of scale is not typically seen as a PRO; rather, it is more related to a demographic survey.

The *ordinal scale of measurement* has the property of both identity and direction. Each value on the ordinal scale has a unique meaning, and it has an ordered relationship to every other value on the scale. An example of an ordinal scale is low/medium/high. An experience as a 9 on a scale from 1 to 10 tells us that it was higher than an experience ranked as a 6. Other examples include level of agreement (no, maybe, yes) and political orientation (left, center, right). Many health measurement scales are, in theory, at the ordinal level of measurement.

TABLE 1.1

Definition of Common Terms Used in the Field of Patient-Reported Outcomes

Ability to detect change—Evidence that a PRO instrument can identify differences in scores over time in individuals or groups who have changed with respect to the measurement concept.

Claim—A statement of treatment benefit. A claim can appear in any section of a medical product's FDA-approved labeling or in advertising and promotional labeling of prescription drugs and devices.

Cognitive interviewing—A qualitative research tool used to determine whether concepts and items are understood by patients in the same way that instrument developers intend. Cognitive interviews involve incorporating follow-up questions in a field test interview to gain a better understanding of how patients interpret questions asked of them. In this method, respondents are often asked to *think aloud* and describe their thought processes as they answer the instrument questions.

Concept—The specific measurement goal (i.e., the *thing* that is to be measured by a PRO instrument). In clinical trials, a PRO instrument can be used to measure the effect of a medical intervention on one or more concepts. PRO concepts represent aspects of how patients function or feel related to a health condition or its treatment.

Conceptual framework of a PRO instrument—An explicit description or diagram of the relationships between the questionnaire or items in a PRO instrument and the concepts measured. The conceptual framework of a PRO instrument evolves over the course of instrument development as empiric evidence is gathered to support item grouping and scores. We review the alignment of the final conceptual framework with the clinical trial's objectives, design, and analysis plan.

Construct validity—Evidence that relationships among items, domains, and concepts conform to *a priori* hypotheses concerning logical relationships that should exist with other measures or characteristics of patients and patient groups.

Content validity—Evidence from qualitative research demonstrating that the instrument measures the concept of interest including evidence that the items and domains of an instrument are appropriate and comprehensive relative to its intended measurement concept, population, and use. Testing other measurement properties will not replace or rectify problems with content validity.

Criterion validity—The extent to which the scores of a PRO instrument are related to a known *gold standard* measure of the same concept. For most PROs, criterion validity cannot be measured because there is no gold standard.

Domain—A subconcept represented by a score of an instrument that measures a larger concept comprised of multiple domains. For example, psychological function is the larger concept containing the domains subdivided into items describing emotional function and cognitive function.

Endpoint—The measurement that will be statistically compared among treatment groups to assess the effect of treatment and that corresponds with the clinical trial's objectives, design, and data analysis. For example, a treatment may be tested to decrease the intensity of symptom Z. In this case, the endpoint is the change from baseline to time T in a score that represents the concept of symptom Z intensity.

Endpoint model—A diagram of the hierarchy of relationships among all endpoints, both PRO and non-PRO, that corresponds to the clinical trial's objectives, design, and data analysis plan.

Health-related quality of life (HRQL)—HRQL is a multidomain concept that represents the patient's general perception of the effect of illness and treatment on physical, psychological, and social aspects of life. Claiming a statistical and meaningful improvement in HRQL implies that (1) all HRQL domains that are important to interpreting change in how the clinical trial's population feels or functions as a result of the targeted disease and its treatment were measured, (2) a general improvement was demonstrated, and (3) no decrement was demonstrated in any domain.

TABLE 1.1 (continued)

Definition of Common Terms Used in the Field of Patient-Reported Outcomes

Instrument—A means to capture data (i.e., a questionnaire) plus all the information and documentation that supports its use. Generally, that includes clearly defined methods and instructions for administration or responding, a standard format for data collection, and well-documented methods for scoring, analysis, and interpretation of results in the target patient population.

Item—An individual question, statement, or task (and its standardized response options) that is evaluated by the patient to address a particular concept.

Item tracking matrix—A record of the development (e.g., additions, deletions, modifications, and the reasons for the changes) of items used in an instrument.

Measurement properties—All of the attributes relevant to the application of a PRO instrument, including the content validity, construct validity, reliability, and ability to detect change. These attributes are specific to the measurement application and cannot be assumed to be relevant to all measurement situations, purposes, populations, or settings in which the instrument is used.

Patient-reported outcome (PRO)—A measurement based on a report that comes directly from the patient (i.e., study subject) about the status of a patient's health condition without amendment or interpretation of the patient's response by a clinician or anyone else. A PRO can be measured by self-report or by interview provided that the interviewer records only the patient's response.

Proxy-reported outcome—A measurement based on a report by someone other than the patient reporting as if that person is the patient. A proxy-reported outcome is not a PRO. A proxy report also is different from an observer report where the observer (e.g., clinician or caregiver), in addition to reporting the observation, may interpret or give an opinion based on the observation. We discourage the use of proxy-reported outcome measures particularly for symptoms that can be known only by the patient.

Quality of life—A general concept that implies an evaluation of the effect of all aspects of life on general well-being. Because this term implies the evaluation of non-health-related aspects of life, and because the term generally is accepted to mean *what the patient thinks it is*, it is too general and undefined to be considered appropriate for a medical product claim.

Questionnaire—A set of questions or items shown to a respondent to get answers for research purposes. Types of questionnaires include diaries and event logs.

Recall period—The period of time patients are asked to consider in responding to a PRO item or question. Recall can be momentary (real time) or retrospective of varying lengths.

Reliability—The ability of a PRO instrument to yield consistent, reproducible estimates of true treatment effect.

Responder definition—A score change in a measure, experienced by an individual patient over a predetermined time period that has been demonstrated in the target population to have a significant treatment benefit.

Saturation—When interviewing patients, the point when no new relevant or important information emerges and collecting additional data will not add to the understanding of how patients perceive the concept of interest and the items in a questionnaire.

Scale—The system of numbers or verbal anchors by which a value or score is derived for an item. Examples include visual analogue scales, Likert scales, and rating scales.

Score—A number derived from a patient's response to items in a questionnaire. A score is computed based on a prespecified, validated scoring algorithm and is subsequently used in statistical analyses of clinical trial results. Scores can be computed for individual items, domains, or concepts, or as a summary of items, domains, or concepts.

(continued)

TABLE 1.1 (continued)

Definition of Common Terms Used in the Field of Patient-Reported Outcomes

Sign—Any objective evidence of a disease, health condition, or treatment-related effect. Signs are usually observed and interpreted by the clinician but may be noticed and reported by the patient.

Symptom—Any subjective evidence of a disease, health condition, or treatment-related effect that can be noticed and known only by the patient.

Target product profile (TPP)—A clinical development program summary in the context of labeling goals where specific types of evidence (e.g., clinical trials or other sources of data) are linked to the targeted labeling claims or concepts.

Treatment benefit—The effect of treatment on how a patient survives, feels, or functions. Treatment benefit can be demonstrated by either an effectiveness or safety advantage. For example, the treatment effect may be measured as an improvement or delay in the development of symptoms or as a reduction or delay in treatment-related toxicity. Measures that do not directly capture the treatment effect on how a patient survives, feels, or functions are surrogate measures of treatment benefit.

Source: Food and Drug Administration (FDA), *Fed. Reg.*, 74(235), 65132, 2009. http://www.fda.gov/ Drugs/DevelopmentApprovalProcess/DrugDevelopmentToolsQualificationProgram/ ucm284399.htm.

The *interval scale of measurement* has the properties of identity, direction, and equal intervals. A perfect example of an interval scale is the Celsius scale to measure temperature. The scale is made up of equal temperature units, so that the difference between 40°C and 50°C is equal to the difference between 50°C and 60°C. If it is known that the distance between 1 and 2 on a 10-point rating scale is the same as that between 7 and 8, then the measurement is based on an interval scale. With an interval scale, the scale informs that not only are different values bigger or smaller, but also how much bigger or smaller. For instance, suppose it is 20°C on Saturday and 24°C on Sunday. It was not only hotter on Sunday but also 4°C hotter. Many PRO scales are assumed to be interval in practice.

Consider an 11-point pain numeric rating scale, which goes from 0 (*no pain*) to 10 (*worst pain imaginable*). Although an ordinal measure in principle, this scale is typically treated as an interval or approximately interval scale for all practical purposes with, for example, a move from 1 to 2 on the scale taken to be the same as a move from 6 to 7. In general, under most circumstances, unless the distribution of scores is drastically skewed, analyzing rating scales as if they were interval is acceptable and is not expected to introduce material bias.

The *ratio scale of measurement* satisfies all four of the properties of measurement: identity, direction, equal intervals, and an absolute zero. The temperature of an object represented by the Kelvin temperature scale would be an example of a ratio scale. The scale is made up of equal temperature units, so that the difference between 300 and 350 K is equal to the difference between 150 and 200 K. Each value on the temperature scale has a unique meaning, temperatures can be rank ordered, units along the temperature scale are equal to one another, and there is an absolute zero when all molecular motion practically stops. Using a ratio scale permits comparisons such as being twice as high, or one-half as much. This is the most important difference from the Celsius temperature scale. If the temperature of one object is 10°C and for another object it is 20°C, then we cannot say that the second object is twice as hot as the first one, but if the temperature is measured in Kelvin, then we can say that the second object is twice as hot as the first one. This interpretation is due to the fact that zero on the Celsius scale was arbitrarily selected as the temperature point, representing the temperature when water is freezing.

Reaction time (how long it takes to respond to a signal of some sort) uses a ratio scale of measurement—time. Although an individual's reaction time is always greater than zero, a zero point in time can be conceptualized and a response of 24 ms can be considered twice as fast as a response time of 48 ms. Other examples of ratio scales include measurements based on a ruler (inches or centimeters), income (e.g., money earned last year), grade-point average, years of work experience, and number of children. Generally, PROs as rating scales are not on a ratio scale, as there is no true zero point and the assignment of a number to a rating scale category is somewhat arbitrary. The 11-point numerical rating scale on pain, for instance, could have been just as easily introduced as going from 0 (*worse pain imaginable*) to 10 (*no pain*), instead of 0 (*no pain*) to 10 (*worse pain imaginable*). The value of 0 on this rating scale does not have any inherent or intrinsic meaning.

Measurements at the interval or ratio level are desirable because of the more powerful statistical procedures, specifically parametric methods, which assume that the response scores follow a normal distribution, available for analyzing mean scores. To have this advantage, often ordinal data are treated as though they were interval data following a normal distribution, and, furthermore, researchers often assume that the intervals are equal. This assumption may be reasonable in many situations when the phenomenon in question can be taken to have an underlying continuous scale. One common and often justifiable practice for analyzing ordinal data is to assign ordered categories consecutive values and then use powerful parametric methods (such as a two-sample *t*-test, analysis of variance, analysis of covariance), which have been shown to be robust to violations of normality (Snedecor and Cochran, 1980; Heeren and D'Agostino, 1987; Stiger et al., 1998; Sullivan and D'Agostino, 2003). The central limit theorem provides further support: Regardless of the true underlying distribution of the individual scores, the sampling distribution of the mean scores (if the same population were hypothetically sampled many times with the same sample size and each time taking a mean score) will increasingly approximate a normal distribution, allowing for parametric methods to be applied successfully (Snedecor and Cochran, 1980).

Although there may be concern that the assignment of integers to the categories is somewhat arbitrary and that the distances between adjacent scores do not represent equal gradations, even moderate differences among various scoring systems are not expected to produce marked changes in results and conclusions in typical circumstances (Baker et al., 1966; Borgatta and Bohrnstedt, 1980; Snedecor and Cochran, 1980). Moreover, the assignment of consecutive integers may be viewed as just a monotonic transformation that is analogous to other types of transformations, such as log and square root transformations, which are commonly employed to help remedy departures from modeling assumptions. Therefore, the statistical approaches discussed in the remainder of the book will generally be parametric tests, which have robust qualities regarding assumptions, enable inferences on the parameters of interest, and are equipped to detect real changes or differences.

1.4.2 Single-Item and Multi-Item Scales

PROs may consist of either one or multiple questions, which are commonly referred to as *items*. The number of PRO items can be related to the complexity of the concept being assessed. Simple concepts can be assessed with a simple scale—that is, a single rating or single-item scale on a particular concept of interest (the *thing* that is measured by the PRO), whose score is estimated by a single response to a single question. Pain is often expressed as a single item, as are particular symptoms like nausea. While a single-item scale is simple and imposes the least respondent burden, a single item may represent an oversimplification and may be less than complete in certain circumstances (Sloan et al., 2002).

As the name implies, multi-item scales are scales formed by more than one item and are used chiefly for concepts considered complex to measure. For extremely complex and abstract concepts, a large number of items are generally needed to assess them adequately. Where multiple items are needed and they are referring to different aspects of the same concept or attribute, they form *domains*. A somewhat complex concept may therefore be assessed with multiple items. For example, adequate assessment of physical function requires a number of items to ensure that all of its relevant aspects are captured for the targeted patient population.

More complex concepts within a PRO instrument require multiple domains as well. Multiple domains would be necessary, for example, for HRQL, where all aspects of health status are considered and each individual concept (domain) would need a set of one or more items; when collectively considered, these domains cover an overall profile or concept of health status referred to as HRQL. The use of multiple items to measure a concept considered not straightforward is important. Combining several related items measuring complementary aspects of the same concept into a domain score results in greater reliability (precision) and translates into more certainty that the concept has been comprehensively assessed (Sloan et al., 2002). A simple concept requiring only one item (e.g., a pain assessment), though, may need multiple administrations to improve its reliability of measurement.

1.4.3 Latent Variables and Manifest Variables

Measurements of PROs often involve unobserved constructs or concepts that are also referred to as latent (hidden) variables. Many psychological aspects, such as depression and anxiety, are not directly observable and are hence considered latent variables. These unobserved phenomena are measured using responses of patients to questionnaire items; these items are referred to as manifest or indicator variables in the psychometric literature (e.g., "How much of the time do you worry?" with response options of "almost always or always," "most times," "sometimes," "a few times," and "almost never or never"). Therefore, in these instances, a health measurement scale becomes an observed entity intended to capture an aspect of some unobservable entity.

1.5 Psychometrics versus Clinimetrics

Psychometrics is a methodological discipline with its roots in psychological research (Lord and Novick, 1968; Nunnally and Bernstein, 1994; Embertson and Reise, 2000), a discipline that has been increasingly applied to other fields such as medicine and health (Fayers and Machin, 2007; Streiner and Norman, 2008; de Vet et al., 2011). Within the field of psychometrics, the measurement theories of classical test theory and item response theory, topics covered in subsequent chapters, have emanated (Crocker and Algina, 1986). A child descendant of classical test theory, generalizability theory involves the identification and measurement of multiple sources of error variances in order to find strategies to reduce the influence of these sources so as to improve reliability. This book does not cover generalizability theory and interested readers who wish to learn about it can consult published sources (Shavelson and Webb, 1991; Brennan, 2001, 2010; Streiner and Norman, 2008; de Vet et al., 2011). Psychometrics usually involves the measurement of a single attribute (construct or concept) with multiple items or variables (each item can be considered a variable) that capture related and distinct aspects of the attribute. Most validation techniques in this book are grounded in psychometric methods.

The term *clinimetrics* has been used to define the construction of clinical indexes, which emphasize clinical expertise and subject matter, in the development of measurement scales (Feinstein, 1987). Clinimetrics involves a description or measurement of symptoms, physical signs, and other distinctly clinical phenomena in medicine. Clinimetrics is typically concerned with incorporating multiple attributes within a single index that can be used for diagnosis or prognosis (predictive) purposes. As such, statistical methods usually center on regression or similar techniques for diagnostic or predictive evaluation. An example is the Apgar method for assessing a newborn infant's condition, as a predictor of neonatal outcome (Apgar, 1953). The Apgar score combines heterogenous elements (heart rate, respiratory effort, reflex irritability, muscle tone, and skin color), which are not intended to be highly interrelated indicators of a baby's condition. Each item is scored from 0 to 2, and a sum-score of 7 or more indicates a good prognosis.

The psychometric paradigm involves variables that indicate (*indicator items*), or are reflective of, the same concept being measured. Data are collected to explore and test the model, and to determine whether the variables fit the model, with emphasis on constructing, validating, and testing models. In contrast, clinimetric indexes behave differently from psychometric scales principally, because the former contain at least some variables that cause (*causal items*) or define what is being measured (rather than being the effect of what is being measured) and use these items to define a summary index of variables that are not necessarily correlated. Details on the differences between psychometrics and clinimetrics, and related themes, are found elsewhere (Fayers and Hand, 1997, 2002; Fayers, 2004; Fayers and Machin, 2007). In this book, we adopt the approach that measurements in medicine and health should be performed using the most adequate methods. When appropriate, we indicate which underlying theories, models, and methods are appropriate and which are not.

1.6 Selection of a PRO Questionnaire

The fulfillment of a study objective requires appropriate scales to measure the PROs included in the objective. Scale development can be an expensive and a time-consuming process. It usually involves a number of considerations: item generation (through expert panels and focus groups), data collection from a sample in the target population of interest, item reduction, scale validation, translation, and cultural adaptation. This whole procedure can easily require at least 1 year. Therefore, the use of a previously validated PRO questionnaire is typically preferable to the development of a new questionnaire for the same purpose.

Updated information on currently available instruments (i.e., questionnaires plus relevant accompanying information and documentation that support them) can be accessed from various sources, including Bowling (2001, 2004), Salek (2004), McDowell (2006), the Patient-Reported Outcomes Measurement Information System (Cella et al., 2010), Patient-Reported Outcome and Quality of Life Instruments Database (http://www.proqolid.org), On-Line Guide to Quality-of-Life Assessment (http://www.OLGA-Qol.com), and Pfizer Patient-Reported Outcomes (http://www.pfizerpatientreportedoutcomes.com). Increasingly, patients are using web-based social networking sites to share and compare their experiences and satisfaction with their pharmaceutical treatments (Baldwin et al., 2011). The PatientsLikeMe's Open Research Exchange™ is designed to provide a system for building new PRO measures and evaluating them with patients from the PatientsLikeMe user community, thereby providing an outline platform where researchers, clinicians, and academics can collaborate to put patients at the center of the clinical research

TABLE 1.2

Brief Checklist for Choosing a PRO Questionnaire

1. *Documentation*—Is there formal written documentation, peer-review publications, or a user's manual to support the claims of the developers?
2. *Development*—Were rigorous procedures, motivated by a clear conceptual basis and a clear aim of the undertaking, adopted and tracked through all stages from item selection to large-scale field testing?
3. *Validity*—Is there sufficient evidence that the scale is measuring what it is intended to measure?
4. *Reliability*—Is there sufficient evidence that the scale is precise in accurately measuring its scores?
5. *Target population*—Is the scale suitable for the target population under study and, if not, is it reasonable to expect the scale to be applicable?
6. *Feasibility*—Does the scale have questions that are easy to understand, have a convenient mode of administration, and no undue patient burden?
7. *Language and cultures*—Are there validated translations of the questionnaire to meet the needs under study?
8. *Scoring*—How is the scoring procedure defined and does it make sense?
9. *Interpretation*—Are there guidelines for interpreting scale scores?

process (www.openresearchexchange.com). The Patient-Centered Outcomes Research Institute (PCORI), authorized by the US Congress, has the objective to help people make informed health-care decisions and to help improve health-care delivery and outcomes that come from research guided by patients, caregivers, and the broader health-care community (www.pcori.org).

With many PROs currently available, the choice of the most appropriate questionnaires becomes vital to the success of a study in which PROs are included as a key endpoint. Table 1.2 highlights some general key considerations for the selection of an appropriate PRO questionnaire. An ISOQOL initiative put forth minimum standards for PRO measures to be used in patient-centered outcomes research (Butt and Reeve, 2012). These recommendations include documentation of the characteristics of the conceptual and measurement model, evidence for reliability, validity, and interpretability of scores, quality translations, and acceptable patient and investigator burden. Further guidance on choosing a suitable PRO questionnaire can be found elsewhere (Fayers and Machin, 2007; Luo and Cappelleri, 2008). However, it may be that a researcher wants to take an existing measure and adapt it for use in a novel patient population, which may or may not require the addition or deletion of items. In either case, psychometric testing would need to be completed to ensure the measure was still valid and reliable for the new patient population. Occasions may arise when an existing measure does not adequately assess the targeted concept of interest and a new measure will need to be developed. This book addresses these concerns by explaining various approaches that may be useful to develop or refine a PRO.

1.7 Summary

In summary, this chapter introduces PROs by putting them into perspective and laying the groundwork for subsequent chapters. PROs are useful in a variety of circumstances pertaining to clinical research, label claims, beyond label claims, clinical practice, and comparative effectiveness research. This chapter also includes terms and their definitions commonly applied in PRO research. The general principles of measurement scales are highlighted; such principles are expounded upon in subsequent chapters. These later chapters give details on the measurement, implementation, and interpretation of PROs by explaining and illustrating approaches or methodologies for evaluating a PRO measure.

References

Aaronson, N.K., Ahmedzai, S., Bergman, B., Bullinger, M., Cull, A., Duez, N.J., A. Filiberti et al. 1993. The European Organization for Research and Treatment of Cancer QLQ-C30: A quality-of-life instrument for use in international trials in oncology. *Journal of the National Cancer Institute* 85:365–376.

Ahmed, S., Berzon, R.A., Revicki, D.A., Lenderking, W.R., Moinpour, C.M., Basch, E., Reeve, B.B., and A.W. Wu on behalf of the International Society for Quality of Life Research. 2012. The use of patient-reported outcomes (PRO) within comparative effectiveness research: Implications for clinical practice and health care policy. *Medical Care* 50:1060–1070.

Alemayehu, D., Sanchez. R.J., and J.C. Cappelleri. 2011. Considerations on the use of patient-reported outcomes in comparative effectiveness research. *Journal of Managed Care Pharmacy* 17:S27–S33.

Apgar, V. 1953. A proposal for a new method of evaluation of the newborn infant. *Anasthetics and Analgesics* 32:260–267.

Baker, B.O., Hardyck, C.D., and L.F. Petrinovich. 1966. Weak measurements vs. strong statistics: An empirical critique of S.S. Steven's proscriptions on statistics. *Educational and Psychological Measurement* 36:291–309.

Baldwin, M., Spong, A., Doward, L., and A. Gnanasakthy. 2011. Patient-reported outcomes, patient-reported information: From randomized controlled trials to the social web and beyond. *Patient* 4:11–17.

Basch, E., Abernethy, A.P., Mullins, C.D., Reeve, B.B., Smith, M.L., Coons, S.J., J. Sloan et al. 2012. Recommendations for incorporating patient-reported outcomes into clinical comparative effectiveness research in adult oncology. *Journal of Clinical Oncology* 30:4249–4255.

Berger, M.L., Bingefors, K., Hedbolm, E.C., Pashos, C.L., and G.W. Torrance. 2007. *Health Care Cost, Quality and Outcomes: ISPOR Book of Terms*. Lawrenceville, NJ: International Society for Pharmacoeconomics and Outcomes Research.

Bergner, M., Babbit, R.A., Carter, W.B., and B.S. Gilso. 1981. The Sickness Impact Profile: Development and final revision of a health status measure. *Medical Care* 19:787–805.

Borgatta, E.F. and G.W. Bohrnstedt. 1980. Level of measurement—Once over again. *Sociological Methods and Research* 9:147–160.

Bottomley, A., Jones, D., and L. Claassens. 2009. Patient-reported outcomes: Assessment and current perspectives of the guidelines of the Food and Drug Administrations and the reflection paper of the European Medicines Agency. *European Journal of Cancer* 45:347–353.

Bowling, A. 2001. *Measuring Disease: A Review of Disease-specific Quality of Life Measurement Scales*, 2nd edition. Buckingham, U.K.: Open University Press.

Bowling, A. 2004. *Measuring Health: A Review of Quality of Life Measurement Scales*, 3rd edition. Buckingham, U.K.: Open University Press.

Brennan, R.L. 2001. *Generalizability Theory*. New York, NY: Springer-Verlag.

Brennan, R.L. 2010. Generalizability theory and classical test theory. *Applied Measurement in Education* 24:1–21.

Brooks R., with the EuroQol group. 1996. EuroQol: The current state of play. *Health Policy* 37:53–72.

Butt, Z. and B. Reeve. 2012. Enhancing the patient's voice: Standards in the design and selection of patient-reported outcomes measures (PROMs) for use in patient-centered outcomes research: Methodology committee report. Submitted to the Patient Centeredness Workgroup, PCORI Methodology Committee, March 30, 2012.

Calvert, M., Blazeby, J., Altman, D.G., Revicki, D.A., Moher, D., and M.D. Brundage for the CONSORT PRO Group. 2013. Reporting of patient-reported outcomes in randomized trials: The CONSORT PRO Extension. *JAMA* 309:814–822.

Cella, D., Riley, W., Stone, A., Rothrock, N., Reeve, B., Yount, S., D. Amtmann et al., on behalf of the PROMIS Cooperative Group. 2010. The patient-reported outcomes measurement information system (PROMIS) developed and tests its first wave of adult self-reported health outcome item banks: 2005–2008. *Journal of Clinical Epidemiology* 63:1179–1194.

Cella, D.F., Tulsky, D.S., Gray, G., Saratian, B., Linn, E., Bonomi, A., M. Silberman et al. 1993. The Functional Assessment of Cancer Therapy Scale: Development and validation of the general measure. *Journal of Clinical Oncology* 11:570–579.

Chassany, O., Sagnier, P., Marquis, P., Fullerton, S., and N. Aaronson for the European Regulatory Issues on Quality of Life Assessment Group. 2002. Patient-reported outcomes: The example of health-related quality of life—A European guidance document for the improved integration of health-related quality of life assessment in the drug regulatory process. *Drug Information Journal* 36:209–238.

Coons, S.J., Kothari, S., Monz, B.U., and L.B. Burke. 2011. The patient-reported outcome (PRO) consortium: Filling measurement gaps for PRO endpoints to support labeling claims. *Clinical Pharmacology & Therapeutics* 90:743–748.

Crocker, L. and J. Algina. 1986. *Introduction to Classical and Modern Test Theory*. Belmont, CA: Wadsworth.

de Haes, J.C.J.M., Olschewski, M., Fayers, P.M., Visser, M.R.M., Cull, A., Hopwood, P., and R. Sanderman. 1996. *Measuring the Quality of Life of Cancer Patients: The Rotterdam Symptom Checklist (RSCL): A Manual*. Groningen, the Netherlands: Northern Center for Healthcare Research.

DeMuro, C., Clark, M., Doward, L., Evans, E., Mordin, M., and A. Gnanasakthy. In press. Assessment of PRO label claims granted by the FDA as compared to the EMA (2006–2010). *Value in Health*. DOI: 10.1016/j.jval.2013.08.2293.

DeMuro, C., Clark, M., Mordin, M., Fehnel, S., Copley-Merriman, C., and A. Gnanasakthy. 2012. Reasons for rejection of patient-reported outcome label claims: A compilation based on a review of patient-reported outcome use among new molecular entities and biologic license applications, 2006–2010. *Value in Health* 15:443–448.

de Vet, H.C.W., Terwee, C.B., Mokkink, L.B., and D.L. Knol. 2011. *Measurement in Medicine*. New York, NY: Cambridge University Press.

Devinsky, O., Vickrey, B.G., Cramer, J., Perrine, K., Hermann, B., Meador, K., and R.D. Hays. 1995. Development of the quality of life in epilepsy inventory. *Epilepsia* 36:1089–1104.

Doward, L.C., Gnanasakthy, A., and M.G. Baker. 2010. Patient reported outcomes: Looking beyond the claim. *Health and Quality of Life Outcomes* 8:89. Open access.

Embertson, S.E. and S.P. Reise. 2000. *Item Response Theory for Psychologists*. Mahwah, NJ: Lawrence Erlbaum Associates.

European Medicines Agency (EMA), Committee for Medicinal Products for Human Use. 2005. Reflection paper on the regulatory guidance for use of health-related quality of life (HRQOL) measures in the evaluation of medicinal products. European Medicines Agency. http://www.ema.europa.eu/ema/ (Accessed on August 31, 2013).

European Medicines Agency (EMA), Committee for Medicinal Products for Human Use. 2009. Qualification of novel methodologies for drug development: Guidance to applicants. European Medicines Agency. http://www.ema.europa.eu/ema/ (Accessed on August 31, 2013).

Fairclough, D.L. 2004. Patient reported outcomes as endpoints in medical research. *Statistical Methods in Medical Research* 13:115–138.

Fairclough, D.L. 2010. *Design and Analysis of Quality of Life Studies in Clinical Trials*, 2nd edition. Boca Raton, FL: Chapman & Hall/CRC.

Fayers, P.M. 2004. Quality-of-life measurement in clinical trials—The impact of causal variables. *Journal of Biopharmaceutical Statistics* 14:155–176.

Fayers, P.M. and D.J. Hand. 1997. Factor analysis, causal indicators, and quality of life. *Quality of Life Research* 6:139–150.

Fayers, P.M. and D.J. Hand. 2002. Causal variables, indicator variables and measurement scales: An example from quality of life. *Journal of the Royal Statistical Society Series A* 165:233–261.

Fayers, P.M. and D. Machin. 2007. *Quality of Life: The Assessment, Analysis and Interpretation of Patient-reported Outcomes*, 2nd edition. Chichester, England: John Wiley & Sons Ltd.

Fehnel, S., DeMuro, C., McLeod, L., Coon, C., and A. Gnanasakthy. 2013. US FDA patient-reported outcome guidance: Great expectations and unintended consequences. *Expert Reviews of Pharmacoeconomics & Outcomes Research* 13:441–446.

Feinstein, A.R. 1987. *Clinimetrics*. New Haven, CT: Yale University Press.

Food and Drug Administration (FDA). 2009. Guidance for industry on patient-reported outcome measures: Use in medical product development to support labeling claims. *Federal Register* 74(235):65132–65133. http://www.fda.gov/Drugs/DevelopmentApprovalProcess/DrugDevelopmentToolsQualificationProgram/ucm284399.htm. (Accessed on August 31, 2013).

Food and Drug Administration (FDA). 2010. Draft guidance for industry on qualification process for drug development tools. *Federal Register* 75(205):65495–65496. http://www.fda.gov/Drugs/DevelopmentApprovalProcess/DrugDevelopmentToolsQualificationProgram/ucm284399.htm. (Accessed on August 31, 2013).

Frost, M., Bonomi, A.E., Cappelleri, J.C., Schünemann, H.J, Moynihan, T.J., Aaronson, A., and the Clinical Significance Consensus Meeting Group. 2007. Applying quality-of-life data formally and systematically into clinical practice. *Mayo Clinic Proceedings* 82:1214–1228.

Gnanasakthy, A., Mordin, M., Clark, M., DeMuro, C., Fehnel, S., and C. Copley-Merriman. 2012. A review of patient-reported outcomes labels in the United States: 2006 to 2010. *Value in Health* 15:437–442.

Hareendran, A., Gnanasakthy, A., Winnette, R., and D. Revicki. 2012. Capturing patients' perspective of treatment in clinical trials/drug development. *Contemporary Clinical Trials* 33:23–28.

Heeren, T. and R. D'Agostino. 1987. Robustness of the two independent samples t-test when applied to ordinal scaled data. *Statistics in Medicine* 6:79–90.

Hunt, S.M., McKenna, S.P., McEwen, J., Williams, J., and E. Papp. 1981. The Nottingham Health Profile: Subjective health status and medical consultations. *Social Science & Medicine* 15A:221–229.

Juniper, E.F., Guyatt, G.H., Feeny, D.H., Ferne, P.J., Griffith, L.E., and M. Townsend. 1996. Measuring quality of life in children with asthma. *Quality of Life Research* 5:35–46.

Lord, F.M. and M.R. Novick. 1968. *Statistical Theory of Mental Test Scores*. Reading, MA: Addison-Wesley.

Luo, X. and J.C. Cappelleri. 2008. A practical guide on interpreting and evaluating patient-reported outcomes in clinical trials. *Clinical Research and Regulatory Affairs* 25:197–211.

Mangione, C.M., Lee, P.P., Gutierrez, P.R., Spritzer, K., Berry, S., and R.D. Hays. 2001. Development of the 25-item National Eye Institute Visual Function Questionnaire (VFQ-25). *Archives of Ophthalmology* 119:1050–1058.

McDowell, I. 2006. *Measuring Health: A Guide to Rating Scales and Questionnaires*, 3rd edition. New York, NY: Oxford University Press.

Melzack, R. 1975. The McGill Pain Questionnaire: Major properties and scoring methods. *Pain* 1:277–299.

Moher, D., Hopewell, S., Schulz, K.F., Montori, V., Gøtzsche, P.C., Devereaux, P.J., Elbourne, D., Egger, M., and D.G. Altman, for the CONSORT Group. CONSORT 2010 explanation and elaboration: Updated guidelines for reporting parallel group randomized trials. *BMJ* 340:c869.

Nunnally, J.C. and I.H. Bernstein. 1994. *Psychometric Theory*, 3rd edition. New York, NY: McGraw-Hill.

Patrick, D.L., Burke, L.B., Powers, J.H., Scott, J.A., Rock, E.P., Dawisha, S., O'Neill, R., and D.L. Kennedy. 2007. Patient-reported outcomes to support medical product labeling claims: FDA perspective. *Value in Health* 10 (Suppl. 2):S125–S137.

Revicki, D.A., Gnanasakthy, A., and K. Weinfurt. 2007. Documenting the rationale and psychometric characteristics of patient reported outcomes for labeling and promotional claims: The PRO evidence dossier. *Quality of Life Research* 16:717–723.

Rosen, R.C., Riley, A., Wagner, G., Osterloh, I.H., Kirkpatrick, J., and A. Mishra. 1997. The International Index of Erectile Function (IIEF): A multidimensional scale for assessment of erectile dysfunction. *Urology* 49:822–830.

Salek, S. 2004. *Compendium of Quality of Life Instruments*, Volume 6. Haslemere, U.K.: Euromed Communications Ltd.

Schulz, K.F., Altman, D.G., Moher, D., for the CONSORT Group. 2010. CONSORT 2010 statement: Updated guidelines for reporting parallel group randomized trials. *BMJ* 340:c332.

Shah, S., Vanclay, F., and B. Cooper. 1989. Improving the sensitivity of the Barthel Index for stroke rehabilitation. *Journal of Clinical Epidemiology* 42:703–709.

Shavelson, R.J. and N.M. Webb. 1991. *Generalizability Theory: A Primer*. Thousand Oaks, CA: Sage Publications.

Sloan, J.A., Aaronson, N., Cappelleri, J.C., Fairclough, D.L., Varricchio, C., and the Clinical Significance Consensus Meeting Group. 2002. Assessing the clinical significance of single items relative to summated scores. *Mayo Clinic Proceedings* 77:488–494.

Smets, E.M.A., Garssen, B., Bonke, B., and J.C.J.M. de Haes. 1995. The Multidimensional Fatigue Inventory (MFI) psychometric qualities of an instrument to assess fatigue. *Journal of Psychosomatic Research* 39:315–325.

Snedecor, G.W. and W.B. Cochran. 1980. *Statistical Methods*, 7th edition. Ames, IA: The Iowa State University Press.

Snyder, C.F., Aaronson, N.K., Choucair, A.K., Elliott, T.E., Greenhalgh, J., Halyard, M.Y., Hess, R., Miller, D.M., Reeve, B.B., and M. Santana. 2012. Implementing patient-reported outcomes assessment in clinical practice: A review of the options and considerations. *Quality of Life Research* 21:1305–1314.

Stiger, T.R., Kosinski, A.S., Barnhart, H.X., and D.G. Kleinbaum. 1998. ANOVA for repeated ordinal data with small sample size? A comparisons of ANOVA, MANOVA, WLS, and GEE methods by stimulation. *Communications in Statistics—Simulations and Computation, Part A*, 27:357–375.

Streiner, D.L. and G.R. Norman. 2008. *Health Measurement Scales: A Practical Guide to Their Development and Use*, 4th edition. New York, NY: Oxford University Press.

Sullivan, L.M. and R.B. D'Agostino Sr. 2003. Robustness and power of analysis of covariance applied to ordinal scaled data as arising in randomized controlled trials. *Statistics in Medicine* 22:1317–1334.

Ware, J.E., Snow, K.K., Kosinski, M., and B. Gandek. 1993. *SF-36 Health Survey Manual and Interpretation Guide*. Boston, MA: The Health Institute, New England Medical Center.

Willke, R.J., Burke, L.B., and P. Erickson. 2004. Measuring treatment impact: A review of patient-reported outcomes and other efficacy endpoints in approved product labels. *Controlled Clinical Trials* 25:535–552.

Zigmond, A.S. and R.P. Snaith. 1983. The Hospital Anxiety and Depression Scale. *Acta Psychiatrica Scandinavica* 67:361–370.

2

Development of a Patient-Reported Outcome

Patient-reported outcomes (PROs) are important assessment tools increasingly used in clinical trials to allow information about such outcomes as symptoms, health-related quality of life (HRQL), and treatment satisfaction to be collected directly from the patient. The rise in the use of PRO measures has occurred because some treatment effects are known only to patients, their perspective is unique, and important information may not be measured if only clinician or biological assessments are made (Kerr et al., 2010). Rigor in the development of the content of a PRO is essential to ensure that the concept of interest is measured accurately, to capture issues of most relevance to the patient, and to subscribe to a language that allows patients to understand and respond without confusion. Items within a questionnaire with little relevance to the patient population being investigated, or if poorly written, will lead to measurement error and bias.

If the questions within a measure are neither understood properly nor very relevant, then an ambiguous response is likely. Therefore, taking time to talk with patients about their symptoms or the impact of a disease or condition on their HRQL is very important before embarking on generation of the questions to measure the concept of interest. Qualitative research with patients is essential for establishing content validity of a PRO measure (Patrick et al., 2011a). Doing so will aid interpretation of scores and provide clarity for communication of findings (Rothman et al., 2007). The steps to consider for conducting qualitative research to establish content validity are discussed later, with the schematic in Figure 2.1 detailing the flow of the process and the main activities required for developing the content of a new measure.

2.1 Population

In developing a new PRO, a researcher should choose subjects who are very closely representative of the intended population of interest (e.g., diagnosis, severity of condition, age, gender). If the measure is to be used in a multinational study, interviews with patients from different countries to enhance the cross-cultural validity and linguistic equivalence of the measure are encouraged (Patrick et al., 2011a). For example, to develop the DFS-Fibro, a daily fatigue measure for use in patients with fibromyalgia, Humphrey et al. (2010) used 20 US, 10 German, and 10 French subjects to increase cross-cultural validity. Generally,

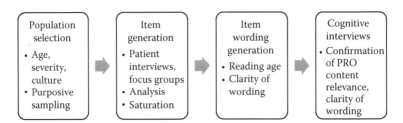

FIGURE 2.1
Process for developing a new PRO instrument.

though, the choice of patient population is based on purposive sampling; the sample of patients best representing a population under investigation should be selected (Kerr et al., 2010).

2.2 Item Generation

2.2.1 Patient Interviews and Focus Groups

To generate the content of a PRO, either individual interviews or group discussion with patients (typically called focus groups) will be required. Choice of individual interviews or focus groups will depend on the sensitivity of the topic to be discussed and whether there is a need for participants to react and feed off each other in discussing a topic. Focus groups require strong moderation to facilitate discussion and ensure no one person dominates the discussion. Individual interviews allow more in-depth discussion and are generally easier to analyze but may take longer to collect data. Generally, a mixture of the two approaches is beneficial.

Qualitative research is a scientific technique that requires a protocol outlining the study details. The protocol should include such things as inclusion/exclusion criteria, number of subjects, prespecification if particular subgroups should be emphasized in recruitment, and information about the questions to be asked by developing an interview guide. Interviews or focus groups should be audio recorded to allow transcription and analysis. The interview guide is essential to ensure consistency of questioning and the questions should be broad and open ended. For example, if a scale to measure sleep disorders is being proposed, examples of questions can include "how long have you had issues with your sleep?", "what kinds of sleep difficulties do you experience?". From these broader questions, a researcher can then probe in more detail such as "you said you had problems with staying asleep, can you describe in more detail what specifically these problems are?". If particular concepts are not raised but have been discussed in other interviews, there may be a need to use more direct questioning, for example, "Does light or noise cause you problems with staying asleep?".

2.2.2 Analysis of Qualitative Data

Once the data have been collected, analysis of the verbatim transcripts is then conducted, involving sorting quotes by concept and could be aided by using software (e.g., ATLAS.ti®). Such software also allows easier analysis by a specific patient characteristic (e.g., gender or disease severity) to determine if there are differences in conceptualization of the issue under discussion. This sorting process will lead to development of a coding scheme, whereby similar concepts are given a code name. For example, if the discussion was about fatigue and how patients described this symptom, then codes might be tiredness, unrested, etc. Quotes from subjects related to these specific terms would then be added under these code names, which allows the researcher to see how such terms were used and how many times the term was used. The codes are usually developed iteratively, changing as the data are analyzed, always through discussion among individuals who are generating the codes to cover the content of the transcripts from the interviews or focus groups. This approach is based on grounded theory methods (Glasser and Strauss, 1999), whereby ideas for the content of a new measure are developed inductively from the qualitative transcripts. Grounded theory is a set of collection and analysis methods that assure that the meaning of a concept is discovered in the words and actions of participants from the ground up – not from application of *a priori* theory or concepts (Lasch et al., 2010). Ground theory involves developing codes to allow the key points of the data to be gathered, which will then be grouped into concepts and from these concepts a theory about the data is developed.

This process is usually completed with independent reviews of the data to ensure that all codes are an accurate reflection of the transcripts; ensuring inter- and intra-rater reliability of the coding scheme is important (Lasch et al., 2010). From this process, a conceptual framework will emerge (see Figure 2.2 for an example)—a visual depiction of the concepts, subconcepts, and items and how they interrelate. Often the conceptual framework has been proposed based on clinician input and a literature review, with qualitative patient interviews serving to refine the model. There are other qualitative research approaches such as phenomenology, ethnography, case study, discourse analysis, and traditional content analysis; a comparison of these approaches is discussed by Lasch et al. (2010). Choice of approach will be dependent on the type of research question(s), but for PRO development, grounded theory is generally preferred (Kerr et al., 2010; Lasch et al., 2010).

Once the codes are agreed upon, usually by two or three reviewers of the transcripts identifying and agreeing on the common themes emerging from the data, these reviewers will then review the transcripts and highlight patient quotes that match or reflect one of the codes. This generates a list of patient statements per code, which allows assessment of how frequently the concept was discussed and by how many subjects, in order to determine whether a concept or category should form part of the new measure. If the concept is deemed important, the verbatim quotes will allow the generation of relevant

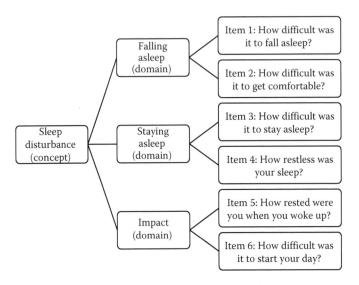

FIGURE 2.2
Example of a conceptual framework.

items, in patient-friendly language, for each concept identified. The conceptual framework will then build to show proposed subconcepts, often called domains, and then items to measure the subconcepts (see Figure 2.2).

While developing the draft items for a new PRO, a researcher should consider the recall period (e.g., immediate, 7 days, 4 weeks), which will be dependent on the concept and the disease being measured. Symptoms are normally best captured daily, whereas questions about HRQL may best be recalled over a longer period (e.g., 7 days). The most appropriate response options should also be thought about and ideally will be consistent to mitigate patient confusion. There are various types of response options, ranging from a simple *yes/no* to Likert scales, which typically have 5–7 response options with descriptors for each response category (e.g., *totally disagree, largely disagree, disagree, disagree to some extent, agree to some extent, largely agree,* and *totally agree*) to an 11 point, 0–10 numeric rating scale that tends to provide wording at the extremes only (e.g., *no pain* to *worst possible pain*). Decisions on how the items were initially decided upon, along with choice of response options and recall period, should be documented using an item-tracking matrix (Patrick et al., 2011b).

2.2.3 Saturation

Knowing when sufficient data have been collected to confidently state that the key concepts of importance for the particular patient group being studied have been captured is generally based on *saturation*. That is, if no new or relevant information is elicited, then there should be confidence that the main concepts of importance to patients have been captured.

An example of the process of determining saturation is as follows:

1. Transcripts of the first 10 interviews are analyzed to identify consistency in the pattern of the responses to the concepts presented during the interview.
2. The second set of 10 interviews will then be analyzed to determine if any new concepts have been identified. If they have not, then no further interviews are required, but if they have, then more interviews should be conducted until nothing new is elicited.

Saturation usually occurs within 20–30 in-depth interviews (Rothman et al., 2009). However, this will be dependent on the complexity of the concept that is being discussed (Patrick et al., 2011b), study design, the purposive sampling strategy used (Kerr et al., 2010), and diversity of the population from which the sample is to be drawn from (Leidy and Vernon, 2008; Patrick et al., 2011b). Table 2.1 shows an example saturation grid. In this example, there was only one new concept elicited in the second set of 10 interviews and no new concepts found during interviews 21–30, which indicated that the list of subconcepts describing *fatigue* was exhausted after 30 interviews. In the first set of interviews subjects described the feeling of fatigue using various adjectives such as tired, exhausted. In the second set of interviews subjects also described their fatigue using similar terms but some went further and described how debilitating it was and had overwhelmed their lives. Use of a saturation grid requires an iterative process whereby the data is analyzed on an ongoing basis to monitor saturation.

There could be situations where, after the third batch of interviews or third focus group, there are one or two new concepts elicited and then the research team has to decide if saturation has been achieved. Conducting a further set of interviews or focus group will address this, but even if new concepts are brought out, the research team will have to decide if these are meaningful and require further investigation or are anomalous or related to other

TABLE 2.1

Example of a Saturation Grid for a Series of Individual Interviews to Understand Fibromyalgia Patients' Experience of Fatigue

Concept	Subconcepts That Emerged from the First 10 Interviews	New Subconcepts That Emerged in Interviews 11–20	New Subconcepts That Emerged in Interviews 21–30
Fatigue	Tiredness		
	Exhausted		
	Lack of energy/no energy		
	Tired despite sleeping well		
		Overwhelmed by tiredness/fatigue	

themes previously elicited. Rather than worry about the number of interviews or focus groups to conduct, Kerr et al. (2010) recommend that data collection and analysis be iterative to allow some assessment of saturation while the data is being collected. They also recommend documenting clearly in the protocol the procedure for assessing saturation and to have flexibility in the study design to allow for additional interviews if necessary.

2.3 Item Wording

Items are generated based on the language used by subjects from the individual interviews or focus groups. At this point, numerous items will be formulated per concept/domain, often with significant overlap in wording because it is not always clear which terminology is most appropriate for the majority of patients. A further study can be conducted to help choose between the various options (cognitive interview study—see Section 2.4). At all times, the reading age of the resulting items for the questionnaire should be considered, and items should be worded carefully and clearly. Reading age should not be expected to be much beyond elementary level. Items measuring two concepts should be avoided because patients may experience one part of the question but not the other and this then makes it difficult for the patient to answer. An example is a question about pain and discomfort—some patients may not experience discomfort, only pain, making it difficult for them to then answer the question.

2.4 Cognitive Interviews

Before psychometric validation of a PRO, it should be reviewed by patients from the target population to evaluate the individual items, the instructions, response options, and recall period for understanding of the content and comprehensiveness. These types of interviews are referred to as cognitive interviews. Patients are asked to complete the measure, and while doing so, they are instructed to speak out what they are thinking and to explain how they are interpreting the content of the measure. Such one-to-one interviews are recommended rather than using a focus group approach. In this way, the interviewer can get a sense of whether the patient can understand the content, the items, the instructions, and response options as intended.

If there are issues with any part of the PRO, the interviewer can ask how they would reword to make it clearer. If a high number of subjects state that they are not happy with an item and would reword it, alternative wording should be considered based on advice from the subjects. For instruments

TABLE 2.2

Checklist of Activities to Conduct to Derive
the Content for a New Measure

Conduct focus groups or individual patient interviews	☐
Analyze the transcripts to generate appropriate content	☐
Saturation of concepts obtained	☐
Cognitive debriefing of content	☐
New measure ready for psychometric testing	☐

with several items in the scale or multiple domains, items that are understood clearly by the majority of subjects should form the core of the new PRO or the PRO domain. Also, response options that make it easiest for the majority of the subjects to respond to should be taken forward. If changes are made to the draft PRO, documenting the reasons using the item-tracking matrix is recommended (Patrick et al., 2011b). Table 2.2 provides a checklist of activities to complete to derive the content of a new measure.

Once the content has been confirmed via the cognitive debriefing exercise, the draft measure is ready for quantitative analysis, more details of which are given in the remaining chapters. Recently though, some have suggested the use of item response theory (see Chapter 6) to help further refine the content of a measure by showing whether or not a measure is covering the continuum of a concept and what part of the response continuum items address before embarking on larger scale psychometric testing (Patrick et al., 2011b; Magasi et al., 2012). If there are gaps in the continuum, then reanalysis of the qualitative data may be required to determine whether additional concepts should be added. This provides confidence that the measure truly is measuring the concept adequately. Indeed, Patrick et al. (2011b) caution that the use of quantitative assessments to validate a new measure in the absence of speaking to patients can lead to an instrument producing scores with unknown meaning, while using qualitative assessment only to develop a PRO "may be rhetorically convincing, but scientifically incomplete."

2.5 Summary

Developing the content of a new measure takes much care, time, and consideration to minimize error in measuring the concept that you are interested in. Not only do we want to be sure that we are measuring what we say we are measuring, we also want to reduce error or ambiguity in the data caused by misunderstanding of the questions or inclusion of irrelevant items, which will lead to the need for larger sample sizes to show an effect if the measure were being used in a research study.

Content validity is an essential part of the development of a new PRO measure and is further elaborated upon in Chapter 3. Indeed, the federal drug authorities are now mandating evidence of content validity before considering a PRO for labeling (FDA, 2009), and the European Medicines Agency (EMA, 2005) also consider content validity important. Taking the time to diligently consider the content of any new measure by exploring the literature, discussing with clinicians who have had many hours of contact with a diverse spectrum of patients, and, most importantly, conducting qualitative research with patients themselves to generate the content of a new measure will pay dividends by producing a robust, valid, and reliable measure.

Interested readers are encouraged to read the International Society of Pharmacoeconomics PRO Good Research Practices Task Force Reports: Part 1, "Eliciting concepts for a new PRO instrument" (Patrick et al., 2011a) and Part 2, "Assessing respondent understanding" (Patrick et al., 2011b) for further detailed information about conducting qualitative research, some of which is detailed in the next chapter covering validation more broadly. A good example of how to develop a new measure is reported in the article by Humphrey et al. (2010) in the development of new fatigue PRO for fibromyalgia patients. For guidance on steps to consider in the modification of existing PRO instruments, readers can consult Rothman et al. (2009).

References

European Medicines Agency (EMA), Committee for Medicinal Products for Human Use. 2005. Reflection paper on the regulatory guidance for use of health-related quality of life (HRQOL) measures in the evaluation of medicinal products. European Medicines Agency. http://www.ema.europa.eu/ema/ (Accessed on August 31, 2013).

Food and Drug Administration (FDA). 2009. Guidance for industry on patient-reported outcome measures: Use in medical product development to support labeling claims. *Federal Register* 74(235):65132–65133. http://www.fda.gov/downloads/Drugs/GuidanceComplianceRegulatoryInformation/Guidances/UCM193282.pdf. (Accessed on August 31, 2013).

Glasser, B.G. and A.L. Strauss. 1999. *The Discovery of Grounded Theory: Strategies for Qualitative Research.* Chicago, IL: Aldine Publishing Company.

Humphrey, L., Arbuckle, R., Mease, P., Williams, D.A., Danneskiold Samsoe, B., and C. Gilbert. 2010. Fatigue in fibromyalgia: A conceptual model informed by patient interviews. *BMC Musculoskeletal Disorders* 11:216–226.

Kerr, C., Nixon, A., and D. Wild. 2010. Assessing and demonstrating data saturation in qualitative inquiry supporting patient-reported outcomes research. *Expert Review of Pharmacoeconomics & Outcomes Research* 10:269–281.

Lasch, K.E., Marquis, P., Vigneux, M., Abetz, L., Arnould, B., Bayliss, M., Crawford, B., and K. Rosa. 2010. PRO development: Rigorous qualitative research as the crucial foundation. *Quality of Life Research* 19:1087–1096.

Leidy, N. and M. Vernon. 2008. Perspectives on patient reported outcomes: Content validity and qualitative research in a changing clinical trial environment. *Pharmacoeconomics* 26:363–370.

Magasi, S., Ryan, G., Revicki, D., Lenderking, W., Hays, R.D., Brod, M., Synder, C., Boers, M., and D. Cella. 2012. Content validity of patient-reported outcome measures: Perspectives from a PROMIS meeting. *Quality of Life Research* 21:739–746.

Patrick, D.L., Burke, L.B., Gwaltney, C.H., Kline Leidy, N., Martin, M.L., Molsen, E., and L. Ring. 2011a. Content validity—Establishing and reporting the evidence in newly developed patient reported outcomes (PRO) instruments for medical product evaluation: ISPOR PRO good research practices task force report: Part 1—Eliciting concepts for a new PRO instrument. *Value in Health* 14:967–977.

Patrick, D.L., Burke, L.B., Gwaltney, C.H., Kline Leidy, N., Martin, M.L., Molsen, E., and L. Ring. 2011b. Content Validity—Establishing and reporting the evidence in newly developed patient reported outcomes (PRO) instruments for medical product evaluation: ISPOR PRO good research practices task force report: Part 2—Assessing respondent understanding. *Value in Health* 14:978–988.

Rothman, M., Burke, L., Erickson, P., Kline Leidy, N., Patrick, D.L., and C. Petrie. 2009. Use of existing patient-reported outcomes (PRO) instruments and their modification: The ISPOR good research practices for evaluating and documenting content validity for the use of existing instruments and their modifications PRO task force report. *Value in Health* 12:1075–1083.

Rothman, M.L., Beltran, P., Cappelleri, J.C., Lipscomb, J., Teschendorf, B., and the Mayo/FDA Patient Reported Outcomes Consensus Meeting Group. 2007. Patient reported outcomes: Conceptual issues. *Value in Health* 10 (Suppl. 2):S66–S75.

3

Validity

This chapter is an introduction to the concepts of validity in the evaluation of a patient-reported outcome (PRO) instrument. In simple terms, validity assesses the extent to which an instrument measures what it is meant to measure. Validity is discussed in terms of content validity and construct validity. As a complementary and supplementary exposition to content validity as introduced and illustrated in Chapter 2, this chapter begins with another round of emphasis on content validity, the cornerstone of validity, this time in the context of and as part of an overall exposition on validity. This chapter then follows with the quantification and evaluation of hypotheses embedded in, and central to, the different aspects of construct validity. This chapter is also the first time that SAS simulations, grounded in practical scenarios, are presented to complement and supplement the exposition given on concepts, methods, and published real-life examples. While the simulations code and its output are intended to be self-contained, readers wanting to go beyond the SAS simulations in this and subsequent chapters can consult other sources (Fran et al., 2002; SAS, 2011a,b, 2012a,b; Wicklin, 2013).

3.1 Content Validity

Content validity is the extent to which an instrument covers the important concepts of the unobservable or latent attribute (e.g., depression, anxiety, physical functioning, self-esteem) the instrument purports to measure. It is "the degree to which the content of a measurement instrument is an adequate reflection of the construct to be measured" (Mokkink et al., 2010). How well does the PRO instrument capture all of the important aspects of the concept from the patient's perspective? Qualitative work with patients is therefore central to supporting content validity.

The content of a PRO measure should be reviewed against the findings of qualitative work to ensure comprehensiveness from the patient's perspective. Although complete or near complete agreement among stakeholders is ideally desired about what a particular construct or concept represents (e.g., physical function for a particular patient group) and what language should be used in the PRO measure, an element of subjectivity inevitably exists among patients, experts in the field of a disease, and other stakeholders in relation to determining content validity. For PRO instruments, however, it is the patient's perspective that reigns in the content validation of a PRO measure.

The importance of content validity in developing PRO instruments is stressed by both the US Food and Drug Administration (FDA, 2009) and the European Medicines Agency (EMA, 2005). The validation of an instrument is an ongoing process and validity relates to both the PRO measure itself and how it is used. When evaluating potential instruments, researchers should consider evidence of content validity for a PRO endpoint—the instrument's ability to measure the stated concepts—in the relevant patient population.

A task force sponsored by the International Society for Pharmacoeconomics and Outcomes Research (ISPOR) has published two reports on content validity (Part 1 and Part 2). Part 1 includes five steps to elicit concepts for new PRO instruments and to document content validity consistent with good research (Patrick et al., 2011a). These five steps cover the following general themes: (1) determine the context of use (e.g., medical product labeling), (2) develop the research protocol for qualitative concept elicitation and analysis, (3) conduct the concept elicitation interviews and focus groups, (4) analyze the qualitative data, and (5) document concept development and elicitation methodology and results.

Part 2 on content validity involves assessing respondent understanding and details the following two themes: (1) the methods for conducting cognitive interviews that address patient understanding of items, instructions, and response options and (2) the methods for tracking item development through the various stages of research and preparing this tracking for submission to regulatory agencies (Patrick et al., 2011b). Several criteria are needed for evaluating new items and a checklist can be applied to whether the criterion is met (Table 3.1). Table 3.2 provides examples of poorly worded and preferred wording or probing to assess patient understanding and content coverage of a PRO instrument.

TABLE 3.1

Sample Criteria for Evaluating New Items

Criteria	Item Meets Criteria: Yes/No
The item captures the concept that is intended.	
The item is relevant to all members of the target population.	
The item is worded in a manner consistent with the expressions used by patients.	
The item reflects different levels of magnitude, e.g., severity, frequency.	
The item represents a single concept, rather than a multidimensional concept.	
The item is not likely to be vulnerable to ceiling or floor effects within the target population, i.e., it will change with treatment.	
The content of the items is appropriate for the recall period.	
The content of the item is appropriate for the mode of administration.	
The response scale corresponds to the item.	

Source: Patrick, D.L. et al., *Value Health*, 14, 978, 2011b.

TABLE 3.2

Examples of Poorly Worded and Preferred Wording or Probing for Cognitive Interviews to Assess Patient Understanding and Content Coverage of a PRO Instrument

Purpose	Poorly Worded	Preferred Wording or Probing
Instructions: To understand respondent's interpretation of the task (s) to be performed.	Are the instructions clear? Yes/No Are the instructions easy to read and understand? Yes/No	Can you tell me in your own words, what this instruction is asking you to do? Can you describe any confusion or difficulty you had in understanding these instructions? Are there any words or phrases that you would change to improve the instructions?
Recall: To identify how patients retrieve information, remember situations or events.	Is this recall period too long? Too short? Just right?	What does (timeframe) mean to you? Describe your experiences with [concept] over the (timeframe). What period of time did you think about when you were completing the questionnaire?
Item stem: To understand the clarity of the question from the respondent's perspective.	Do you like this question? Is this question clear? Is this question easy to understand?	What does [item content] mean to you? Using your own words, how would you explain what this question means?
Response options: To understand how participants interpret the response options and make decisions around response choice.	What response did you choose? Is this the best response for you?	Please read each response choice and tell me what it means to you. In thinking about your experience with [Item x], which response best describes your experience? What caused you to choose this response? Would you ever choose A? Why or why not? Can you describe an experience where you might choose D?
Content coverage: To determine if the content in the instrument is comprehensive/to assure that there are no missing concepts.	Is the instrument comprehensive? Do the questions cover all aspects of [the concept]?	What other experiences do you have with [the concept] that are not covered in this questionnaire?

(continued)

TABLE 3.2 (continued)

Examples of Poorly Worded and Preferred Wording or Probing for Cognitive Interviews to Assess Patient Understanding and Content Coverage of a PRO Instrument

Purpose	Poorly Worded	Preferred Wording or Probing
Format: To identify respondent difficulties with the presentation of the questionnaire or diary.	Is the format okay? Do you have any suggestions for improving the format? Were the skip patterns clear?	Observe the respondent completing the questionnaire. Note facial expressions, indications of reading difficulty, flipping pages or screens back and forth. Listen for comments about difficulty reading or questions that indicate lack of clarity or ease of use. Observe how the respondent completed this portion of the questionnaire. Note if skip patterns were correctly followed. What suggestions do you have for changing the questionnaire so it is easier to complete?
Length: To determine if the length of time it takes to complete the questionnaire is reasonable (does not burden subject).	Is the questionnaire too long? Too short?	What did you think about the amount of time it took you to complete the questionnaire?

Source: Patrick, D.L. et al., *Value Health*, 14, 978, 2011b.

A component of content validity is face validity, "the degree to which a measurement instrument, indeed, looks as though it is an adequate reflection of the construct to be measured" (Mokkink et al., 2010). It concerns whether items in an instrument appear on the face of it to cover the intended topics clearly and unambiguously. For instance, if a questionnaire is designed to assess physical function in the elderly, questions on certain items about activities that are no longer performed by the elderly are not considered to be suitable and hence not face valid. Being a first impression, face validity has no standards with regard to how it should be assessed and quantified. While the greater part of content validity consists of ensuring that comprehensive and thorough development procedures are rigorously followed and documented, face validity surfaces specifically after an instrument has been constructed.

Comprehensive coverage is the hallmark of content validity. The entire range of relevant issues should be covered by the PRO instrument in the target population (Cieza and Stucki, 2005). If the intention is to measure physical functioning in stroke patients in the elderly, the activity items on a questionnaire should be relevant to the stroke population and should ensure that no important activities for stroke patients are missed. If a questionnaire is to measure poststroke patients, the quality-of-life index may be a suitable choice, as it includes self-care and simple activities of daily living that are particularly relevant to severely disabled patients (Spitzer et al., 1981). If, on the other hand, a questionnaire is needed to measure physical functioning in depressive adolescents, the Nottingham Health Profile (NHP) may be the more appropriate choice, because adolescents have the potential to be very physically active and the NHP can accommodate this (Hunt et al., 1985).

Content validity (including face validity) for PROs is optimized by including a wide range of patients from the target population in the development process. In addition to the qualitative work, quantitative evaluation of items is useful and desirable during the content validity stage in order to assess how well items address the entire continuum of patient experience on the concept, regardless if the concept is a symptom, behavior, or feeling. A preliminary quantitative assessment using classical test theory or item response theory can be considered (provided of course that the sample size is not too small and that there are a sufficient number of items to warrant examination for certain assessments). During the content validation stage, a numerical descriptive approach can examine directionality of responses and serve as a barometer on how well items address the entire continuum of the targeted concept (construct) of interest.

Specifically, such an exploratory descriptive assessment can enrich content validity by addressing the frequency of the categories across the range of item responses, the distribution of total scores, floor and ceiling effects, the relationship between item response options and the total score, and the extent that the hypothesized item difficulty order is represented by observed responses. An additional set of recommendations for reporting and interpreting content validity in psychological assessment is elaborated elsewhere (Haynes et al., 1995). After a PRO instrument emanates from the content validity phase, full psychometric testing of the instrument can be conducted during subsequent stages of validation.

In addition to guidelines for the content validity of new PRO instruments in the drug approval process, guidelines on content validity have been recommended for existing PRO instruments and their modification in the drug approval process (Rothman et al., 2009). Both sets of guidelines are worth considering even when a label claim is not being sought.

Steps involved in identifying and evaluating an existing PRO measure include the following: (1) name and define the concept; (2) draft the claim, target population, target product profile, and endpoint model; (3) identify candidate measures; (4) identify or formulate a conceptual framework for the instrument(s); (5) assemble and evaluate information on development methods; (6) conduct any needed qualitative research; (7) assess adequacy of content validity for purpose; and (8) determine the need for modifications or new instrument development (Rothman et al., 2009).

Various scenarios can be considered in the content validation of an existing PRO instrument (Rothman et al., 2009). For example, if an existing PRO instrument is used in a new patient population, qualitative analyses with the new patients and extensive literature search can be part of the remediation strategy. If a focus group appraisal of the existing PRO instrument identifies the same concepts but with different item wording, cognitive interviews can be conducted to assure patient understanding is consistent with the concept and to modify the instrument should there be patient misunderstanding. If a short form of an existing PRO instrument is used, patient interviews or focus groups can be conducted with representative patients to determine the importance that patients placed on the omitted items relative to those retained in the shorter version.

3.2 Construct Validity

Attributes such as height or weight are readily observable and measurable. A person's blood pressure is typically expressed in terms of systolic pressure over diastolic pressure and is measured in millimeters of mercury (e.g., 120/80). Physical attributes like these are measured concretely. As movement shifts into the realm of more psychological attributes like anxiety and pain, however, the attributes of interest become more abstract and cannot be directly observed or realized. The measurement of anxiety can be observed, though, through behaviors that are consequences of anxiety, such as uneasiness, sweaty palms, and pacing back and forth.

Words like hyperactivity, assertiveness, and fatigue (as well as anxiety, depression, and pain) refer to abstract ideas that humans construct in their minds to help them explain observed patterns or differences in their behavior, attitudes, or feelings. A construct is an unobservable (latent) postulated attribute that helps to characterize or theorize about the human experience or condition through observable attitudes, behaviors, and feelings. Because such constructs are not directly measurable with an objective device (such as a ruler, weighing scale, or stethoscope), PRO instruments are designed to measure these more abstract concepts.

Construct validity can be defined as "the degree to which the scores of a measurement instrument are consistent with hypotheses (for instance, with regard to internal relationships, relationships with scores of other instruments or differences between relevant groups)" (Mokkink et al., 2010). Construct validity involves constructing and evaluating postulated relationships involving a scale intended to measure a particular concept of interest. The PRO measure under consideration should indeed measure the postulated construct under consideration. If there is a mismatch between the targeted PRO scale and its intended construct, then the problem could be that the scale is good but the theory is wrong, the theory is good but the scale is not, or both the theory and the scale are useless or misplaced. Assessment of construct validity can be quantified through descriptive statistics, plots, correlations, and regression analyses.

Mainly, assessments of construct validity make use of correlations, changes over time, and differences between groups of patients. Construct validation is a lengthy, ongoing process. In practical applications, a part of construct validation appraises whether items on a PRO domain (or subscale) relate to a single latent construct or to multiple latent constructs, whether items are homogeneous in measuring equally strongly the same latent construct, and to what extent do items from one subscale on one latent construct correlate with latent constructs from other subscales. All aspects of validity are essentially some form of construct validity. In what follows, the chief aspects of validity are highlighted.

3.2.1 Convergent Validity and Divergent Validity

Convergent validity addresses how much the target scale relates to other variables or measures to which it is expected to be related, according to the theory postulated. For instance, patients with higher levels of pain might be expected to also have higher levels of physical impairment and this association should be sizeable. How sizeable? It depends on the nature of the variables or measures. Generally, though, a correlation between 0.4 and 0.8 would seem reasonable in most circumstances as evidence for convergent validity. The correlation should not be too low or too high. A correlation that is too low would indicate that different things are being measured; a correlation that is too high would indicate that the same thing is being measured and hence one of the variables or measures is redundant.

In contrast, *divergent validity* addresses how much the target scale relates to other variables or measures to which it is expected to have a weak or no relation (according to the theory postulated). For instance, little or no correlation might be expected between pain and intelligence scores.

As an example of convergent validity and divergent validity, consider the Self-Esteem and Relationship (SEAR) questionnaire, a 14-item psychometric instrument specific to erectile dysfunction (ED) (Althof et al., 2003; Cappelleri et al., 2004). Here the focus is on measuring its convergent validity and divergent validity through its two domains, the 8-item Sexual Relationship Satisfaction domain and the 6-item Confidence domain, using two generic questionnaires: the 22-item Psychological General Well-Being (PGWB) index and the 36-item Medical Outcomes Short-Form (SF-36). Evidence for convergent validity was based on a Pearson correlation of 0.40 or higher; evidence for divergent validity was based on a Pearson correlation less than 0.30. Correlations between 0.30 and 0.40 were taken as no evidence to dismiss either convergent validity or divergent validity. Results were based on 98 men who self-reported a clinical diagnosis of ED in the past year (49 treated with sildenafil at least once, 49 were not treated) and 94 men who self-reported no clinical diagnosis of ED in the past year.

Divergent validity (or at least no evidence to dismiss it) on the Sexual Relationship Satisfaction domain of the SEAR questionnaire was hypothesized and confirmed by its relatively low correlations with all domains on the PGWB and SF-36 (Table 3.3). For the Confidence domain of the SEAR questionnaire, divergent validity (or at least no evidence to dismiss it) was hypothesized and confirmed by its relatively low correlations with physical factors of the SF-36 (Physical Functioning, Role-Physical, Bodily Pain, Physical Component Summary). Convergent validity (or at least no evidence to dismiss it) was hypothesized and confirmed with relatively moderate correlations with the SF-36 Mental Component Summary and the Role-Emotional and Mental Health domains, as well as with the PGWB index score and the PGWB domains on Anxiety, Depressed Mood, Positive Well-Being, and Self-Control (Table 3.3). No other hypotheses were made.

This study also provided an example of item-level discriminant tests, a form of the multitrait–multimethod approach (Campbell and Fiske, 1959), as a validation method that combines both convergent validity and divergent validity (Table 3.4). Specifically, each item had a corrected item-to-total correlation greater than 0.4 with its domain total score (*corrected* for by excluding the item under consideration from its domain score). In terms of item-level discriminant validity tests, based on the item-to-total correlations, 11 of the 14 items were classified as successful in the sense that the correlation of

TABLE 3.3

Correlations of SEAR Questionnaire Domain Scores with PGWB Scale and SF-36 Scores

	SEAR Domain: Sexual Relationship	SEAR Domain: Confidence
PGWB Scale	*Correlations with PGWB Scale*	
Anxiety	0.18	0.32
Depressed Mood	0.20	0.37
Positive Well-Being	0.30	0.47
Self-Control	0.21	0.41
General Health	0.28	0.29
Vitality	0.26	0.34
PGWB Index	0.28	0.44
SF-36	*Correlations with SF-36*	
Physical Functioning	0.13	0.30
Role-Physical	0.21	0.30
Bodily Pain	0.21	0.32
General Health	0.38	0.40
Vitality	0.34	0.36
Social Functioning	0.15	0.34
Role-Emotional	0.24	0.44
Mental Health	0.21	0.45
Physical Component Summary	0.27	0.38
Mental Component Summary	0.27	0.45

Source: Cappelleri, J.C. et al., *Int. J. Impot. Res.*, 16, 30, 2004.

TABLE 3.4

Item-to-Total Correlations and Item-Level Discriminant Validity on the SEAR
Questionnaire

	Item-to-Total Correlations[a]	
Item	Domain: Sexual Relationship Satisfaction	Domain: Confidence
1. I felt relaxed about initiating sex with my partner	**0.68**	0.50
2. I felt confident that during sex my erection would last long enough	**0.74**	0.56
3. I was satisfied with my sexual performance	**0.85**	0.54
4. I felt that sex could be spontaneous	**0.62**	0.49
5. I was likely to initiate sex	**0.63**	0.44
6. I felt confident about performing sexually	**0.82**	0.57
7. I was satisfied with our sex life	**0.82**	0.60
8. My partner was unhappy with the quality of our sexual relations	**0.57**	0.34
9. I had good self-esteem	0.48	**0.68**
10. I felt like a whole man	0.56	**0.73**
11. I was inclined to feel that I am a failure	0.37	**0.50**
12. I felt confident	0.51	**0.71**
13. My partner was satisfied with our relationship in general	0.55	**0.63**
14. I was satisfied with our relationship in general	0.52	**0.68**

Source: Cappelleri, J.C. et al., *Int. J. Impot. Res.*, 16, 30, 2004.

[a] Under item-to-total correlations, bold numbers represent corrected item-to-total correlations of Items 1–8 with scores on the Sexual Relationship Satisfaction domain and Items 9–14 with scores on the Confidence domain. Other (not bold) numbers are uncorrected item-to-total correlations, with the item included instead of excluded from the domain total.

each was significantly higher ($p < 0.05$) with its corresponding domain score
(which excludes the item) than with the other domain score (which includes
the item). The remaining 3 items (Items 4, 11, and 13) were classified as likely
successes in the sense that the correlation of each trended higher with its corresponding domain score than with the other domain score.

3.2.2 Known-Groups Validity

Known-groups validity is based on the principle that the measurement scale of
interest should be sensitive to differences between specific groups of subjects
known to be different in a relevant way. As such, the scale is expected to
show differences, in the predicted direction, between these known groups.
The magnitude of the separation between known groups is more important
than whether the separation is statistically significant, especially in studies
with small or modest sample sizes where statistical significance may not be
achieved. For instance, if a PRO instrument is intended to measure visual
functioning, mean scores on it should be able to differentiate sufficiently

between subjects with different levels of visual acuity (mild, moderate, severe). A scale that cannot distinguish between groups with known differences is hardly likely to be of much value. In the literature, known-groups validity is sometimes referred to as discriminant validity and sometimes as divergent validity, so readers should be careful how these terms are defined.

The *sensitivity* and *responsiveness* of a scale are aspects of known-groups comparisons and hence of validity. In terms of known-groups validity, sensitivity is the ability of a scale to detect differences between patients or groups of patients. A scale is useless for group assessment or evaluation unless it can reflect differences between poor and good prognosis patients or between a beneficial treatment and a less beneficial one. If a treatment in a multiple treatment clinical trial is known to be beneficial (relative to a control treatment) on what the PRO instrument is measuring, and the scale shows this, the scale provides evidence of sensitivity in measuring the construct of interest. Related to sensitivity, responsiveness refers to the ability of the scale to detect within-individual changes when a patient improves or deteriorates; for instance, the two groups could be related samples of the same patients taken before and after an intervention. A measurement scale is futile for patient monitoring unless it can reflect changes in a patient's condition.

Known-groups validity of the SEAR questionnaire was based on a single self-assessment of ED severity (none, mild, moderate, severe) from 192 men (Cappelleri et al., 2004). Figure 3.1 shows the means and 95% confidence intervals for scores on the 8-item Sexual Relationship Satisfaction domain,

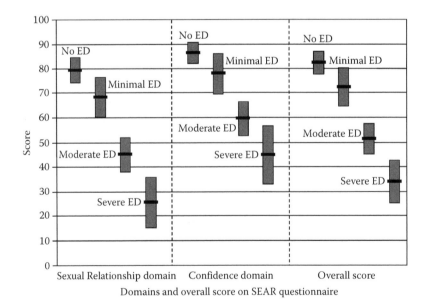

FIGURE 3.1
Mean scores and 95% confidence intervals on the SEAR questionnaire for four self-reported levels of ED. (From Cappelleri, J.C. et al., *Int. J. Impot. Res.*, 16, 30, 2004.)

the 6-item Confidence domain, and the 14-item Overall score of the SEAR questionnaire. For each, a score of 0 is least favorable and a score of 100 is most favorable.

Mean scores across levels of ED severity differed significantly ($p = 0.0001$) and, as expected, increased (i.e., improved) approximately linearly and noticeably with decreases in severity ($p = 0.0001$). Not only where each pair of mean scores statistically different ($p < 0.05$), the difference in mean scores on the SEAR questionnaire was in the predicted direction and tangible between each pair of adjacent categories on ED severity. The difference in mean scores between adjacent categories ranged from 8.4 (the difference in mean scores between no ED and mild ED on the Confidence domain) to 23.4 (the difference in mean scores between mild ED and moderate ED on the Sexual Relationship Satisfaction domain).

3.2.3 Criterion Validity

Criterion validity involves assessing an instrument against the true value or against another standard indicative of the true value of measurement. It can be defined as "the degree to which the scores of a measurement instrument are an adequate reflection of a gold standard" (Mokkink et al., 2010). Criterion validity can be divided into concurrent validity and predictive validity.

Concurrent validity involves an assessment of scores from the targeted measure (e.g., the PRO measure of interest) with the scores from the gold standard at the same time.

Predictive validity involves an assessment of how well the target measure predicts the gold standard in the future. A natural question to ask is, if a suitable criterion already exists, why go through the often laborious process of developing a new measure? There are several valid reasons: a current criterion measure may be too expensive, invasive, dangerous, and time-consuming; the new measure may not have its outcomes known until it is too late; or the new measure may be measuring something similar but not exactly the same as what is taken or perceived as the gold standard. This last reason is generally why PRO measures are developed: an existing instrument does not quite measure what is needed, despite it being taken or perceived previously as the gold standard. For example, a health-related quality-of-life instrument may be too general and therefore a disease-specific PRO measure is developed. Yet the disease-specific measure is then often correlated to the health-related quality-of-life instrument because this generic instrument was previously considered the gold standard when nothing more suitable was available.

3.2.3.1 Concurrent Validity

As an example of *concurrent validity* on a PRO instrument, consider the 6-item erectile function domain on the 15-item International Index of

Erectile Function (Rosen et al., 1997; Cappelleri et al., 1999). The erectile function domain has a range of scores from 6 to 30, where higher scores are more favorable, for men who have had sexual activity and attempted sexual intercourse over the past 4 weeks (the range is from 1 to 30 for men who did not necessarily have sexual activity or attempted sexual intercourse, provided that they had an opportunity to engage in sexual relations). Concurrent validity on the erectile function domain was examined with the gold standard being a complete, documented clinical diagnosis on ED. A total of 1151 men had a score on the erectile function domain: 1035 had an established clinical diagnosis of ED and 116 were without any history of ED and clinically judged as having normal erectile function (Cappelleri et al., 1999). For the purpose of the diagnostic evaluation, 1035 men with ED were assessed at baseline, during the pretreatment phase, in a clinical trial; the 116 men without ED were assessed once and were not part of a clinical trial.

A logistic regression model was fit with true ED status (yes, no) as the dependent variable and the erectile function domain score as a continuous predictor. The logistic model yielded an estimated odds ratio of 0.54 (95% confidence interval, 0.48–0.60). Hence, for every one-point increase in the erectile function score, the odds of having ED (relative to not having ED) decreased by about half.

From the logistic regression model, a receiver operating characteristic (ROC) curve was obtained by knowing a subject's actual diagnosis (ED, no ED) as the binary outcome (dependent) variable and, relative to each of the 25 candidate cutoff scores (6–30), the subject's predicted diagnosis based on the erectile function score as the continuous predictor (independent) variable (Figure 3.2). (An ROC curve is a graphical plot that illustrates how well different threshold levels of a predictor discriminate with respect to a binary outcome.) A score less than or equal to a given cutoff score classifies a subject (retrospectively) as having ED and a score greater than the same cutoff classifies a subject as not having ED.

Figure 3.2 shows the ROC curve. For each cutoff point (6–30), the true positive rate and the false positive rate were obtained and plotted on the ROC curve. The more steep the curve is (i.e., the closer the curve is to the upper left corner of the ROC space), and hence the more upwardly sloping the curve is, the better the accuracy of the predictive diagnostic.

The true positive rate—that is, the sensitivity—was the proportion of subjects truly with ED that were correctly classified as such by their erectile function scores. Note that *sensitivity* as defined here for concurrent validity is different from *sensitivity* as defined earlier for known-groups validity. The false positive rate—that is, 1 minus the specificity—was the proportion of subjects truly without ED that were incorrectly classified as having ED by their erectile function scores. By implication, the specificity was the proportion of subjects truly without ED that were correctly classified as not having ED according to their erectile function scores.

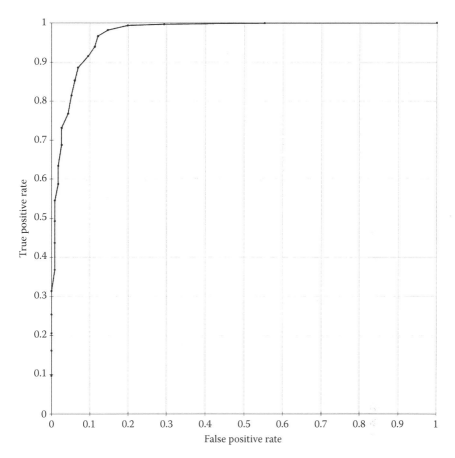

FIGURE 3.2
Receiver operating characteristic curve of the erectile function domain. (From Cappelleri, J.C. et al., *Drug Inf. J.*, 33, 179, 1999.)

The area under the curve (AUC) was estimated to be 0.97. This AUC (also known as the *c*-statistic) can be interpreted as there being a 97% chance that a randomly chosen subject with ED had a lower erectile function score (and hence was more likely to be diagnosed as having had ED) than a randomly chosen subject without ED.

An inverse relationship exists between sensitivity and specificity: as one goes up, the other goes down. Because sensitivity and specificity were considered equally important, the cutoff that gave the highest (arithmetic or unweighted) mean value of sensitivity and specificity was selected. Based on this criterion, a cutoff score of 25 on the erectile function domain resulted in the best or maximal separation between men with ED and without ED. Hence men who scored 25 or less would be classified as having ED, while men who scored above 25 (26–30) would be classified as not having ED (Table 3.5). Of the 1035 men with true ED, 1000 (97%) were classified correctly by the erectile

TABLE 3.5

Cross-Tabulation of Erectile Function Scores (PRO Measure) and Clinical Diagnosis (Gold Standard)

| | Gold Standard | | |
Erectile Function Domain	Clinical Diagnosis of ED	Clinical Diagnosis of No ED	Total
ED (≤25)	1000 (true positive)	14 (false positive)	1014
No ED (26–30)	35 (false negative)	102 (true negative)	137
Total	1035	116	1151

ED, erectile dysfunction.

function domain as having ED, resulting in a sensitivity of 0.97 or 97%. Of the 116 men truly without ED, 102 (88%) were classified correctly by the erection function domain as not having ED, resulting in a specificity of 0.88 or 88%.

3.2.3.2 Predictive Validity

As an application of predictive validity, consider three patient-reported quality-of-life (QOL) questionnaires from the field of oncology, with progressive-free survival (PFS) taken as the gold standard for this purpose (Cella et al., 2009). The first questionnaire, the Functional Assessment of Cancer Therapy-General (FACT-G), is a 27-item instrument with scores ranging from 0 (worst cancer-related quality of life) to 108 (best cancer-related quality of life). The second questionnaire, the Functional Assessment of Cancer Therapy–Kidney Symptom Index (FSKI)–Disease-Related Subscale (FKSI-DRS), is a 9-item scale with scores ranging from 0 (most severe symptoms) to 36 (no symptoms). The third instrument, the EuroQol-Visual Analogue Scale (EQ-VAS), is a 100-point visual analog scale (0 = worst imaginable health state; 100 = best imaginable health state). Thus, for all three of these QOL variables, higher scores indicate better outcomes, that is, better QOL or fewer/less severe symptoms.

For these three PROs, only baseline data (cycle 1, day 1, administered prior to the start of study treatment) were used for the purpose of their predictive validity with respect to PFS. A Cox proportional-hazards model, a type of time-to-event model, was fitted to the data to test whether the baseline QOL scores predicted PFS, the outcome or dependent variable (Cella et al., 2009). As moderate-to-high Pearson's correlations were found between the baseline scores of the three QOL variables (range: 0.61–0.69), three separate models were fitted, each distinguished by its own baseline QOL variable.

Each model included one baseline QOL variable, treatment group (sunitinib or interferon-α), and additional covariates on baseline demographic and clinical factors (age, gender, baseline Eastern Cooperative Oncology Group score, number of Memorial Sloan-Kettering Cancer Center risk factors, prior nephrectomy and radiotherapy, number of metastases, and sites of metastases (lung, liver, bone, and lymph nodes)). Therefore, each resulting hazard ratio (HR) corresponding to a given variable was adjusted for the effects of the other variables on PFS. The HR for the baseline QOL variable was the key measure of treatment effect and was calculated as the hazard (*risk*) of PFS per minimum important difference (MID) in each of the three baseline QOL variables (FACT-G, MID = 5; FKSI-DRS, MID = 2; EQ-VAS, MID = 10). (A MID on a PRO instrument may be defined as the smallest difference between treatment groups considered important to patients; see Chapter 11.)

All three baseline QOL variables were individually predictive of PFS. Higher baseline scores of FACT-G (per 5-point change), FKSI-DRS (per 2-point change), and EQ-VAS (per 10-point change) were significantly associated with longer PFS (respectively, HR: 0.93, 0.89, and 0.91; p-value: ≤ 0.001, $p \leq 0.001$, and 0.008). These data therefore suggest that the risk of tumor progression or death at any given time was approximately 7%, 11%, and 9% lower for every MID increase respectively on the FACT-G, FKSI-DRS, and EQ-VAS.

3.3 Simulated Example Using SAS: Convergent and Divergent Validity

As an illustration on assessments of convergent and divergent validity, an example described in Section 3.2.1 is used with respect to the Confidence domain of the SEAR questionnaire. An assessment of its convergent and divergent validity was made by correlations with domains of the SF-36. For the Confidence domain, convergent validity (or at least no evidence to dismiss it) was hypothesized and confirmed with a relatively moderate correlation value of 0.45 with the SF-36 Mental Component Summary (MCS) (Table 3.3). Divergent validity (or at least no evidence to dismiss it) was hypothesized and supported by its lower correlation value of 0.38 with the SF-36 Physical Component Summary (PCS) (Table 3.3).

To simulate values of the 192 subjects (98 men who self-reported a clinical diagnosis of ED in the past year and 94 men who self-reported no clinical diagnosis of ED in the past year) to mimic the example in Section 3.2.1, we first need to create a dataset describing correlations between scores on the SEAR Confidence domain, SF-36 PCS, and SF-36 MCS (see Figure 3.3). In the simulation exercise, the correlations of the Confidence domain with the SF-36 PCS and SF-36 MCS are defined to be 0.3 and 0.5, respectively. In the simulation, the correlation between PCS and MCS is defined to be 0.4. Note also that we need to define not only the number of observations but also the means and standard deviations for each of the three variables.

The SIMNORMAL procedure in SAS is used to simulate values for the SEAR Confidence domain, SF-36 PCS, and SF-36 MCS for every subject. The CORR procedure (the last procedure in Figure 3.3) outputs the correlation matrix from the simulated dataset (see Figure 3.4). As expected, the

```
data _corr_(type=corr);
input
_TYPE_ $   _NAME_ $      Conf              PCS           MCS;
datalines;
  CORR        Conf        1                0.3           0.5
  CORR        PCS         0.3              1             0.4
  CORR        MCS         0.5              0.4           1
  MEAN         .          47               50            50
  STD          .          15               12            16
  N            .          192              192           192

  ;
run;

proc simnormal data=_corr_ out=_sim_corr_ numreal=192 seed=456789;
var Conf PCS MCS;
run;

proc corr data=_sim_corr_  ;
var Conf PCS MCS;
Run;
```

FIGURE 3.3
Generating values of SEAR Confidence domain, SF-36 PCS, and SF-36 MCS based on a multi-variate normal distribution.

```
The CORR Procedure
   3  Variables:   Conf    PCS    MCS

                             Simple Statistics
Variable      N       Mean      Std Dev      Sum     Minimum     Maximum

Conf         192    46.05100   14.08713     8842    13.55376    84.74691
PCS          192    49.43078   12.22950     9491     2.47412    82.52488
MCS          192    48.56976   16.20312     9325     8.95680    98.87201

Pearson Correlation Coefficients, N = 192
          Prob > |r| under H0: Rho=0
                 Conf            PCS            MCS

Conf        1.00000         0.33566        0.47791
                            <.0001         <.0001

PCS         0.33566         1.00000        0.38458
            <.0001                         <.0001

MCS         0.47791         0.38458        1.00000
            <.0001          <.0001
```

FIGURE 3.4
Correlation matrix for simulated dataset (CORR procedure output).

correlations based on the simulated dataset (Figure 3.4) are close to the values initially assigned to them (see the data step in Figure 3.3).

3.4 Factors Affecting Response

Numerous factors may influence a response, making it less than a totally accurate reflection of reality (Streiner and Norman, 2008). These factors, for example, include how questions are framed and the cognitive complexity or ambiguity of the questions (e.g., "Compared to how you were a year ago..."). Regardless of the content of the item, patients may find it convenient to respond in a certain way (e.g., choosing the middle category on all questions or, alternatively, favoring the more desirable end of the scale) or in a socially acceptable manner. Factors that influence responses affect their validity, reliability or reproducibility (Chapter 4), and subsequent interpretations (Chapter 11).

Response shifts can also affect validity, reliability, and interpretation (Schwartz and Sprangers, 1999). Over time the meaning of the self-reported constructs may be subject to change because the standards or perceptions used to assess them have changed. For instance, a group of patients with chronic pain may have adapted nicely over time and now report a higher quality of life than those who are objectively healthier. This group of patients with chronic pain may have learned to cope with a constant level of pain for a long time and hence may even report diminishing levels of pain over time, even though their pain receptors are receiving the same signals as previously. On the other hand, low test–retest reliability among patients with a very disabling disease may reflect a meaningful behavioral change toward increased frustration and angst rather than measurement error, despite no change in their disease state.

A debate exists on whether or not to adjust for response shift. To a certain extent, response shift can be avoided by a careful formulation of questions, which can be made more specific with less room for varied interpretation by patients—for example, rather than asking about the ability to take long walks, asking about a 10-mile walk instead. Researchers who regard response shift as bias would prefer an adjustment. Methods for adjustment include qualitative and quantitative methods (Schwartz and Sprangers, 1999; Schwartz, 2010; de Vet et al., 2011). Qualitative methods involve interviewing patients directly, asking patients how they interpret questions and how they choose their answers.

Several quantitative methods have been also proposed to adjust for response shift. Among them are the *then-test* and confirmatory factor analysis. For the *then-test*, the patient first completes a questionnaire on health status (the pretest) and, after some time when the patient's health status has changed, a second questionnaire is completed (the posttest). The *then-test* method is a retrospective assessment of the pretest period, assessed at the same time as the posttest; the difference between the *then-test* and the actual pretest (assessed during the actual pretest period) is referred to as the response shift effect. Confirmatory factor analysis (Chapter 5) can also be used to detect response shift by first testing the assumption of measurement invariance over time and then examining whether the relationships among variables are similar over time.

Other researchers believe that an adjustment is not always necessary. If perceived health status is the objective to be assessed, then adjustment for response shift may not be necessary. In some cases, as in the case of physical rehabilitation when a patient's physical condition cannot be improved, achieving response shift may be the actual aim of treatment—for example, by learning new ways of movement, resetting goals or accepting limitations. Response shift is usually less important for treatment comparisons in a clinical trial because the magnitude of response shift is expected to apply equally to all treatment arms.

3.5 Summary

This chapter covers different facets of validity. Content validity is the extent to which an instrument measures the important aspects of concepts that developers or patients purport it to assess. Construct validity is the degree to which the scores of a measurement instrument are consistent with hypotheses. Different aspects of construct validity are considered: convergent validity and divergent validity, whereby a PRO scale is assessed in relation to other variables to which it is expected to be related or not related; known-groups validity, whereby a PRO scale is assessed with respect to differences between specific groups of subjects known to be different in a relevant way; and criterion validity, whereby a PRO scale is assessed against the true value or against some other standard indicative of the true value of measurement. Convergent validity and divergent validity are further studied via a simulated example. Finally, factors affecting response and hence validity are highlighted.

References

Althof, S.E., Cappelleri, J.C., Shpilsky, A., Stecher, V., Diuguid, C., Sweeney, M., and S. Duttagupta. 2003. Treatment responsiveness of the Self-Esteem And Relationship (SEAR) questionnaire in erectile dysfunction. *Urology* 61:888–893.

Campbell, D.T. and D.W. Fiske. 1959. Convergent and discriminant validation by the multitrait-multimethod matrix. *Psychological Bulletin* 56:81–105.

Cappelleri, J.C., Althof, S.E., Siegel, R.L., Shpilsky, A., Bell, S.S., and S. Duttagupta. 2004. Development and validation of the Self-Esteem And Relationship (SEAR) questionnaire in erectile dysfunction. *International Journal of Impotence Research* 16:30–38.

Cappelleri, J.C., Rosen, R.C., Smith, M.D., Quirk, F., Maytom, M.C., Mishra, A., and I.H. Osterloh. 1999. Some developments on the International Index of Erectile Function (IIEF). *Drug Information Journal* 33:179–190.

Cella, D., Cappelleri, J.C., Bushmakin, A., Charbonneau, C., Li, J.Z., Kim, S.T., Chen, I., Michaelson, M.D., and R.J. Motzer. 2009. Quality of life predicts progression-free survival in patients with metastatic renal cell carcinoma treated with sunitinib vs. interferon-alfa. *Journal of Oncology Practice* 5:66–70.

Cieza, A. and G. Stucki. 2005. Content comparison of health related quality of life (HRQOL) instruments based on the international classification of functioning, disability and health (ICF). *Quality of Life Research* 14:1225–1237.

de Vet, H.C.W., Terwee, C.B., Mokkink, L.B., and D.L. Knol. 2011. *Measurement in Medicine: A Practical Guide.* New York, NY: Cambridge University Press.

European Medicines Agency (EMA), Committee for Medicinal Products for Human Use. 2005. Reflection paper on the regulatory guidance for use of health-related quality of life (HRQOL) measures in the evaluation of medicinal products. European Medicines Agency. http://www.ema.europa.eu/ema/ (Accessed on August 31, 2013).

Food and Drug Administration (FDA). 2009. Guidance for industry on patient-reported outcome measures: Use in medical product development to support labeling claims. *Federal Register* 74(235):65132–65133. http://www.fda.gov/Drugs/DevelopmentApprovalProcess/DrugDevelopmentToolsQualificationProgram/ucm284399.htm.

Fran, X., Felsovalyi, Â., Sivo, S.A., and S.C. Keenan. 2002. *SAS® for Monte Carlo Studies: A Guide for Quantitative Researchers.* Cary, NC: SAS Institute Inc.

Haynes, S.N., Richard, D.C.S., and E.S. Kubany. 1995. Content validity in psychological assessment: A functional approach to concepts and methods. *Psychological Assessment* 7:238–247.

Hunt, S.M., McEwen, J., and S.P. McKenna. 1985. Measuring health status: A new tool for clinicians and epidemiologists. *Journal of the Royal College of General Practitioners* 35:185–188.

Mokkink, L.B., Terwee, C.B., Patrick, D.L., Alonso, J., Stratforth, P.W., Knol, D.L., Bouter, L.M., and H.C.W. de Vet. 2010. International consensus on taxonomy, terminology, and definitions of measurement properties for health-related patient-reported outcomes: Results of the COSMIN study. *Journal of Clinical Epidemiology* 63:737–745.

Patrick, D.L., Burke, L.B., Gwaltney, C.J., Leidy, N.K., Martin, M.L., Molsen, E., and L. Ring. 2011a. Content validity—Establishing and reporting the evidence in newly developed patient-reported outcomes (PRO) instruments for medical product evaluation: ISPOR PRO Good Research Practices Task Force Report: Part 1—Eliciting concepts for a new PRO instrument. *Value in Health* 14:978–988.

Patrick, D.L., Burke, L.B., Gwaltney, C.J., Leidy, N.K., Martin, M.L., Molsen, E., and R. Ring. 2011b. Content validity—Establishing and reporting the evidence in newly developed patient-reported outcomes (PRO) instruments for medical product evaluation: ISPOR PRO Good Research Practices Task Force Report: Part 2—Assessing respondent understanding. *Value in Health* 14:978–988.

Rosen, R.C., Riley, A., Wagner, G., Osterloh, I.H., Kirkpatrick, J., and A. Mishra. 1997. The International Index of Erectile Function (IIEF): A multidimensional scale for assessment of erectile dysfunction. *Urology* 49:822–830.

Rothman, M., Burke, L., Erickson, P., Leidy, N.K., Patrick, D.L., and C.D. Petrie. 2009. Use of existing patient-reported outcome (PRO) instruments and their modification: The ISPOR Good Research Practices for Evaluating and Documenting Content Validity for the Use of Existing Instruments and Their Modification PRO Task Force Report. *Value in Health* 12:1075–1083.

SAS Institute Inc. 2011a. *SAS/STAT® 9.3 User's Guide*, 2nd edition. Cary, NC: SAS Institute Inc.

SAS Institute Inc. 2011b. *SAS/ETS 9.3 User's Guide*. Cary, NC: SAS Institute Inc.

SAS Institute Inc. 2012a. *Base SAS® 9.3 Procedure Guide*, 2nd edition. Cary, NC: SAS Institute Inc.

SAS Institute Inc. 2012b. *SAS/OR® 9.3 User's Guide: Mathematical Programming*. Cary, NC: SAS Institute Inc.

Schwartz, C.E. 2010. Applications of response shift theory and methods to participation: A brief history of a young field. *Archives of Physical Medicine and Rehabilitation* 91 (Suppl. 1):S38–S43.

Schwartz, C.E. and M.A. Sprangers. 1999. Methodological approaches for assessing response shift in longitudinal health-related quality-of-life research. *Social Science & Medicine* 48:1531–1548.

Spitzer, W.O., Dobson, A.J., Hall, J., Chesterman, E., Levi, J., Shepherd, R., Battista, R.N., and B.R. Catchlove. 1981. Measuring the quality of life of cancer patients: A concise QL-index for use by physicians. *Journal of Chronic Diseases* 34:585–597.

Streiner, D.L. and G.R. Norman. 2008. *Health Measurement Scales: A Practical Guide to Their Development and Use*, 4th edition. New York, NY: Oxford University Press.

Wicklin, R. 2013. *Simulating Data with SAS®*, Cary, NC: SAS Institute Inc.

4

Reliability

This chapter is an introduction to the concept of reliability in the evaluation of a patient-reported outcome (PRO) instrument. While validity assesses the extent to which an instrument measures what it is meant to measure (Chapter 3), reliability assesses how precise or stable the instrument measures what it measures and is typically discussed in terms of reproducibility.

An essential requirement of all measurements in clinical practice and research is that they be reliable. Reliability is defined as "the degree to which measurement is free from measurement error" (Mokkink et al., 2010). A measurement is never or seldom perfect. An observed score from a measurement reported by a patient has error associated with it and therefore does not equate to its true score. The true score is the limit that the mean score will be approaching if the measurements were hypothetically performed an infinite number of times. Reliability refers to the precision of the score observed, to its reproducibility, and not to its validity. Note that an instrument can be reliable but not valid, neither reliable nor valid, or both reliable and valid. Validity is limited by reliability. If responses are inconsistent, it necessarily implies invalidity as well (note that the converse is not true: consistent responses do not necessarily imply valid responses).

As part of scale validation, two types of reliability can be considered: *internal reliability* for multi-item scales and *repeatability reliability*. Both concepts are mathematically related. Internal reliability, also known as internal consistency, is based on item-to-item correlations and the number of items in multi-item scales. Repeatability reliability, which is applicable to single-item scales as well as multi-item scales, is based upon the analysis of variances between repeated measurements on the same set of subjects, where the measurements are repeated over time (*test–retest reliability*), made by different observers (*interrater reliability*), or involve different variants of the same attribute or construct (*equivalent-forms reliability*).

If a patient is in a stable condition, an instrument should yield reproducible results when it is repeated on that patient. Under this condition, when patients complete the same PRO questionnaire on multiple occasions (time points), the level of agreement between the PRO scores at multiple occasions is a measure of the reliability of the PRO measure.

Such *test–retest reliability* is a critical feature of measurement theory. The PRO instrument is measured at one time (test) and then at least at one other time (retest). Selecting the right period between test and retest, or between times or occasions, is crucial. Too long a period would increase the chance of a true change in the status of the patient; too short a period would allow subjects to recall their responses.

Poor test–retest reliability may indicate a problem with the nature of the construct, the items (or scales) themselves, or the nature of the target population. For example, the assessment of current pain may show low test–retest reliability because the intensity of pain may vary over time (values of the construct are changing). In such a case, it would be more appropriate to take average values of pain across time. Even if a patient's underlying condition or disease is not fluctuating over time, test–retest reliability may be compromised when the items are poor or with special populations such as the very young, the very old, and patients with cognitive impairment (e.g., Alzheimer's disease).

Interrater reliability, like test–retest reliability, involves absolute agreement or relative agreement but between at least two raters instead of at least two time points, as with test–retest reliability. Absolute agreement refers to the comparison scores agreeing completely, where relative agreement refers to the comparison scores agreeing closely when ranked. For the purpose of PRO measurement, interest typically centers by definition on the patient's self-assessment and not on rater or observer assessment. Therefore, for reliability of a self-administered questionnaire like a PRO measure, interrater reliability is usually of lesser concern than test–retest reliability. When instruments are interviewer administered, however, an assessment of interrater reliability becomes critical.

Equivalent-forms reliability involves absolute agreement or relative agreement between scores from two or more instruments that are designed to measure the same attribute (not to be confused with convergent validity, which addresses how much the target scale correlates with another [similar] measure to which it is expected to be related, as described in Chapter 3). For example, a new PRO instrument could be compared against a standard measure or against a measure that is longer and more time consuming. When appropriate, the same methods applied to test–retest reliability can be applied to equivalent-forms reliability. However, equivalent-forms reliability (and also interrater reliability) may tend to focus on prediction or estimation using linear regression analysis (relative agreement) rather than absolute agreement.

4.1 Intraclass Correlation Coefficient for Continuous Variables

Reliability is inversely related to measurement error. Measurement error includes random variation within subjects, systematic variation other than that between patients, or both types of variation, depending on the study design and objective. Measurement error is caused by any factor that affects a measurement score and pushes the observed scores up or down randomly or systematically in ways not related to true differences among individuals, adding variability to the measurements. Useful information about measurement error requires that it be put in context and contrasted with the expected variation or true differences between the individuals assessed.

Consider the case of a PRO score taken as a continuous measurement. This situation includes cases when the PRO is not strictly a continuous measure per se (e.g., it may be an ordinal measure) but is considered appropriate for it to be conceptualized and analyzed like a continuous variable. From classical test theory, it turns out that reliability can be formally defined as the ratio of variability between patients to total variability (the sum of patient variability plus measurement error). In other words, for a PRO measure, reliability expresses how well patients with true systematic differences can be distinguished from each other in spite of, or after accounting for, the presence of measurement error.

For data taken as continuous, the intraclass correlation coefficient (ICC) is a reliability parameter that measures the strength of agreement between repeated measurements on the same set of patients by assessing the proportion of total variance (with total variance being the sum of between-patient variance plus within-subject variance) in the observed measurements that is due to true differences between patients as reflected in the between-patient variability in the observed scores:

$$\text{ICC for a single score} = \frac{\text{Between-patient variability}}{\text{Between-patient variability} + \text{Within-patient variability}} \qquad (4.1)$$

$$\text{ICC for a single score} = \frac{\sigma_p^2}{\sigma_p^2 + \sigma_e^2}, \qquad (4.2)$$

where

σ_p^2 symbolizes the variance for the systematic differences between patients

σ_e^2 symbolizes within-patient variance (also described as measurement error variance), and the sum of these two variances gives the total variance in the observed score

In practice, both types of variances of these components $\left(\sigma_p^2 \text{ and } \sigma_e^2\right)$ are estimated from a sample, and the values of ICC can be obtained and estimated from an analysis of variance model (Fayers and Machin, 2007; de Vet et al., 2011). The theoretical range on an ICC is from 0 to 1. Higher values indicate more reliability. If an ICC is large (close to 1), then measurement error is low relative to between-patient variability, indicating high reliability. If an ICC is low (close to 0), then measurement error variability dominates over between-patient variability, indicating low reliability.

Consider the ICC given in Equation 4.2 as pertaining to test–retest reliability, or precision, of a single measurement. In medicine, certain patient-rated measurements (as well as clinician-rated measurements) may fluctuate over time, an example being chronic pain. It is common practice in these instances to average the results of the measurements, for example, by taking the average (i.e., arithmetic or simple mean) of the last seven diary measurements of pain to arrive at an average weekly pain score, in order to increase reliability. In this case, the ICC pertains to the test–retest reliability of the averaged measurements and its formula becomes

$$\text{ICC for an average score} = \frac{\text{Between-patient variability}}{\begin{array}{c}\text{Between-patient variability} \\ + (\text{Within-patient variability})/m\end{array}} \quad (4.3)$$

$$\text{ICC for an average score} = \frac{\sigma_p^2}{\sigma_p^2 + (\sigma_e^2/m)}, \quad (4.4)$$

where m is the number of measurements taken to compute the average score. Equations 4.3 and 4.4 can be transformed equivalently into what is known as the Spearman–Brown prophecy formula:

$$\text{ICC for an average score} = \frac{m * \text{ICC}}{[1 + (m-1) * \text{ICC}]}, \quad (4.5)$$

where ICC comes from Equation 4.2. In general, for group comparisons, ICC values of at least 0.70 indicate acceptable reliability; for individual comparisons, values should be at least 0.90.

It should be noted that there are several formulas for ICC giving different values; there is not just one type of ICC. All types of ICC are grounded in ratio of variances obtained through an analysis of variance model. The different forms of ICC differ with respect to whether the objective is to obtain absolute agreement or merely relative agreement (i.e., ranking) between measurements, whether the components of variability involve only those pertaining to patients (and not, in addition, to other components of systematic variability such as raters or occasions), and whether inferences on any of these components pertain only to their current levels sampled (fixed-effect component) or to a random sample of all possible levels of a component (random-effect component).

The difference between absolute agreement and relative agreement measures is defined in terms of how the systematic variability due to a component other than from between patients (such as time or rater) is treated. If that variability is considered irrelevant, it is not included in the denominator of an ICC estimate (by excluding that variability from measurement error) and a measure of relative agreement is produced. If such systematic differences among levels of a component are considered relevant, a component's variability contributes to the denominator of an ICC estimate (by including that variability as part of measurement error) and a measure of absolute agreement is produced. In medicine, attention mainly centers on absolute agreement because interest is on obtaining the same set of results in an absolute sense rather than in a relative sense. Equation 4.2 on ICC for a single score reflects absolute agreement, as does Equation 4.4 on the ICC for an average score, with measurement error (σ_e^2) reflecting all residual sources of within-patient variability (i.e., all variation beyond between-patient variability).

Details about different types of ICCs, including their confidence interval estimation, can be found in several publications (Shrout and Fleiss, 1979; McGraw and Wong, 1996; Shoukri and Pause, 1999; Zou and McDermott, 1999; Fan and Thompson, 2001; Cappelleri and Ting, 2002; Schuck, 2004; Tian and Cappelleri, 2004; Weir, 2005; Gilder et al., 2007; Streiner and Norman, 2008; Ting et al., 2009; de Vet et al., 2011). They are relevant for interrater reliability and equivalent-forms reliability as well as test–retest reliability.

4.2 ICC Example

In sexual medicine, erection hardness is a fundamental component of erectile function (EF) and is a very specific and an easily monitored outcome. The erection hardness score (EHS) is a single-item PRO measure for scoring erection hardness (Mulhall et al., 2007). Interest here centers on the test–retest reliability of EHS. As part of a randomized placebo-controlled trial, 307 men with erectile dysfunction (ED) were asked to rate the hardness of their erection based on five response categories: 0 = penis does not enlarge, 1 = penis is larger but not hard, 2 = penis is hard but not hard enough for penetration, 3 = penis is hard enough for penetration but not completely hard, and 4 = penis is completely hard and fully rigid (Mulhall et al., 2007).

Analyses illustrated here were based on EHS data from event logs (at each event of sexual intercourse) collected before treatment intervention, during the 2-week screening phase, and at baseline. To assess test–retest reliability, an ICC was estimated in SAS based on a repeated-measures analysis of EHS responses using a one-way random effects model based on absolute agreement, where patients are assumed to be randomly drawn from, and where inferences are to be made to, all possible patients of a certain kind (Singer, 1998; Shoukri and Pause, 1999). All pretreatment data collected during the 2-week period between the screening visit and the baseline visit were used. No postrandomization data were used in the analysis of test–retest reliability.

The ICC of a single EHS response was estimated using Equation 4.2, which measures the degree of absolute agreement. The ICC for an average (mean) EHS response was estimated using the Spearman–Brown prophecy formula (Equation 4.5), which approximates the reliability of an averaged measurement.

The between-patient variance estimate was 0.58 and the measurement error (within-patient) variance estimate was 0.56. Based on these values, the estimated ICC of a single EHS response was approximately 0.51 (i.e., 0.58/(0.58+0.56)). As expected, reliability increased with the number of EHS responses (Figure 4.1), and the cutoff for acceptable reliability ($\geq$0.7) was attained when three EHS responses were averaged, which gave an estimated test–retest reliability of 0.76.

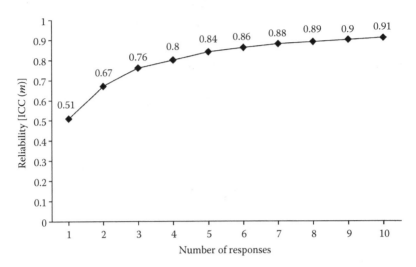

FIGURE 4.1
Reliability of the EHS: ICC based on an average number of responses (*m*). (From Mulhall, J.O. et al., *J. Sex. Med.*, 4, 1626, 2007.)

4.3 ICC Simulated Example

To illustrate the implementation of ICC estimation, we first need to understand how a simulated dataset should be created. Consider a simulated example with 307 subjects, the number given previously in the ICC example (Section 4.2). The outcome variable is taken as the EHS response (*Y*) and assumed to be collected during 2 weeks between screening and baseline, as in the ICC example. Every subject has up to 14 observations, again as in the published and real example from Section 4.2. The model for the response assumes that all within-patient changes during the 2-week period are caused by random variability for subject *i* at measurement occasion *j*. This model can be expressed as

$$Y_{ij} = a + p_i + e_{ij}, \tag{4.6}$$

where
  Y_{ij} is the EHS response for subject *i* at the measurement occasion *j* (*i* = 1, 2, ..., 307; *j* = 1, 2, ..., n_i; n_i represents the number of observations for subject *i*, which could be from only one observation to 14 observations)
  a is the overall mean
  p_i is the between-patient error (assumed to be from a normal distribution with mean 0 and variance σ_p^2, i.e., $p_i \sim N(0, \sigma_p^2)$)
  e_{ij} is the within-patient error or measurement error (assumed to be from a normal distribution with mean 0 and variance σ_e^2, i.e., $e_{ij} \sim N(0, \sigma_e^2)$)

Figure 4.2 represents the corresponding simulated dataset. It is important
to note that the between-patient error is generated by the SAS code line

$$ep = rannor(\mathbf{1})*sqrt(\&sp);$$

and will have the same value for all observations for subject i as noted
in Equation 4.6 and represented by the term p_i. In contrast, the other error
term, e_{ij}, will be different at every occasion for every subject (and is represented
by rannor($\mathbf{3}$)*sqrt(&se)). Then the SAS code that models EHS outcome becomes

$$y = \&a + ep + rannor(\mathbf{3})*sqrt(\&se);$$

which is the equivalent of Equation 4.6.

Figure 4.3 represents the implementation in SAS of the analysis to obtain
ICC estimation. The MIXED procedure in SAS is used to estimate the

```
/*
For this example, there are 307 subjects (NumberOfRows) and every
subject has up to 14 repeated measures (NumberOfRepeatedMeasures).
Between-subject and within-subject variances were defined with
values of 0.1 and 0.08, respectively.
*/

options nofmterr nocenter pagesize=2000 linesize=256;

%Let NumberOfRows              = 307;
%Let NumberOfRepeatedMeasures  = 14;

%Let a = 2; /*value for the overall mean*/
%Let sp = 0.1; /*value for the between-subject variance*/
%Let se = 0.08; /*value for the within-subject variance*/

/*
The rannor(arbitrary seed value) function returns a (pseudo)
random number from a (standard) normal distribution with mean 0
and standard deviation 1.
The ranuni(arbitrary seed value) function returns a (pseudo)
random number from a uniform distribution on the interval [0, 1].
The Int(argument) function returns the integer portion of the argument.
*/

Data _icc_;
    Do ID=1 To &NumberOfRows;

    ep= rannor(1)*sqrt(&sp) ;

        Do i=1 To (1+Int(&NumberOfRepeatedMeasures*ranuni(2)));
            y = &a + ep + rannor(3)*sqrt(&se) ;
            output;
        End;

    End;
Keep i y ID;
Run;
```

FIGURE 4.2
Generating dataset for the ICC analysis.

```
Proc Mixed data=_icc_;
Class ID ;
Model y= ;
Random Int / subject=ID ;
Run;
```

FIGURE 4.3
Implementation of the model to assess between-patient and within-patient variances.

```
Covariance Parameter Estimates

Cov Parm     Subject    Estimate

  Intercept     ID        0.1096
  Residual                0.07666
```

FIGURE 4.4
Covariance parameter estimates.

between-patient and within-patient variances needed to calculate ICC (for details on modeling using MIXED procedure, readers are referred to Chapter 8).

Figure 4.4 represents the corresponding partial output. The value of 0.1096 for "Intercept" represents the between-patient variance (which was 0.1 in the simulation) and the value of 0.07666 for "Residual" represents the within-patient variance (which was 0.08 in the simulation). Then the ICC becomes

$$ICC = \frac{0.1096}{(0.1096 + 0.07666)} = 0.588.$$

The true ICC for this dataset is ICC = 0.1/(0.1 + 0.08) = 0.556, which is quite close to the value of 0.588 estimated from the MIXED procedure.

4.4 ICC in Context

For PRO data taken as continuous, the Pearson correlation coefficient is another form of the reliability coefficient. The Pearson correlation measures association between two variables, whereas the particular form of the intraclass correlation discussed here measures the agreement between them. A high association between two variables does not automatically guarantee good agreement between them. In practice, though, the Pearson correlation and the intraclass correlation tend to be quite close. Nonetheless, the intraclass correlation is preferred as, unlike the Pearson correlation, it will yield a value of 1.0 only if all the observations on each patient are identical; the Pearson correlation can yield a value of 1.0 even when all the observations on each patient are not identical.

Another important characteristic of a scale is its *standard error of measurement* (SEM). It can be defined as follows: If a subject is measured on the same outcome repeatedly when in a stable condition (i.e., no real changes in the outcome are anticipated and there are no changes external to the subject's environment that could influence the outcome), the standard deviation of the repeated measurements on the outcome is the SEM.

From this definition, it can be shown that the value of σ_e (see Equation 4.6) is the value of SEM. Often, when SEM is discussed, the following formula is introduced (Wyrwich, 2004; Weir, 2005; Streiner and Norman, 2008):

$$SEM = \sigma\sqrt{1-R}, \tag{4.7}$$

where

σ is the standard deviation of the observed scores
R is an index of reliability such as ICC

According to Equation 4.6, note that even for a single occasion the standard deviation σ includes both between-subject variance and within-subject variance. Generally speaking, for the case of repeated measures and even for just one measurement, this formula translates to

$$SEM = \sqrt{\sigma_p^2 + \sigma_e^2}\ \sqrt{1-ICC}. \tag{4.8}$$

If the ICC in Equation 4.8 is replaced with the ICC in Equation 4.2, then Equation 4.8 in expectation (or based on known population values) will be reduced to

$$SEM = \sigma_e \tag{4.9}$$

when based on their true population values. Thus Equation 4.7 is simply an attempt to extract the within-patient standard deviation, σ_e, by using the already estimated ICC and standard deviation of observed scores using just *one* cross-sectional measurement, assuming that this standard deviation can serve as an unbiased estimator of $\sqrt{\sigma_p^2 + \sigma_e^2}$. Note that during the estimation of the ICC we already obtained SEM (which is the within-subject standard deviation, σ_e).

Let's illustrate the approach based on Equation 4.7. Figure 4.5 provides the SAS code to calculate the standard deviation (SD) for every occasion

```
Proc Sort Data=_icc Out=_icc_sorted;
By i;
Run;
Proc Means Data=_icc_sorted;
Var y;
By i;
run;
```

FIGURE 4.5
Estimation of the standard deviation during 14 days.

TABLE 4.1

Estimation of SEM by Day Using
Formula SEM $= \sigma\sqrt{1-\text{ICC}}$

Day	SD, σ	SEM, $\sigma\sqrt{1-0.588}$
1	0.41845	0.268591
2	0.426394	0.27369
3	0.416009	0.267025
4	0.445538	0.285978
5	0.413828	0.265625
6	0.452765	0.290617
7	0.403538	0.25902
8	0.430295	0.276195
9	0.39166	0.251396
10	0.382354	0.245422
11	0.407343	0.261462
12	0.41653	0.267359
13	0.42228	0.27105
14	0.417958	0.268276
Average	*0.417*	*0.268*

Abbreviations: ICC, intraclass correlation coefficient; SD, standard deviation; SEM,
standard error of measurement.

when EHS scores were assessed (during 14 days) using the dataset "_icc_"
created earlier in Section 4.3.

Table 4.1 summarizes the results by time point (first column). The third
column gives the estimation of the SEM using value of the earlier estimated ICC (0.588) and the estimated standard deviation at each point. The
estimated average value of the third column is 0.268, which accurately corresponds to the estimated value of $\sigma_e = \sqrt{0.07666} = 0.277$. It is also worth
noting that the estimated average value of the standard deviations (second column) is 0.417, which also corresponds well to the estimated value of
$\sqrt{\sigma_p^2 + \sigma_e^2} = \sqrt{0.1096 + 0.07666} = 0.432$.

When using Equation 4.7, a researcher should be sure that it applies only
to the case when an estimation of σ comes from the set of subjects equivalent
(or at least similar) to the set of subjects used for ICC estimation. This requirement is needed because the value of σ from the new dataset should be representative of the value of $\sqrt{\sigma_p^2 + \sigma_e^2}$ from the dataset used for ICC estimation.
Otherwise, this formula will produce an incorrect assessment of the SEM.

4.5 Bland and Altman Plot for Continuous Variables

Consider again the case of PRO scores taken as a continuous outcome. The
Bland and Altman plot is a graphical approach to illustrate agreement
between two measurements on the same set of individuals (Bland and

Altman, 1986). This plot can be used to visually evaluate (absolute) agreement between two methods of clinical assessments (assessed on the same scale of measurement) at the same time, such as agreement between two raters or between two measures intended to measure the same thing. As an assessment of test–retest reliability, the Bland–Altman method can also be used for measuring agreement between two measurements of the same measure repeated at two different times on the same set of individuals. Here, the method involves the calculation of the mean within-patient difference on scores between two occasions, the corresponding standard deviation of the difference (SD), and 95% limits of agreement [mean difference ± 1.96(SD)].

The mean difference represents the mean systematic difference, or the magnitude of consistent bias, between scores at the two time points; the smaller the mean difference, the higher the agreement. Based on a paired *t*-test, the mean difference ideally should not differ statistically from zero. Presentation of the 95% limits of agreement provides visual judgment of how well two repeated assessments agree. Under the assumption that the difference scores approximate a normal distribution, approximately 95% of them will fall between the limits of agreement. The smaller the range between these two limits, the better the agreement is. The question of how small is small depends on the clinical context and whether a difference between the two occasions as extreme as that described by the 95% limits of agreement would meaningfully affect the interpretation of the results.

As an illustrative example, Figure 4.6 shows a Bland–Altman plot for baseline and screening scores on a hypothetical PRO measure on 106 patients. For each patient, the mean of the scores assessed at screening and baseline (taken to represent the true value) is plotted on the horizontal axis, and the within-patient difference between these scores (taken to represent

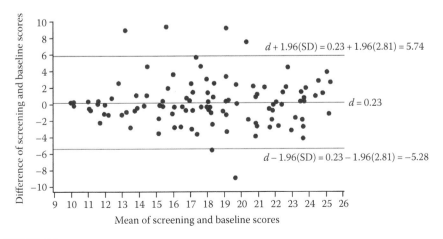

FIGURE 4.6
Illustration of Bland–Altman plot on a patient-reported outcome assessed at screening and baseline.

measurement error) is plotted on the vertical axis. The figure contains three horizontal lines. The middle line represents the mean systematic difference (d) of 0.23 between screening and baseline scores. This estimated mean difference is not statistically different from zero, as the value of 0 falls within the 95% confidence interval for the mean difference [$d \pm 1.98(2.81/\sqrt{106}) = -0.31$ to 0.77]. As shown in Figure 4.6, the limits of agreement are 5.74 (upper line) to −5.28 (lower line) and can be considered small enough to be confident that screening and baseline scores have a good agreement.

Figure 4.6 shows that there is no relationship between the difference in values across the two visits (which represents measurement error) and the mean of values across the two visits (which represents the true value), meaning that the calculated value for the limits of agreement holds for the whole range of measurement (an assumption of the Bland and Altman method as well as ICC and SEM). (If this assumption were violated, the data can be transformed accordingly before testing for reliability.) For these data, the estimated ICC of 0.79 is consistent with the Bland–Altman plot in reflecting good test–retest reliability.

4.6 Simple Kappa and Weighted Kappa Coefficients for Categorical Variables

4.6.1 Simple Kappa for Binary Data

For categorical data, the kappa statistic is a measure of agreement between two nominal variables having two or more categories (Cohen, 1960). Consider the case of a binary nominal variable, with levels such as presence or absence. Kappa can apply, for instance, to test–retest reliability of a PRO measure given on two separate occasions (such as whether or not a patient reports the presence of fatigue on two separate occasions), to interrater reliability pertaining to agreement between two observers on a single occasion (such as whether or not the raters agree with the presence of a disease), or to equivalent-forms reliability between two methods of diagnosing a disease on a single occasion (such as whether or not the two methods agree with the presence of a disease). The kappa coefficient explicitly adjusts for agreement that occurs by chance alone and thus can be defined as chance-corrected agreement. The kappa coefficient does this by examining the proportion of responses in the agreement cells (e.g., yes/yes, no/no) in relation to the proportion in these cells that would be expected by chance, given the total counts at the margins of the table.

For example, reconsider the data in Table 3.5 on the diagnosis of ED based on two methods: a gold standard (clinical) diagnosis and a PRO-based diagnosis (EF domain of the International Index of Erectile Function [IIEF]). For convenience, these data are reproduced here in Table 4.2 and are intended to

TABLE 4.2

Cross-Tabulation of Erectile Function Scores (PRO Measure) and Clinical Diagnosis (Gold Standard)

	Gold Standard		
Erectile Function Domain	**Clinical Diagnosis of ED**	**Clinical Diagnosis of No ED**	**Total**
ED ($\leq$25)	1000 (true positive)	14 (false positive)	1014
No ED (26–30)	35 (false negative)	102 (true negative)	137
Total	1035	116	1151

Abbreviation: ED, erectile dysfunction.

convey equivalent-forms reliability. The overall agreement observed is simply $(1000 + 102)/1151 = 0.96$ (or 96%). However, it is expected that a certain number of agreements would arise by chance alone. Specifically, expected agreement can be calculated from the margins (total counts) in Table 4.2. The top-left cell would be $(1014) \times (1035)/1151 = 911.8$ expected observations and the bottom-right cell would be $(137) \times (116)/1151 = 13.8$ expected observations.

Kappa corrects for chance agreement as follows:

$$k = \frac{p_o - p_e}{1 - p_e}, \qquad (4.10)$$

where

p_o is the observed proportion of agreements
p_e is the proportion expected by chance

In the case of Table 4.2,

$$k = \frac{((1000 + 102)/1151) - ((911.8 + 13.8)/1151)}{1 - ((911.8 + 13.8)/1151)} = 0.78. \qquad (4.11)$$

Thus, the kappa coefficient (or the proportion of chance-corrected agreement) between the EF domain of the IIEF and the clinical diagnosis was 0.78, which is substantial given that the maximum value of kappa is 1.

4.6.2 Weighted Kappa for Ordinal Data

The simple kappa coefficient only considers total or full agreement and does not provide partial credit or agreement for responses that are in proximity or nearby, for instance, that differ by only one or two categories for variables with more than two levels or categories. An extension of (simple) kappa, weighted kappa does consider partial agreement for ordinal variables (Cohen, 1968).

The formula for weighted kappa is

$$k = 1 - \frac{\Sigma w_{ij} P_{o(ij)}}{\Sigma w_{ij} P_{e(ij)}},$$

(4.12)

where

w_{ij} is the weight assigned to cell (i, j) (row $i = 1, 2, ..., N$; column $j = 1, 2, ..., N$)

$P_{o(ij)}$ and $P_{e(ij)}$ are, respectively, the observed and expected proportions in cell (i, j)

The sigma sign (Σ) represents summation over all (i, j) cells. Weighted kappa is then the sum of weighted proportions corrected for chance. Note that the calculation of weighted kappa focuses on disagreement in the sense that the second term in Equation 4.12 shows that the cells of total agreement found along the diagonal of the contingency table (top-left through bottom-right, or equivalently, when $i = j$) have weights of zero and the two opposite extreme corners (cells $(1, N)$ and $(N, 1)$) have maximum weights.

While in principle the weights could be assigned arbitrary values between 0 and 1, the difficulty of arbitrary weights is the lack of a uniform or fair comparison with another weighted kappa reported by other researchers for the same variables on the same topic. A different weighting scheme can be considered such as linear (or absolute) weights, which bases disagreement weights on the absolute difference between categories: the same category gets a weight of 0, an adjacent category apart a weight of 1, two categories apart a weight of 2, three categories apart a weight of 3, four categories apart a weight of 4, and so on. In general, however, a weighted scheme of quadratic weights, which bases disagreement weights on the square of the amount of the discrepancy, is often used: the same category gets a weight of 0, an adjacent category apart a weight of 1, two categories apart a weight of 4, three categories apart a weight of 9, four categories apart a weight of 16, and so on.

Table 4.3 shows a five-by-five contingency table on "true" and predictive severity grades of ED among men with ED before treatment intervention (at baseline) enrolled in a clinical trial for ED and men with no ED who were sampled separately and not part of a clinical trial (Cappelleri et al., 1999). Predictive grading of ED was based on a range of EF domain scores on the IIEF—namely, no ED (EF scores 26–30), mild (22–25), mild to moderate (17–21), moderate (11–16), and severe (6–10). "True" grading was based on a more complicated algorithm (Cappelleri et al., 1999). The grading system was based on a sample of 1013 men who attempted sexual activity within the past 4 weeks of responding.

Then, using frequencies rather than percentages (by multiplying the proportions in Equation 4.12 by the total sample size of 1013) to heighten understanding, the weighted kappa (as a metric of equivalent-forms reliability) based on quadratic weights for these data was

$$k = 1.0 - \frac{(0 \times 239) + (1 \times 77) + \cdots + (1 \times 4)(0 \times 92)}{(0 \times 103.3) + (1 \times 103.9) + \cdots + (1 \times 8.7)(0 \times 10)} = 1 - 0.2 = 0.8.$$

(4.13)

TABLE 4.3

Number of Men Classified by "True" Grading and Predictive Grading for Erectile Dysfunction

"True" Grading of Erectile Dysfunction	Predictive Grading of Erectile Dysfunction					
	Severe	Moderate	Mild to Moderate	Mild	No ED	Total
Severe	239	77	18	7	1	342
	(103.3)	(103.9)	(68.2)	(31.1)	(35.8)	
	0	1	4	9	16	
Moderate	52	152	58	8	1	271
	(81.9)	(82.1)	(54.0)	(24.6)	(28.4)	
	1	0	1	4	9	
Mild to Moderate	11	59	91	32	4	197
	(59.5)	(59.7)	(39.3)	(17.9)	(20.6)	
	4	1	0	1	4	
Mild	4	19	35	41	8	107
	(32.3)	(32.8)	(21.3)	(9.7)	(11.2)	
	9	4	1	0	1	
No ED	0	0	0	4	92	96
	(32.3)	(29.1)	(19.1)	(8.7)	(10.0)	
	16	9	4	1	0	
Total	306	307	202	92	106	1013

Note: For each cell, the top entry is the observed frequency, the middle entry (in parenthesis) is the expected frequency, and the bottom entry is the quadratic weight.

As Table 4.3 shows, men were classified correctly in their "true" level of ED more often than any other level. Men who were misclassified tended to be assigned into a category adjacent to the "correct" or "true" category, rather than to a more remote category.

Simple kappa and weighted kappa statistics share the same type of interpretation as the ICC for agreement. Kappa statistics in principle lie between −1 and 1. If simple or weighted kappa exceeds chance agreement, kappa would be positive. In contrast, a negative kappa means that the observed agreement between two assessments is less than what would occur by chance. If kappa equals 1, then there is complete agreement between the two assessments (e.g., the diagnostic measure is as accurate as the gold standard). Simple kappa and weighted kappa can be interpreted as follows: ≤0, poor; 0–0.2, slight agreement; 0.21–0.40, fair agreement; 0.41–0.60, moderate; 0.61–0.80, substantial; and 0.81–1.00, almost perfect (Landis and Koch, 1977). Kappa has also been interpreted with less than 0 being no agreement and 0–0.2 being poor agreement (Elliott and Woodward, 2010).

4.7 Internal Consistency Reliability: Cronbach's Alpha Coefficient

As noted previously, assessment of reliability consists of determining that a scale or measurement yields reproducible and consistent results. Reproducibility and consistency apply to two related but different facets of scale reliability. As discussed in previous sections, one way involves *repeatability reliability* (equivalent-forms reliability, interrater reliability, and especially test–retest reliability for PRO scales) where a measurement, whether based on a single item or multiple items, should yield reproducible or similar values if it is assessed repeatedly on the same patient when the patient's condition has remained stable or not changed materially.

The second way to assess reliability is called *internal consistency reliability* and applies to consistency of responses to items on the same multi-item scale, where the items are intended to tap into the same construct (or complementary interrelated aspects of it). This form of reliability, which is related to convergent validity, uses item correlations to assess the homogeneity (similarity) of items on a multi-item scale at a particular time and refers to the extent to which the items are interrelated.

Cronbach's alpha coefficient is the most widely used method to assess internal consistency (Cronbach, 1951). As a measure of scale consistency, Cronbach's alpha can be shown to be a form of an ICC. It can also be shown to underestimate the true reliability of an observed summed score for a single latent variable of interest and is therefore considered a conservative measure. Values of Cronbach's alpha are between 0 and 1.

Cronbach's alpha presumes that the multi-item scale reflects a single concept (latent variable) and is therefore unidimensional. As a consequence of multidimensionality, for instance, consider a scale taken as the sum of body weight and height (Fayers and Machin, 2007). Although this sum would have very high test–retest repeatability (assuming that each measurement, and hence their sum, is stable over time), Cronbach's alpha would not be correspondingly high because body weight and height are only moderately correlated and represent two distinct dimensions.

As such, as is the case with most psychometric methods (including those in this book), Cronbach's alpha assumes that items in a scale are parallel tests: all items in any one multi-item scale are reflective of the same postulated latent variable, with each item presumed to be measuring the same thing (or complementary aspects of the same thing). Cronbach's alpha is therefore applicable to items that are indicator variables, which indicate or reflect the concept of interest (as the concept differs, the items move in tandem to reflect that difference), and not to items that are causal variables, which are merely consequences of (say) certain symptom clusters arising wholly from the disease or treatment.

For instance, in cancer patients, the symptoms of hair loss and nausea may be both associated with chemotherapy and therefore may be highly correlated, even though they are not measuring any underlying concept per se. Here, as symptoms, hair loss and nausea are triggered or caused by chemotherapy treatment, rather than being reflective of some underlying attribute that induces or influences hair loss and nausea independently from treatment (or disease). Patients may or may not experience other symptoms like constipation and bleeding, and these symptoms may not have a strong correlation with hair loss and nausea. When a scale contains causal variables, such as a symptom cluster, it is not uncommon for the scale to have low internal consistency. The methods in this chapter are usually inappropriate for clinimetric or other scales containing causal items.

For summated scales of n items, Cronbach's alpha can be formulated as

$$\text{Cronbach's alpha} = \frac{n}{n-1}\left(1 - \frac{\text{Sum of item variances}}{\text{Sum of variances and covariances}}\right)$$

$$\text{Cronbach's alpha} = \frac{n}{n-1}\left(1 - \frac{\sum Var(X_i)}{Var(S)}\right), \tag{4.14}$$

where
$Var(X_i)$ is the variance of the ith item
Σ represents the summation over the n items
$S = \Sigma X_i$ is the summed or total score

When the items are uncorrelated, the very last term in Equation 4.14 becomes 1 [$\Sigma Var(X_i) = Var(S) = Var(\Sigma X_i)$] and Cronbach's alpha becomes zero. At the other extreme, when the items are identical and hence perfectly correlated, Cronbach's alpha can be shown to equal 1 (as the very last term reduces to n/n^2).

In general, a measure's reliability equals the proportion of total variance among its items that is due to the latent variable and is thus considered communal or shared variance. The formula for Cronbach's alpha in Equation 4.14 expresses such reliability by specifying the portion of total variance for the item that is unique (not shared), subtracting this from 1 to determine the proportion that is communal, and multiplying this quantity by a correction factor [$n/(n-1)$] to adjust for the number of items contributing to the prior calculations on the variances.

Equation 4.14 is the covariance-based formula for Cronbach's alpha. Another common formula for computing Cronbach's alpha is based on correlations rather than covariances (and, by implication, variances as the variance is the covariance of an item with itself). This correlation-based formula is

$$\text{Cronbach's alpha} = \frac{n\bar{r}}{1+(n-1)\bar{r}},\tag{4.15}$$

where
  n remains the number of items
  $\bar{r}$ is the average interitem correlation

Equation 4.15, which is the Spearman–Brown prophecy formula, shows that Cronbach's alpha is a function of both the average interitem correlation and the number of items on a multi-item scale; as either of these increases, so does Cronbach's alpha. Therefore, a scale may have high Cronbach's alpha not necessarily because its items are homogeneous, or march in step, but rather because it has a large number of items, which has been a criticism of Cronbach's alpha.

The correlation-based formula (Equation 4.15) stems directly from the covariance-based formula (Equation 4.14) under the assumption that each item variance is standardized to equal one (DeVellis, 2012). As such, the correlation-based formula provides a standardized score for Cronbach's alpha, while the covariance-based formula provides a raw (unstandardized) score. The raw score formula preserves information as covariances between items are based on values that retain their original scaling. If items have markedly different variances, items with larger variances will have greater weight in the computation of Cronbach's alpha in the raw score formula. The standardized formula, which does not retain the original scaling metric of items, places all items on a common metric and thereby weights them equally in the computation of the Cronbach's alpha. Which of the two formulas is preferred depends on the specific context and whether equal weighting is desired.

What values of Cronbach's alpha are considered acceptable? Benchmark values have been provided. Alpha coefficients of at least 0.7 are generally regarded as acceptable for psychometric scales, although it is often recommended that values should be above 0.8 (good) or even 0.9 (excellent) for an assessment at the group level (Nunnally and Bernstein, 1994; Fayers and Machin, 2007; Streiner and Norman, 2008; de Vet et al., 2011). A well-accepted guideline, therefore, for the value of Cronbach's alpha is between 0.70 and 0.90. But this general recommendation is also meant to take into account the length of the scale and the set of interitem correlations.

It is not unusual to see alpha coefficients greater than 0.9 for measures with several items; our experience suggests that good scales can have alpha coefficients between 0.90 and 0.95. If a multi-item domain has a more modest number of four items, then an alpha coefficient of at least 0.7 would be considered acceptable (with an assumed average interitem correlation of 0.4, the correlation-based Equation 4.15 gives a value of 0.73). Multi-item domains with more than four items can be considered to have acceptable alpha values in the 0.75–0.95 range. Because Cronbach's alpha is affected by the pairwise correlation of items and the number of items in the multi-item scale, values that are extremely high (say, above 0.95) may suggest redundancy in the multi-item scale or simply too many items (even for relatively low inter-item correlations) or both. When the alpha value is higher when the item is excluded, consideration should be given to deleting this item to improve the overall reliability of the scale. For individual patient assessment, greater internal consistency is required and it is recommended that values should be above 0.9 (Fayers and Machin, 2007).

As an example, in an observational study of 192 men (98 who reported a clinical diagnosis of ED in the past year and 94 who reported no clinical diagnosis of ED in the past year), Cronbach's alpha was determined for the Self-Esteem And Relationship questionnaire (Cappelleri et al., 2004). Cronbach's alpha for the Sexual Relationship Satisfaction domain, the Confidence domain, and Overall score were 0.91, 0.86, and 0.93, respectively. Cronbach's alpha for the Self-Esteem subscale and Overall Relationship Satisfaction subscale of the Confidence domain were 0.82 and 0.76, respectively.

4.8 Simulated Example of Cronbach's Alpha

Later in Section 5.4.1, a simulated dataset is created with 100 observations (100 subjects), who are assessed on a scale with 10 items and two latent factors. In the current section, we are using the same dataset "_tmp_3" to illustrate the assessment of the Cronbach's alpha. Assuming that all the steps described in Section 5.4.1 have been performed, Figure 4.7 represents implementation of the calculations to estimate Cronbach's alpha using the CORR procedure. Figures 4.8 and 4.9 represent partial output. For example, for Factor 1, Cronbach's alpha is 0.77, indicating good internal consistency reliability. But a closer examination of the results also shows that Item 5 has

```
Proc Corr Data=_tmp_3 alpha;
Var v1 v2 v3 v4 v5 v6;
Title "Factor 1";
Run;
Proc Corr Data=_tmp_3 alpha;
Var v7 v8 v9 v10;
Title "Factor 2";
Run;
```

FIGURE 4.7
Estimation of Cronbach's alpha using the CORR procedure.

```
Factor 1
The CORR Procedure

6  Variables:      v1          v2          v3          v4          v5          v6

Cronbach Coefficient Alpha

Variables                    Alpha
-------------------------
Raw                          0.770257
Standardized                 0.777430

Cronbach Coefficient Alpha with Deleted Variable

                  Raw Variables                      Standardized Variables

Deleted      Correlation                           Correlation
Variable     with Total          Alpha             with Total          Alpha
-----------------------------------------------------------------------------
v1           0.690511            0.691274           0.693356            0.700013
v2           0.539495            0.729969           0.546471            0.738470
v3           0.602754            0.713105           0.607316            0.722852
v4           0.597554            0.716570           0.605328            0.723369
v5           0.201242            0.817681           0.200725            0.819245
v6           0.524476            0.733695           0.526666            0.743460
```

FIGURE 4.8
Cronbach's alpha for Factor 1.

```
Factor 2
The CORR Procedure

4  Variables:      v7          v8          v9          v10

Cronbach Coefficient Alpha

Variables                    Alpha
-------------------------
Raw                          0.665692
Standardized                 0.671065

Cronbach Coefficient Alpha with Deleted Variable

                  Raw Variables                      Standardized Variables

Deleted      Correlation                           Correlation
Variable     with Total          Alpha             with Total          Alpha
-----------------------------------------------------------------------------
v7           0.414288            0.625428           0.417465            0.627412
v8           0.521430            0.548029           0.526836            0.553708
v9           0.561541            0.511821           0.564526            0.527030
v10          0.324583            0.687001           0.314506            0.691923
```

FIGURE 4.9
Cronbach's alpha for Factor 2.

a relatively small corrected item-to-total correlation of 0.201242 (i.e., a small correlation between Item 5 and the total score of Factor (or domain) 1 that excludes Item 5). This finding indicates that Item 5 should be considered for exclusion from this domain and, by excluding this item, the Cronbach's alpha increases to 0.82 (0.817681). For the assessment of internal consistency reliability, this exercise highlights the importance of examining not only Cronbach's alpha on all items in a scale but also corrected item-to-total correlations and Cronbach's alpha with each item deleted. Note that, for Factor 2, Cronbach's alpha is 0.67, indicating less than desirable internal consistency reliability (less than 0.7).

4.9 Summary

This chapter covers two main forms of reliability. As one form, repeatability reliability is described as a way to examine and quantify the degree to which measurement is stable and free from measurement error. Three types of repeatability reliability are discussed: ICC, Bland–Altman plot, and kappa coefficients. They are highlighted in terms of inter-rater reliability and, especially, test–retest reliability and equivalent-forms reliability. As a second form of reliability, internal consistency reliability is described as a way to quantify the consistency of responses to items on the same multi-item scale. General concepts are supplemented with specific examples throughout the chapter.

References

Bland, J.M. and D.G. Altman. 1986. Statistical methods for assessing agreement between two methods of clinical assessment. *Lancet* i:307–310.

Cappelleri, J.C., Althof, S.E., Siegel, R.L., Shpilsky, A., Bell, S.S., and S. Duttagupta. 2004. Development and validation of the Self-Esteem And Relationship (SEAR) questionnaire in erectile dysfunction. *International Journal of Impotence Research* 16:30–38.

Cappelleri, J.C., Rosen, R.C., Smith, M.D., Mishra, A., and I.H. Osterloh. 1999. Diagnostic evaluation of the erectile function domain of the International Index of Erectile Function. *Urology* 54:346–351.

Cappelleri, J.C. and N. Ting. 2002. A modified large-sample approach to approximate interval estimation for a particular intraclass correlation coefficient. *Statistics in Medicine* 22:1861–1877.

Cohen, J. 1960. A coefficient of agreement for nominal scales. *Educational and Psychological Measurement* 20:37–46.

Cohen, J. 1968. Weighted kappa: Nominal scale agreement with provision for scaled disagreement or partial credit. *Psychological Bulletin* 70:213–220.

Cronbach, L.J. 1951. Coefficient alpha and the internal structure of tests. *Psychometrika* 16:297–334.

DeVellis, R.F. 2012. *Scale Development: Theory and Applications*, 3rd edition. Thousand Oaks, CA: SAGE Publications Inc.

de Vet, H.C.W., Terwee, C.B., Mokkink, L.B., and D.L. Knol. 2011. *Measurement in Medicine: A Practical Guide*. New York, NY: Cambridge University Press.

Elliott, A.C. and W.A. Woodward. 2010. *A Guide to Mastering SAS for Research*. Hoboken, NJ: John Wiley & Sons Ltd.

Fan, X. and B. Thompson. 2001. Confidence intervals about score reliability coefficients, please: An EPM guidelines tutorial. *Educational and Psychological Measurement* 61:517–531.

Fayers, F.M. and D. Machin. 2007. *Quality of Life: The Assessment, Analysis and Interpretation of Patient-reported Outcomes*, 2nd edition. Chichester, England: John Wiley & Sons Ltd.

Fleiss, J.L. and J. Cohen. 1973. The equivalence of weighted kappa and the intraclass correlation coefficient as measures of reliability. *Educational and Psychological Measurement* 33:613–619.

Gilder, K., Ting, N., Tian, L., Cappelleri, J.C., and R.C. Hanumara. 2007. Confidence intervals on intraclass correlation coefficients in a balanced two-factor random design. *Journal of Statistical Planning and Inference* 137:1199–1212.

Landis, J.R. and G.G. Koch. 1977. The measurement of observer agreement for categorical data. *Biometrics* 33:159–174.

McGraw, K.O. and S.P. Wong. 1996. Forming inferences about some intraclass correlation coefficients. *Psychological Methods* 1:30–46.

Mokkink, L.B., Terwee, C.B., Patrick, D.L., Alonso, J., Stratforth, P.W., Knol, D.L., Bouter, L.M., and H.C.W. de Vet. 2010. International consensus on taxonomy, terminology, and definitions of measurement properties for health-related patient-reported outcomes: Results of the COSMIN study. *Journal of Clinical Epidemiology* 63:737–745.

Mulhall, J.O., Goldstein, I., Bushmakin, A., Cappelleri, J.C., and K. Hvidsten. 2007. Validation of the erectile hardness score. *Journal of Sexual Medicine* 4:1626–1634.

Nunnally, J.C. and I.H. Bernstein. 1994. *Psychometric Theory*, 3rd edition. New York, NY: McGraw-Hill.

Schuck, P. 2004. Assessing reproducibility for interval data in health-related quality of life questionnaires: Which coefficient should be used? *Quality of Life Research* 13:571–586.

Shoukri, M.M. and C.A. Pause. 1999. *Statistical Methods for Health Sciences*, 2nd edition. New York, NY: CRC Press.

Shrout, P.E. and J.L. Fleiss. 1979. Intraclass correlations: Uses in assessing rater reliability. *Psychological Bulletin* 86:420–428.

Singer, J. 1998. Using SAS PROC MIXED to fix multilevel models, hierarchical models, and individual growth models. *Journal of Educational and Behavioral Statistics* 24:323–355.

Streiner, D.L. and G.R. Norman. 2008. *Health Measurement Scales: A Practical Guide to Their Development and Use*, 4th edition. New York, NY: Oxford University Press.

Tian, L. and J.C. Cappelleri. 2004. A new approach for interval estimation and hypothesis testing of a certain intraclass correlation coefficient: The generalized variable method. *Statistics in Medicine* 23:2125–2135.

Ting, N., Cappelleri, J.C., and A.G. Bushmakin. 2009. Two confidence interval approaches on the dependability coefficients in a two-factor crossed design. *Journal of Biopharmaceutical Statistics* 19:610–624.

Weir, J.P. 2005. Quantifying the test-retest reliability using the intraclass correlation coefficient and the SEM. *Journal of Strength and Conditioning Research* 19:231–240.

Wyrwich, K.W. 2004. Minimal important difference thresholds and the standard error of measurement: Is there a connection? *Journal of Biopharmaceutical Statistics* 14:97–110.

Zou, K.H. and M.P. McDermott. 1999. Higher-moment approaches to approximate interval estimation for a certain intraclass correlation coefficient. *Statistics in Medicine* 18:2051–2061.

5

Exploratory and Confirmatory Factor Analyses

The methods presented in previous chapters were primarily concerned with examining item-to-item correlations or correlations among multi-item or single-item domains. Items in multi-item scales in the previous chapter are often based upon and confirmed by factor analysis. A *factor* is a latent variable, that is, an unobserved or hidden variable; the term *factor* may be defined and interchanged with the terms *domain*, *construct*, or *concept*. A latent variable is a hypothetical construct that is not directly observed, but whose existence is inferred from the way that it influences the observed or manifest variables. Examples of a latent variable include depression and anxiety.

Suppose we would want to capture the structure of the Hospital Anxiety and Depression Scale (HADS), a questionnaire with 14 variables (or items), each measured on a 4-point ordinal scale. It would be desirable to capitalize on a statistical technique so that, if anxiety has a high value, then the seven items assessing anxiety would also have a high value. Furthermore, these items should show an appreciable correlation with each other.

The statistical technique that can govern and quantify those interrelationships is factor analysis. Factor analysis is a multivariate statistical method designed to detect and analyze patterns based on the correlations among quantitative variables. Its use is to identify groups of variables with strong correlations among all variables within the same group and weaker correlations with variables in different groups. In the context of PRO measurement, these "groups" can be considered "domains" and "variables" can be considered "items" from a PRO questionnaire. The purposes of factor analysis are mainly for the structural development and validation of scales.

In factor analysis, a set of measured variables is transformed into a smaller set of latent (unobserved) factors that manifest themselves via the measured variables. An objective is to identify the number and the nature of the factors that are responsible for covariation in the data and to determine the domain structure of a questionnaire (which items represent which domains), which is usually done with exploratory factor analysis (EFA). The domain structure may be unidimensional or multidimensional with several factors or domains (sometimes also called subscales). A further objective may be to confirm an existing domain structure in a separate, independent group of individuals from the same population, which confirmatory factor analysis (CFA) addresses.

Exploratory and confirmatory factor analyses are two major approaches to factor analysis, and several references are available describing them in depth (Bollen, 1989; Hatcher, 1994; Kaplan, 2000; Pett et al., 2003; Brown, 2006; Fayers and Machin, 2007; Cappelleri and Gerber, 2010; Kline, 2010). In this chapter, the two approaches are described in varying degrees of detail (giving more emphasis to areas we consider more important) and then illustrated with simulated examples and also real-life examples taken from the areas of smoking cessation, erectile dysfunction, and obesity.

Exploratory and confirmatory factor analyses are best exemplified through the power of visual displays. In this chapter, manifest variables (or, in PRO terms, observable items) are represented by squares. Latent (or unobserved) variables are represented by ovals. Relationships between variables are expressed as lines (paths) with one or two arrow heads. Two-headed arrows represent covariances or variances. If the heads of the arrow point to a different variable, it is a covariance; if both heads point to the same variable, it is a variance. One-headed arrows represent regressions; the variable pointed to is the endogenous variable, regressed on the independent variable. Endogenous (*dependent*) variables are causally affected or directly influenced by the other variables in the model. Exogenous (*independent*) variables affect other variables in the model and are not affected by any variable in the model.

5.1 Exploratory Factor Analysis

5.1.1 Role of Exploratory Factor Analysis

In EFA, there is initial uncertainty as to the number of factors being measured, as well as which items are representing these factors. EFA is suitable for generating hypotheses about the structure of distinct concepts and which items represent a particular concept as embodied by a factor or domain. EFA can further refine an instrument by revealing what items may be dropped from the questionnaire, because they contribute little to the presumed underlying factors. Most statistical packages are equipped to execute EFA.

EFA is often confused with principal component analysis (PCA). Both EFA and PCA are variable reduction procedures, reducing a number of variables to a smaller number, and have been applied to determine item reduction and factor structure in the analysis of patient-reported outcomes (PROs). But the two procedures are generally different and not conceptually identical. In EFA, the observed variables are linear combinations of the underlying factors. In PCA, however, the principal components are linear combinations of the observed variables.

In EFA, factors are extracted to account only for the common item variance while the unique variance remains unanalyzed. In PCA, on the other hand, components are extracted to account for the total variance in the dataset, both common and unique, and not just the common variance. Because PCA makes no attempt to separate the common component from the unique component of each item's (variable's) variance, and EFA does, EFA is the appropriate method in identifying the factor structure of the data for PROs (and, more generally, in the behavioral and social sciences). The most widely used method in EFA to extract the factors is principal axis factoring, an approach that focuses on shared variance and not on sources of error that are unique to individual measurements. Another approach employed is the maximum likelihood method, which provides a significance test for solving the *number of factors* problem.

5.1.2 EFA Model

A factor is a latent or unobserved entity. Such a latent construct affects certain observed variables (or manifest variables) that can be measured directly. Figure 5.1 depicts a typical EFA model where responses to questions 1–6 are represented as six squares labeled V1–V6. This path model suggests that there are two underlying factors, called anxiety and depression, but initially it is not known which items represent which domains. If variables V1, V2, and V3 are related and measure the same latent variable called anxiety, then this construct (anxiety) exerts a powerful influence on the way subjects respond to questions 1, 2, and 3 (notice the arrows going from the oval factor to the square variables). Similarly, the Items V4, V5, and V6 are related to each other and influenced mainly by the underlying Factor 2, depression. In Figure 5.1, only one factor is hypothesized to have a *substantial* loading for every variable; for example, V1 displays a substantial loading Lf1v1 from Factor 1 but not from Factor 2 (Lf2v1 is not considered a meaningful or sizeable loading).

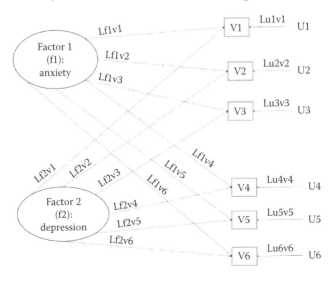

FIGURE 5.1
Exploratory factor analysis model.

The anxiety factor (Factor 1) in Figure 5.1 is known as a common factor, as is the depression factor (Factor 2). A common factor is a factor that influences more than one observed variable; it is a latent variable that is common to the set of manifest variables. Notice that in the EFA model in Figure 5.1 the two common factors (anxiety and depression) are not the only factors that influence the observed variables. For example, three factors actually influence variable V1: the common Factor 1, the common Factor 2, and a third factor labeled U1. Here U1 is a unique factor that only influences V1 and represents all of the independent and unmeasured factors that are unique to V1 (including the unique error component). The unique factor U1 affects only V1, U2 affects only V2, and so on. For variable V1, this relationship in the EFA model can be written as

$$V1 = Lf1v1 \times f1 + Lf2v1 \times f2 + Lu1v1 \times U1. \tag{5.1}$$

In Figure 5.1, each of the arrows from a common factor to an observed variable is identified with a specific coefficient such as (Lf1v1, Lf1v2, Lf1v3, Lf1v4, Lf1v5, and Lf1v6) for the first factor (f1). These coefficients represent factor loadings or path coefficients that represent the size of the effect that the underlying factor has on the variability of the scores of each observed variable. If the factor variables and observed variables are standardized to have unit variance (a variance of 1), those coefficients (loadings) are analogous to the standardized regression coefficients (regression weights) obtained in regression analysis.

5.1.3 Number of Factors

How does a researcher determine the number of factors that accounts for the relationships among the observed variables? That is, how many underlying dimensions (or subscales or domains) are there in the instrument? A widely used approach on how many domains or factors to retain is the scree test. The scree test is a rule-of-thumb criterion and involves the plot of the eigenvalues associated with each factor (i.e., the amount of incremental variance that is accounted for by a given factor) associated with each factor. The objective of a scree plot is to look for a break between factors with relatively large eigenvalues and those with smaller eigenvalues; factors that appear before the break are taken to be meaningful and retained. Researchers often refer to the break as the elbow in the curve of the scree plot.

Parallel analysis is another, more objective way to determine the number of factors to retain (O'Connor, 2000; Hayton et al., 2004). This method allows the identification of factors that are beyond chance. Parallel analysis can be described as a series of three steps.

The first step is to generate a random dataset (as implemented in Section 5.4.3) with the same number of observations and variables as the real data being analyzed. Another part of this step is to randomly populate this dataset by values representing all possible response values of each item from the real dataset.

In the second step, the newly generated random dataset is analyzed in order to extract the eigenvalues, with all eigenvalues saved for every simulation. The first two steps should be repeated a sufficient number of times to create a stable distribution for every parallel eigenvalue.

In the third step, the eigenvalues from the actual dataset are compared with the 95th percentile of the simulated eigenvalues. The first actual eigenvalue would be compared with the 95th percentile of the first random eigenvalue, the second actual eigenvalue would be compared with 95th percentile of the second real eigenvalue, and so forth. Factors retained are only those whose eigenvalues in the actual dataset are greater than the 95th percentile of eigenvalues from the random data. An example of applying parallel analysis for a PRO is the Power of Food Scale (PFS, Cappelleri et al. 2009; see also simulated example later in this chapter).

In addition to the scree plot and parallel analysis, two other criteria can be used to evaluate the number of factors and their content for suitability: (1) items that load on a given factor should have a shared conceptual meaning and (2) items should have high standardized factor pattern loadings or, equivalently, standardized regression coefficients (≥ 0.40 in absolute value) on one factor and low loadings on the other factors (Hatcher, 1994; Cappelleri and Gerber, 2010).

5.1.4 Factor Rotation

A rotation is a transformation that is performed on the factor solution for the purpose of making the solution easier to interpret. In EFA, an orthogonal rotation is one in which the (common) factors are treated as uncorrelated, which is a very strong assumption and not a reasonable one for most PROs with more than one dimension; of the methods for orthogonal rotation, varimax is the most widely used. A more realistic approach is to use an oblique rotation, which allows the factors to be correlated or associated, and, of the methods for oblique rotation, promax is the most widely used. This approach is more realistic because the general expectation in measurement is that subscales of PRO instruments tend to be at least somewhat correlated as they reflect underlying facets or aspects of a larger underlying construct. Thus, because factors tend to be correlated, an oblique rotation is often preferred over an orthogonal rotation. In particular, promax makes relatively low variable loadings even lower by relaxing the assumption that factors should be uncorrelated with each other. Not surprisingly, given its nature, promax usually results in similar but simpler and more interpretable factors than those derived from varimax (Fayers and Machin, 2007).

5.1.5 Sample Size

Factor analysis is a large-sample procedure, and a valid factor analysis typically involves hundreds of subjects. Regarding the minimum sample size needed, complete agreement among authorities of factor analysis is absent. Recommendations for the minimum number of subjects have ranged from 100 to 400 or more, depending on considerations such as the distribution of items and correlations between items (Fayers and Machin, 2007). Some researchers have suggested that the minimum sample size be at least five times the number of variables (or items) being analyzed. We prefer that, as a suggested rule of thumb, the sample size be at least 10 times the number of variables being analyzed. Therefore, for a 20-item questionnaire, at least 100 subjects and preferably 200 subjects would meet our suggested sample size for a study. As rough or crude approximations, this rule regarding the number of subjects per item constitutes a lower bound and may need to be modified depending on the amount of variability in the observed items, the number of items expected to load on each factor, and other considerations such as the magnitude of the correlations between the items.

5.1.6 Assumptions

The fundamental assumption underlying factor analysis is that one or more underlying factors can account for the patterns of covariation among a number of observed variables. Covariation exists when two variables vary together. Therefore, before conducting a factor analysis, it is important to analyze data for patterns of correlation. If no correlation exists, then a factor analysis is needless. If, however, at least moderate levels of correlation among variables are found, factor analysis can help uncover underlying patterns that explain these relationships.

EFA is generally intended for analyzing interval-scale data. An interval scale is one whose distance between any two adjacent points is the same. The Celsius temperature scale is an example of an interval measurement. The distance between 40°C and 41°C is exactly the same as the distance between 10°C and 11°C. Although factor analysis in principle is designed for interval-scale data, many researchers in practice also use the technique to successfully analyze ordinal data. An ordinal scale is a ranking scale in which the differences between ranks are not necessarily equal. A Likert scale (e.g., strongly agree, agree, neither agree nor disagree, disagree, strongly disagree) on which the responses are assigned a numerical value is an example of ordinal measurement.

Textbooks often state that, in principle, another assumption of EFA is that each observed variable be approximately normally distributed and, moreover, that each pair of observed variables be approximately bivariate normal distribution. However, in practice, we found this assumption is not critical to a successful implementation of factor analysis. The Pearson correlation coefficient, the key driver of EFA, is robust against violations of the normal assumption when the sample size exceeds 25 (Hatcher, 1994).

Tests for deciding on goodness-of-fit and the number of factors using maximum likelihood factor analysis, a less common variant of factor analysis, assume multivariate normality that is required for significance tests.

Given that a factor-analytic model assumes that data are continuous (interval level) and normally distributed, a natural question is whether factor analysis is well suited for the analysis of PROs, where most variables are (strictly speaking) often neither continuous measures nor normally distributed. While more research is welcomed on the consequences of violating these two assumptions, empirical results and simulation studies suggest that factor analysis is relatively robust to reasonable degrees of departure from interval-level data and normality (Fayers and Machin, 2007).

Factor analysis is a linear procedure of each observed item or variable regressed on a set of factors, so a linearity assumption is also required as in the case of multiple linear regression. Factor analysis is expected to be sufficiently robust when that relationship is approximately linear or does not deviate markedly from linearity.

5.2 Confirmatory Factor Analysis

5.2.1 Exploratory Factor Analysis versus Confirmatory Factor Analysis

Like EFA, the purpose of CFA is to examine latent factors that account for variation and covariation among a set of observed items or variables. Observed items (variables) are also known, in psychometric terminology, as indicators. Both types of factor analysis are based on the common factor model and thus they share many of the same concepts, terms, assumptions, and estimation methods. In CFA, as well as in EFA, factor loadings are coefficients that indicate the importance of a variable to each factor. These coefficients are important because they signify the nature of the variables that most strongly relate to a factor; the nature of the variables helps to capture the nature and meaning of a factor.

However, while EFA is generally an exploratory or hypothesis-generating procedure, CFA is usually a hypothesis-confirming technique relying on a researcher's hypothesis that requires prespecification of all relevant aspects of the factor model: the number of factors, the pattern of item–factor relationships, the pattern of factor–factor relationships, and so forth. While EFA explores the patterns in the correlations of items, CFA tests whether the correlations conform to an anticipated or expected scale structure given in a particular research hypothesis. Thus, CFA is suited in later phases of scale development or validation after the underlying structure of the data has been tentatively established by prior empirical analyses using EFA as well as by a theoretical understanding and knowledge of the subject matter.

Confirmatory factor analysis (like other forms of structural equation models) cannot prove causation. Rather, a major purpose of CFA is to determine whether the causal inferences of a researcher are consistent with the data. If the confirmatory factor model does not fit the data, then revisions are needed because then one or more of the model assumptions are incorrect or need refinement. Even if the CFA model is consistent with the data, this still does not prove causation. Instead, it shows that the assumptions made are not contradicted and may be valid, without ruling out that other models and assumptions also may fit the data.

5.2.2 Structural and Measurements Models

Structural equation modeling is a comprehensive statistical approach to testing hypotheses about relations among indicator (observed) and latent (unobserved) variables. Indicator variables are also considered manifest variables because only through them can latent variables manifest their current states. A structural equation model can be viewed as consisting of two components: (1) a measurement model that describes the relationships between the latent factors and their indicator variables and (2) a structural model that describes relationships between the latent factors themselves.

In the case of CFA, the structural part only generally specifies that latent variables are correlated, with no indication of causality. The measurement model not only covers a prespecified number of unobserved factors (latent variables) being assessed but also covers a theoretical framework of which observable (manifest) variables are affected and not affected by which factors. A measurement model in a CFA can initially spring from an EFA or from a conceptual model based on subject matter knowledge. Within a structural equation modeling framework, variations exist regarding the structural or causal component around the common theme that involves tests for a specified relationship between concepts (constructs) of interest and, in doing so, allows for testing hypotheses on which factors affect other factors. One particular variation involves statistical mediation models, the topic of Chapter 9.

5.2.3 Standard Model versus Nonstandard Model

A standard CFA model refers to a system in which all variables constituting the structural portion of the model are latent factors with multiple indicators. Here, multiple manifest variables are used as indicators of each latent factor. It may not be possible, however, to include multiple measures for each construct in the structural model. It may be necessary to use a single indicator as part of a CFA because of the nature of the variable (e.g., vomiting) or the unavailability of multiple measures of a construct. This type of CFA model may have some structural variables as single observable indicators and others as latent factors with multiple indicators, and is referred to as a nonstandard model.

5.2.4 Depicting the Model

Creating a diagram of the confirmatory factor model with its postulated latent variables and corresponding indicator variables is a natural way to begin a CFA. In Figure 5.2, we consider the same model described earlier

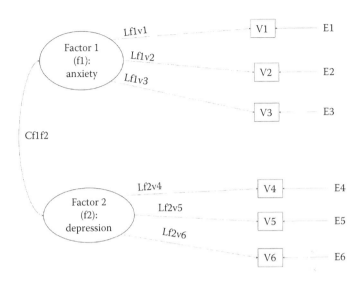

FIGURE 5.2
Confirmatory factor analysis model.

in this chapter (see Figure 5.1). Now, though, Factor 1 is postulated to affect only three indicator variables V1, V2, and V3, represented by rectangles, and Factor 2 is postulated to affect only indicator variables V4, V5, and V6. The two factors are connected by a curved two-headed arrow, meaning that they are allowed to covary. This particular connection between factors is analogous to the oblique solution in EFA discussed earlier in this chapter.

Figure 5.2 is an example of a basic standard model in which each indicator variable is assumed to be affected by only one factor. In Figure 5.2, notice also that no covariances exist between any of the indicators. The reason for this is that only variables that are not influenced or predicted by other variables in a model (like Factors 1 and 2 in Figure 5.2) are allowed to covary. These variables are called exogenous variables. Variables predicted to be casually affected by other variables, such as the indicators V1–V6 in Figure 5.2, are not allowed to have covariances. These variables are called endogenous variables.

5.2.5 Identifying Residual Terms for Endogenous Variables

A residual term for a variable represents all the factors that influence variability in the variable other than variables that precede and predict that variable. A residual term must be identified for each endogenous variable in the model and, because all of the indicator variables are endogenous variables (i.e., affected by factor variables), a residual term must be created for each indicator. In Figure 5.2, the residual term begins with the letter *E* and ends with the same numerical suffix as its corresponding indicator. Thus, the residual for V1 is E1, the residual for V2 is E2, and so forth. Each indicator is affected only by the underlying common factor on which it loads, along with a residual term. Indicator V1 is affected only by Factor 1 and E1, V4 is affected only by Factor 2 and E4, and so on. This relationship for variable V1, for instance, in the CFA model can be written as

$$V1 = Lf1v1 \times f1 + E1. \tag{5.2}$$

Comparison of this Equation 5.2 with the Equation 5.1 highlights the main methodological difference between EFA and CFA: in EFA all factors potentially affect all indicator variables (to varying degrees), but in CFA only one factor is hypothesized to affect any indicator variable.

5.2.6 Identifying All Parameters to Be Estimated

Three types of parameters need to be estimated in Figure 5.2: variances of the residual variables, covariances between the two factors, and factor loadings. Variances of exogenous variables, such as residual terms (E1, E2, ..., E6) and latent factors (f1 and f2) should be identified. For residual terms variances should be estimated. But latent variables, which, as a hypothetical construct (rather than a real-world observed variable), have no established metric or scale. Instead, the latent factors can be given unit variances by fixing their variances at 1. Note that variances are not estimated for endogenous variables.

Next, the covariance between the factors needs to be estimated. In Figure 5.2, the symbol *Cf1f2* represents this covariance estimate. Finally, the factor loadings need to be estimated. Factor loadings are basically path coefficients for the paths leading from a factor to an indicator variable. In Figure 5.2, the *L* symbol for "Loading" appears on the causal arrow from factor variable to indicator variable—for example, Lf1v1 represents the path coefficient from Factor 1 to V1 and Lf2v6 represents the path coefficient from Factor 2 to V6. Factor loadings are estimated for every causal path from factor to indicator. If the path coefficient (factor loadings) is relatively large and significantly different from zero, it means that the indicator is doing a good job in measuring the factor.

5.2.7 Assessing Fit between Model and Data

A measurement model in CFA postulates the existence of a specific number of latent factors and also which indicator variables are affected by (load on) each factor. The model is tested in a sample of subjects drawn from a population of interest. If the model provides a reasonably good approximation to reality, the model should adequately account for the observed relations in the sample dataset—that is, the model should provide a *good fit* to the data.

A host of model-fit indices exists. Among the most common are the following: Goodness-of-Fit Index (GFI), Comparative Fit Index (CFI), Normed Fit Index (NFI), Non-Normed Fit Index (NNFI), and Root-Mean-Square Error of Approximation (RMSEA). For the first four of these indices, values above 0.90 generally indicate an acceptable fit (Hatcher, 1994). For the RMSEA, values below 0.10 can be considered desirable and 90% confidence intervals for the true RMSEA are often obtained (Steiger, 1999).

Tests of statistical significance for the unstandardized and standardized factor loadings should also be conducted. Unstandardized factor loadings can be interpreted in the same way as unstandardized regression coefficients, where the metric of the indicator variable is passed onto the latent factor, so that a one-unit change in the factor is associated with an estimated change in the indicator. Also relevant are the magnitudes of the standardized factor loadings, where the metrics of both the indicators and the factors are standardized to have means of 0 and variances of 1, and their interpretation is the same as those given to standardized regression coefficients. Thus, they reflect an increase in one standardized score in the factor that is associated with a given change in one standardized score in the indicator. Being measured in standard deviation units, standardized factor loadings with values of 0.40 or larger (in absolute values) can be considered noteworthy and sizeable.

Some researchers also report a model chi-square statistic (the null hypothesis of perfect model fit). The model chi-square statistic with a low enough p-value (say, less than 0.05) suggests rejection of the null hypothesis of perfect fit. This hypothesis, however, is likely to be implausible because it is unrealistic to expect a model to have perfect fit. Moreover, the chi-square statistic is known to increase its sensitivity and get larger (and hence be more probable to lead to rejection of the null hypothesis) with larger correlations and larger sample sizes, even for a very good fitting model where the differences between observed and predicted covariances are slight.

Regarding the sample size required for CFA, rules of thumb have been offered including a minimum number of subjects per each parameter to be estimated (e.g., at least 10 subjects per parameter). The same caution given about such rules of thumb for EFA also applies to CFA. It is safe to say that, in general, hundreds of subjects would be needed. Statistical power and sample sizes for CFA are explained in more detail elsewhere (Brown, 2006).

Among the features of CFA is the ability to compare and test nested models, akin to the comparison and evaluation of nested models in regression analysis. For example, one model may allow the latent factors to be correlated while another model may assume that they are orthogonal and not correlated. A likelihood ratio test can be performed to compare the two models on whether the null hypothesis of no correlation between factors can be rejected in favor of the alternative hypothesis of nonzero correlation between at least one pair of factors.

5.3 Causal Indicators versus Effect Indicators

Exploratory and confirmatory factor analyses for multi-item scales, as well as most classical approaches to measurement scale evaluations including Cronbach's alpha and item-to-total correlations, are based on the assumption of parallel tests (Fayers and Machin, 2007; Steiner and Norman, 2008). Hence each item should be distinct from the others but should be similar and consistent with them in reflecting all important and related aspects of the same underlying attribute or construct; item responses should differ only as a consequence of random error. Multiple items on a PRO scale reflect the level of the intended construct; that is, the items are assumed to indicate the level of, and tap into, the postulated construct. Therefore, for example, a high level of cognitive ability implies that the patient most likely has high levels of vocabulary, problem solving, mathematical ability, and other characteristics indicative of high cognitive ability. The level or amount of each item (e.g., the patient's score on mathematical ability) is assumed to be the result of the hypothesized underlying construct (e.g., cognitive ability). Each of those multiple items taps into the postulated construct and is called an effect indicator, because each relays the status of the construct.

On the other hand, exploratory and confirmatory factor analyses (and other traditional psychometric barometers such as Cronbach's alpha and item-to-total correlation) should not be applied when items, not being effect indicators, are considered causal indicators because they cause the construct rather than the construct causes them (Fayers and Machin, 2007; Streiner and Norman, 2008). Effect indicators can be considered as homogeneous items that constitute a scale, whereas causal indicators can be considered as heterogeneous items that constitute an index.

Consider an index on activities of daily living. A patient with an impaired rotator cuff, for instance, may have difficulty brushing her teeth but not with dressing. Another patient with rotator cuff damage may have a different story. This patient may have difficulty to comb his hair but have no difficulty tying his shoelaces. A patient with poor activity of daily living does not necessarily imply difficulty tying his shoelaces. But a patient who has difficulty raising her hand to comb her hair may be sufficient to cause a poor level of daily activity. Activities of daily living, which are caused by and idiosyncratic to treatment or disease, may show the reverse pattern for patients with rheumatoid arthritis. Symptoms and side effects also tend to be causal indicators.

Interitem correlations among causal indicators may or may not be sizeable and they may be positively correlated, negatively correlated, or not correlated at all. Even if the correlations are positive and substantial, the reason may be external circumstances such as treatment or disease and not any natural or inherent relationship that the causal indicators have with the construct (independent or irrespective of treatment, disease, study population, or anything else external).

Effect indicators may be in one questionnaire, causal indicators in another questionnaire, or both sets of indicators may be in the same questionnaire. Traditional psychometric approaches to scale design, validation, scoring, and analysis will often be invalid and misleading when the items are causal indicators. In the design of a questionnaire with items as causal indicators, it becomes most important to ensure that there is item saturation so that a comprehensive coverage of all important causal indicators are included and that none are excluded. Omitting a causal indicator is omitting part of the construct. Because the items may be uncorrelated or poorly correlated, it cannot be assumed that what is missed if one item is omitted will be covered by the other items that remain. Such is not the case generally with effect indicators, where only a sufficient number of items would be needed to represent the construct.

Causal indicators are usually heterogeneous and therefore it may not make sense to preserve psychometric unidimensionality, as would typically be the case for the homogeneous set of effect indicators. Unlike the conventional psychometric approach where responses on effect indicators on a scale are combined through a simple sum or average, simple summated-scaling method on an index (where items are heterogeneous) cannot always or necessarily be assumed for responses on causal indicators. Weights that reflect item importance may have to be incorporated whenever causal indicators are combined. A minimum number of symptoms or a certain combination of symptoms may be required for an effective analysis of symptom data.

Causal indicators can be modeled through causal paths using structural equation models. For example, symptoms as causal indicators can be modeled separately as individual observed or manifest variables or as a summed index score (rather than having a multi-item cluster intended to measure latent symptomology), alongside multi-item domains of effect indicators, in a confirmatory factor analysis.

5.4 Simulated Examples Using SAS: Exploratory Factor Analysis

5.4.1 Simulated Dataset

A simulated dataset is used to illustrate the implementation of EFA. In this example, consideration is given to a scale with 10 items and two latent factors. The first step is to simulate values of the latent factors. The SAS code in Figure 5.3 generated the simulated dataset with 100 observations (100 subjects) with two random values representing latent scores of the two factors for each subject.

Based on this dataset, we can now simulate 10 item values, which will represent responses to a fictional 10-item scale (see Figure 5.4). Note that columns representing latent scores are dropped from the dataset.

To be lifelike, the variables v1–v10 are transformed as if every item was measured on the visual analog scale from 0 to 10 (see Figure 5.5 for the SAS code and Figure 5.6 for how a final simulated dataset will look like). Note

```
/*
Create dataset "_tmp_1" by simulating 100 subjects and two factors.
*/
Data _tmp_1;
    Do ID=1 to 100;
    F1=ranuni(1); F2=ranuni(2); output;
    End;
Keep F1 F2;
Run;
```

FIGURE 5.3
Simulating values of the latent factors.

```
/*
Create dataset "_tmp_2": Based on factor values we create 10 items
(v1, v2,...,v9, v10).
First 6 items (v1, v2, v3, v4, v5, v6) represent Factor 1 (F1) and
last 4 items (v7, v8, v9, v10) represent Factor 2 (F2).
Note that we deleted values for Factor 1 and Factor 2 (Drop F1
F2;) from the dataset
*/
Data _tmp_2;
Set _tmp_1;
    v1 = F1 * 0.8366 + 0.2479 * rannor(1);
    v2 = F1 * 0.7902 + 0.3129 * rannor(2);
    v3 = F1 * 0.9034 + 0.2289 * rannor(3);
    v4 = F1 * 0.8580 + 0.2137 * rannor(4);
    v5 = F1 * 0.6392 + 0.4690 * rannor(5);
    v6 = F1 * 0.8366 + 0.2479 * rannor(6);
    v7 = F2 * 0.7902 + 0.3129 * rannor(7);
    v8 = F2 * 0.9034 + 0.2289 * rannor(8);
    v9 = F2 * 0.8580 + 0.3137 * rannor(9);
    v10 = F2 * 0.6392 + 0.4690 * rannor(10);
Drop F1 F2;
Run;
```

FIGURE 5.4
Simulating responses of the observed items.

```
Proc Stdize data=_tmp_2 out=_tmp_3 method=Range mult=10 add=0;
        var v1-v10;
Run;
Proc Means data=_tmp_3;
Run;
```

FIGURE 5.5
Transforming responses onto scale from 0 to 10.

v1	v2	v3	v4	v5	v6	v7	v8	v9	v10
6.4681845669	4.344841039	3.2417072261	2.5496701347	10	2.4009131469	7.3671581567	8.277509487	6.685460368	6.20864186
4.1971342436	4.9332288554	5.2118981102	4.0539194549	3.9193353102	3.2617487515	4.7043401795	3.2919716423	1.7584318993	5.080774051
8.950843863	9.6622222598	6.8736232345	10	4.8183797353	5.7611604196	7.9597991161	9.0626121641	7.6269219965	8.567651558
4.9344453948	4.8951584036	4.4143752535	5.7700262798	8.225370468	3.3579861471	6.7767394298	4.9954596672	7.5713358087	4.689625902
1.9442646785	0.2481626724	0.9190424038	4.1237381504	5.426043327	1.9326989536	4.7566278512	1.0058503087	5.591118974	0.813679636
7.3239786391	6.9148853761	4.7656758017	7.5232361085	4.9965735376	6.5490269454	3.986587495	6.7754540504	5.6245508959	8.767847158
6.5988034481	9.675760691	5.3569929432	7.1505917367	7.4052134402	5.6010415003	4.279776688	0	4.6861459407	5.411705644
7.9028801125	8.0886994516	5.995750809	7.3525736063	8.6157536037	8.5391575097	6.2394543037	2.3922930104	2.8780565085	5.908337238
6.3052138367	3.2492380761	2.0658231721	4.2792712221	6.8744989431	5.2245985732	5.1614880465	6.4103735711	8.2718366504	3.402411196
7.4855599936	10	6.8975629512	6.4362684534	6.3575872171	6.0432813047	0.7681569325	2.2088203701	3.7367144233	6.711530083
6.6508536134	7.5838271822	5.9084671728	6.8960267572	3.0728873038	5.443671182	5.2047771076	3.1872362736	1.8530501784	4.863539214
7.0307465602	7.273404844	6.5558429667	5.5806424504	8.888622498	7.0630611887	3.0999436913	3.4163713788	1.3946818813	2.697308407
6.4029880422	6.0576012258	5.3719890971	4.5723510042	3.2115072242	4.5305474913	6.0328687613	7.6513357584	5.2172923061	7.253309325
6.5174714614	6.8222839112	5.844352784	5.5792712321	7.1231042334	7.4556675399	6.9403108068	4.3939216117	4.1942754491	7.849043347
4.9286656472	6.5399854761	5.7105471567	5.9741158045	5.5965166488	1.9813125674	7.0000726142	5.8271233897	4.9654077696	7.836311601

FIGURE 5.6
Final simulated dataset (data for the first 15 subjects are shown).

```
                       The MEANS Procedure

      Variable     N        Mean        Std Dev     Minimum      Maximum
      -------------------------------------------------------------------
         v1        100     5.1842797    2.0968628       0      10.0000000
         v2        100     5.8380213    2.1356512       0      10.0000000
         v3        100     4.3975432    2.1810920       0      10.0000000
         v4        100     5.5372705    2.0294069       0      10.0000000
         v5        100     5.4451246    2.3647852       0      10.0000000
         v6        100     4.8122062    2.2599504       0      10.0000000
         v7        100     5.1127352    1.6239322       0      10.0000000
         v8        100     5.2905349    2.0283544       0      10.0000000
         v9        100     5.4549849    2.2786728       0      10.0000000
        v10        100     5.1838519    2.2449005       0      10.0000000
      -------------------------------------------------------------------
```

FIGURE 5.7
Mean values and ranges for indicator variables.

that this is the standard way a dataset should be structured for exploratory and confirmatory factor analyses in most statistical software systems used today. Results of the MEANS procedure (SAS, 2011) show that all items have values from 0 to 10, with their means close to 5 (see Figure 5.7).

5.4.2 Implementation

Figure 5.8 represents implementation of the EFA using the FACTOR procedure (SAS, 2012). Although only one step is shown to do the EFA, in real life a researcher will need to run this code at least twice. First, this code will be run just to output eigenvalues, which represents the amount of variance captured by a given factor. (Note: Number of factor [nfactors = 1] is not important at this first run.) After an examination of the scree plot, a second run of the same code is needed, but the number of factors will be based on the results of the scree plot test, that is, the parameter **nfactors** should be equal to the number of factors from the scree test.

```
Proc Factor data=_tmp_3
        method=prin
        PRIORS=SMC
        scree
        rotate=PROMAX
        nfactors=1
        reorder outstat=_all_;
Var v1-v10;
Run;
```

FIGURE 5.8
Implementation of the exploratory factor analysis using SAS.

```
Eigenvalues of the Reduced Correlation Matrix: Total = 3.2976679
Average = 0.32976679

        Eigenvalue    Difference      Proportion     Cumulative
   1    2.41159624    1.07993602        0.7313         0.7313
   2    1.33166022    1.08897029        0.4038         1.1351
   3    0.24268993    0.12048113        0.0736         1.2087
   4    0.12220880    0.09714281        0.0371         1.2458
   5    0.02506599    0.10047638        0.0076         1.2534
   6   -.07541039     0.01842389       -0.0229         1.2305
   7   -.09383428     0.10778847       -0.0285         1.2021
   8   -.20162275     0.01657619       -0.0611         1.1409
   9   -.21819894     0.02828797       -0.0662         1.0747
  10   -.24648691                      -0.0747         1.0000
```

FIGURE 5.9
Eigenvalues.

Figure 5.9 represents output of the FACTOR procedure with calculated eigenvalues. Figure 5.10 shows a break just before Factor 3, suggesting that only the first 2 factors should be kept. After establishing the number of factors, we need to run SAS code from Figure 5.8 again but the parameter **nfactors** will now be equal to 2.

The next step is to analyze the rotated factor pattern (in SAS output it can be found under "Rotated Factor Pattern [Standardized Regression Coefficients]"). For an item to be considered as a part of a particular factor, its standardized regression coefficient should be at least 0.4 for this factor and less than 0.4 for other factors (Hatcher, 1994; Cappelleri and Gerber, 2010). If an item has standardized regression coefficients less than 0.4 for all factors, we consider this item weak. If an item has two or more standardized regression coefficients of at least 0.4, we consider this item ambiguous relative to the extracted factors. This item, though, can still be kept as a part of the scale

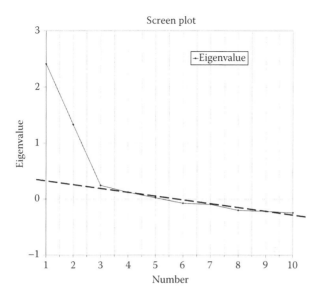

FIGURE 5.10
Scree plot test.

```
Rotation Method: Promax (power = 3)
Rotated Factor Pattern (Standardized Regression Coefficients)

                Factor1              Factor2

    v1         0.75658              0.00624
    v4         0.72723             -0.02364
    v3         0.69066              0.04131
    v2         0.64343              0.02937
    v6         0.59002             -0.02074
    v5         0.22672             -0.08067
    v9        -0.06590              0.66847
    v8         0.03143              0.65132
    v7        -0.04409              0.53648
    v10        0.04363              0.41376
```

FIGURE 5.11
Rotated factor pattern.

if that item can be justified as a singular aspect of a measure rather than one belonging to a particular multi-item domain.

The rotated factor pattern (see Figure 5.11) indicates that variables (v1, v4, v3, v2, v6) should be assigned to Factor 1, and variables (v9, v8, v7, v10) to Factor 2. Indicator variable v5 was a part of Factor 1 in the simulation. Nonetheless, because this variable had the smallest loading and biggest error term (when simulating values for v5), variable v5 is considered weak and should be deleted from the model. However, indicator variable 10, with the same simulated loading and error term as indicator variable v5, is retained because of the loading being above 0.4 on Factor 2.

5.4.3 Parallel Analysis

As powerful and simple to use as a scree test is, it is not always obvious when working with real-life data to identify *the break* (or discontinuity) on the scree plot, which can be somewhat subjective. On the other hand, parallel analysis provides an objective way of identifying the number of factors to retain in the model. The methodology was described earlier in Section 5.1.3. In this section, we demonstrate how this approach can be implemented using SAS.

The first step in parallel analysis is (a) to create a random dataset of the same size as the original dataset and (b) to have response values for every indicator variable (item) in the range as in the original dataset. In our example, we have 100 observations (subjects) and all responses for all indicator variables were continuous values from 0 to 10. The first SAS data step (see Figure 5.12) creates a dataset with 100 observations and every variable is assigned a random value from 0 to 10. The next step is to calculate eigenvalues; this step is identical to the first step in any factor analysis. The following step is to save the calculated eigenvalues. After at least 1000 simulations are performed, the MEANS procedure can be used to calculate the 95th percentiles for the simulated eigenvalues (see Figure 5.13 for results).

Now the results from the parallel analysis (i.e., results presented by the Figure 5.13) are overlaid onto the original eigenvalues (from the Figure 5.9). Figure 5.14 shows that only the first 2 eigenvalues can be considered to be beyond chance (only the first 2 observed eigenvalues exceeded the 95th percentile of eigenvalues from the random data), and, by doing so, parallel analysis enabled an accurate revelation of two factors for consideration.

5.5 Simulated Examples Using SAS: Confirmatory Factor Analysis

5.5.1 Simulated Dataset

A different simulated dataset is used to illustrate the implementation of CFA. In this example, consideration is given to a scale with 12 items and three latent factors. The first step is to simulate values of the latent factors.

```
proc printto log='NUL:' print='NUL:';
Run;

%macro Parallel_Analysis(NumberOfSimulations);

%do i=1 %to &NumberOfSimulations;
/* -----------------------------------------------------------
Create dataset "_tmp_2" with random 10 items (v1, v2, …, v10).
values for every item will be randomly taken from the range
of values from 0 to 10.
*/
Data _tmp_2;
Do id=1 to 100;
    v1  = 10*ranuni(0);
    v2  = 10*ranuni(0);
    v3  = 10*ranuni(0);
    v4  = 10*ranuni(0);
    v5  = 10*ranuni(0);
    v6  = 10*ranuni(0);

    v7  = 10*ranuni(0);
    v8  = 10*ranuni(0);
    v9  = 10*ranuni(0);
    v10 = 10*ranuni(0);
    output;
End;
Drop ID;
Run;

    Proc Factor data=_tmp_2
        method=prin
        PRIORS=SMC
        OUTSTAT=_stat_;
    Var v1-v10;
    Run;

    Data _stat_1;
    Set  _stat_;
    Where _TYPE_="EIGENVAL";
    Keep v1-v10;
    Run;

/**        Summarize Datasets                   **/
PROC APPEND BASE=EIGENVAL DATA=_stat_1;
Run;

%End;
```

FIGURE 5.12
Implementation of parallel analysis.

(continued)

```
%mend Parallel_Analysis;

/* Run 1000 simulations */
%Parallel_Analysis(1000);

/* Calculate 95th percentile for every eigenvalue */
proc means data=EIGENVAL P95;
run;

proc printto;
Run;
```

FIGURE 5.12 (continued)
Implementation of parallel analysis.

```
The MEANS Procedure

Variable          95th Pctl
- - - - - - - - - - - - - - - - - - - - - - -
v1                0.8344861
v2                0.5913913
v3                0.4249913
v4                0.2926755
v5                0.1711588
v6                0.0806229
v7               -0.0175551
v8               -0.1074904
v9               -0.1902815
v10              -0.2754632
- - - - - - - - - - - - - - - - - - - - - - -
```

FIGURE 5.13
Parallel analysis results: 95th percentiles.

The following SAS code (Figure 5.15) generated the simulated dataset with 500 observations (i.e., 500 subjects) and three random values representing latent scores of the three factors. Note that values for latent factors were based on the same variable *i*. As a result, those variables will be inherently correlated.

To simplify comparison of results of the CFA with the values of loadings and variances used in the simulations, we transformed values of the factors to have a mean of 0 and standard deviation of 1 (see Figure 5.16). Figure 5.17 represents output from the CORR procedure (SAS, 2011). The three factors are highly correlated, with correlations ranging from 0.7 to 0.8.

Based on this dataset "_Factors_s", we can now simulate 12 item values, which will represent responses to a 12-item scale (see Figure 5.18). Note that only responses for the observed variables (variables v1, v2, v12) are kept.

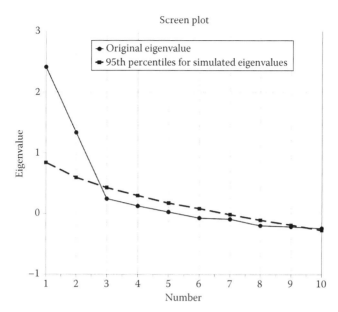

FIGURE 5.14
Original eigenvalues overlaid by the results of the parallel analysis.

```
/* -----------------------------------------------------------------
Create dataset "_Factors_": simulating 500 subjects and 3 factors.
*/

Data _Factors_;

        Do i= 1 to 500;
        F1=i*2 + 200*rannor(1);
        F2=i*5 + 400*rannor(2);
        F3=i*8 + 500*rannor(3);
        Output;
        End;

        Drop i;
    Run;
```

FIGURE 5.15
Simulating values of the latent factors.

5.5.2 Implementation

Figure 5.19 represents one of the ways to implement a CFA using the CALIS procedure (SAS, 2011). We highly recommend that the input dataset for CFA analysis contain only responses to indicator variables (i.e., only columns v1, v2,..., v12). If, just by chance, this dataset has a column with name f1, e01,

```
/* --------------------------------------------------------------
Standardize factor values to have mean of 0 and STD of 1.
*/
Proc Stdize data=_Factors_ out=_Factors_s method=STD;
    var F1 F2 F3;
Run;

Proc Corr data=_Factors_s;
Run;
```

FIGURE 5.16
Standardizing factor values.

```
The CORR Procedure

3  Variables:      F1        F2        F3

                        Simple Statistics

Variable       N      Mean     Std Dev     Sum     Minimum     Maximum

F1           500        0     1.00000       0    -2.69369     3.04441
F2           500        0     1.00000       0    -2.33175     2.61871
F3           500        0     1.00000       0    -2.39998     2.03519

   Pearson Correlation Coefficients, N=500
            Prob > |r| under H0: Rho=0

              F1               F2               F3

F1        1.00000          0.70213          0.74934
                           <.0001           <.0001

F2        0.70213          1.00000          0.78446
          <.0001                            <.0001

F3        0.74934          0.78446          1.00000
          <.0001           <.0001
```

FIGURE 5.17
Factor means and correlations.

or another name used in the description of the model, this could lead to incorrect results. As the input dataset has only variables (v1, v2,..., v12), it means that all other variables in the model are the parameters, which need to be identified and hence estimated. We need to estimate 12 loadings (lv01f1, lv02f1,..., lv12f3), 12 variances for the error terms (vare01, vare02,..., vare12), and 3 covariances between latent factors (cf1f2, cf1f3, cf2f3). Variances of the latent factors are fixed at 1 (f1 = **1**, f2 = **1**, f3 = **1**).

```
/*
Create dataset "_items_": Based on factor values we create 12
items (v1, v2, ..., v11, v12).
First 4 items (v1, v2, v3, v4) represent Factor 1 (F1), Items v5,
v6, v7, and v8 represent Factor 2 (F2), and Items v9, v10, v11, and
v12 represent Factor 3 (F3).
Note that we keep only columns v1, v2, ...,v12 (statement Keep v1-v12;)
in the dataset to "emulate" how the dataset would look like in practice.
*/

    Data _items_;
    Set   _Factors_s;

    v1= 0.5*F1 + sqrt(.21)*rannor(1);
    v2= 0.6*F1 + sqrt(.31)*rannor(2);
    v3= 0.7*F1 + sqrt(.42)*rannor(3);
    v4= 0.4*F1 + sqrt(.55)*rannor(4);

    v5= 0.45*F2 + sqrt(.51)*rannor(5);
    v6= 0.55*F2 + sqrt(.71)*rannor(6);
    v7= 0.88*F2 + sqrt(.42)*rannor(7);
    v8= 0.99*F2 + sqrt(.5 )*rannor(8);

    v9=  0.75*F3 + sqrt(.351)*rannor(9);
    v10= 0.85*F3 + sqrt(.671)*rannor(10);
    v11= 0.58*F3 + sqrt(.742)*rannor(11);
    v12= 0.89*F3 + sqrt(.35 )*rannor(12);

    Keep v1-v12;
    Run;
```

FIGURE 5.18
Simulating responses of the observed items.

Figure 5.20 demonstrates that the model fits the data exceedingly well; for example, Bentler's CFI is equal to 0.9995 (values more than 0.9 indicate an acceptable fit). It should be noted that it is not enough for the model to have only Bentler's CFI be more than 0.9. Additionally, all loadings from Figure 5.21 should be statistically significant (*t*-values should be more than 1.96 in absolute values). And all standardized loadings (see Figure 5.22) should be equal to or more than 0.4. At least these three conditions should be satisfied to indicate that this particular model fits the data.

With these simulated data, we can also find how close the estimated parameters are to the values assigned to those parameters when data were simulated. From Figure 5.21, for example, the loading from factor 1 to variable 1 is 0.4695, and in the simulation a value of 0.5 was taken as a loading from factor 1 to variable 1 (see Figure 5.18: `v1 = `**`0.5`**`*F1 + sqrt(`**`.21`**`)*rannor(`**`1`**`);`). The loading from factor 1 to variable 2 is 0.6062 and in the simulation a value of 0.6 was specified. The same pattern of concordance was accorded to all other loadings.

```
Proc Calis COV data=_items_ G4=1000 GCONV=1E-10 Method=ML ALL;

     LINEQS
        v1    = lv01f1 f1 + e01,
        v2    = lv02f1 f1 + e02,
        v3    = lv03f1 f1 + e03,
        v4    = lv04f1 f1 + e04,

        v5    = lv05f2 f2 + e05,
        v6    = lv06f2 f2 + e06,
        v7    = lv07f2 f2 + e07,
        v8    = lv08f2 f2 + e08,

        v9    = lv09f3 f3 + e09,
        v10   = lv10f3 f3 + e10,
        v11   = lv11f3 f3 + e11,
        v12   = lv12f3 f3 + e12
        ;

     STD
     f1=1, f2=1, f3=1,
     e01 =    vare01  ,
     e02 =    vare02  ,
     e03 =    vare03  ,
     e04 =    vare04  ,
     e05 =    vare05  ,
     e06 =    vare06  ,
     e07 =    vare07  ,
     e08 =    vare08  ,
     e09 =    vare09  ,
     e10 =    vare10  ,
     e11 =    vare11  ,
     e12 =    vare12
     ;

     COV
     f1  f2  =   cf1f2 ,
     f1  f3  =   cf1f3 ,
     f2  f3  =   cf2f3
     ;

  Run;
```

FIGURE 5.19
Implementation of the confirmatory factor analysis using SAS.

Figure 5.23 represents the variances of the exogenous variables. From this figure we can see that modeled variances are also close to the variances used to simulate the data. For example, the variance of the error term for variable 1 is 0.19699, and in the simulation the value of 0.21 was specified (see again Figure 5.18: v1 = **0.5***F1 + sqrt(**.21**)*rannor(**1**);).

Finally, Figure 5.24 represents the correlations among exogenous variables. Comparing these results with the results of the CORR procedure

```
The CALIS Procedure
Covariance Structure Analysis: Maximum Likelihood Estimation

Fit Function                                             0.1046
Goodness of Fit Index (GFI)                              0.9827
GFI Adjusted for Degrees of Freedom (AGFI)               0.9736
Root Mean Square Residual (RMR)                          0.0215
Standardized Root Mean Square Residual (SRMR)            0.0235
Parsimonious GFI (Mulaik, 1989)                          0.7594
Chi-Square                                              52.2049
Chi-Square DF                                                51
Pr > Chi-Square                                          0.4269
Independence Model Chi-Square                           2403.9
Independence Model Chi-Square DF                             66
RMSEA Estimate                                           0.0069
RMSEA 90% Lower Confidence Limit                              .
RMSEA 90% Upper Confidence Limit                         0.0297
ECVI Estimate                                            0.2157
ECVI 90% Lower Confidence Limit                              .
ECVI 90% Upper Confidence Limit                          0.2587
Probability of Close Fit                                 1.0000
Bentler's Comparative Fit Index                          0.9995
Elliptic Corrected Chi-Square                           53.0900
Pr > Elliptic Corrected Chi-Square                       0.3936
Normal Theory Reweighted LS Chi-Square                  52.6696
Akaike's Information Criterion                          -49.7951
Bozdogan's (1987) CAIC                                 -315.7401
Schwarz's Bayesian Criterion                           -264.7401
McDonald's (1989) Centrality                             0.9988
Bentler & Bonett's (1980) Non-normed Index              0.9993
Bentler & Bonett's (1980) NFI                           0.9783
James, Mulaik, & Brett (1982) Parsimonious NFI          0.7559
Z-Test of Wilson & Hilferty (1931)                      0.1844
Bollen (1986) Normed Index Rho1                          0.9719
Bollen (1988) Non-normed Index Delta2                    0.9995
Hoelter's (1983) Critical N                                 658
```

FIGURE 5.20
Fit statistics.

(see Figure 5.17), we can also conclude that predicted correlations are close to the values of the correlations of the simulated latent variables, as expected.

5.5.3 Nonstandard Measurement Model

As pointed out earlier (Section 5.2.3), in the case of the nonstandard measurement model at least one indicator variable plays the role of the "latent factor", or the latent factor only manifests via this one indicator variable. Previously we simulated dataset "_items_" with 12 items and three factors

```
v1        =      0.4695*f1          +    1.0000 e01
Std Err          0.0272 lv01f1
t Value         17.2396
v2        =      0.6062*f1          +    1.0000 e02
Std Err          0.0361 lv02f1
t Value         16.8149
v3        =      0.6957*f1          +    1.0000 e03
Std Err          0.0383 lv03f1
t Value         18.1637
v4        =      0.3727*f1          +    1.0000 e04
Std Err          0.0356 lv04f1
t Value         10.4822

v5        =      0.4810*f2          +    1.0000 e05
Std Err          0.0382 lv05f2
t Value         12.6028
v6        =      0.6073*f2          +    1.0000 e06
Std Err          0.0450 lv06f2
t Value         13.4839
v7        =      0.8601*f2          +    1.0000 e07
Std Err          0.0418 lv07f2
t Value         20.5704
v8        =      0.9652*f2          +    1.0000 e08
Std Err          0.0477 lv08f2
t Value         20.2205

v9        =      0.7655*f3          +    1.0000 e09
Std Err          0.0380 lv09f3
t Value         20.1460
v10       =      0.8710*f3          +    1.0000 e10
Std Err          0.0501 lv10f3
t Value         17.3989
v11       =      0.5658*f3          +    1.0000 e11
Std Err          0.0458 lv11f3
t Value         12.3434
v12       =      0.9256*f3          +    1.0000 e12
Std Err          0.0418 lv12f3
t Value         22.1520
```

FIGURE 5.21
Manifest variable equations with estimates.

(see Section 5.5.1). Let us now assume that the third factor is affecting only one indicator variable, v9. Figure 5.25 shows that we use a dataset created in Section 5.5.1 and now keep only the first 9 items. The equations representing first 2 factors are the same, but instead of Factor 3 with four indicator variables we now have only the single indicator variable v9. For this indicator variable, we need to define its variance (v9=varv9) and also the correlations among latent factors f1 and f2 and the manifest variable v9.

```
v1   =   0.7267*f1     +   0.6869 e01
                lv01f1
v2   =   0.7129*f1     +   0.7013 e02
                lv02f1
v3   =   0.7564*f1     +   0.6541 e03
                lv03f1
v4   =   0.4825*f1     +   0.8759 e04
                lv04f1

v5   =   0.5558*f2     +   0.8313 e05
                lv05f2
v6   =   0.5879*f2     +   0.8089 e06
                lv06f2
v7   =   0.8114*f2     +   0.5845 e07
                lv07f2
v8   =   0.8015*f2     +   0.5980 e08
                lv08f2

v9   =   0.7917*f3     +   0.6109 e09
                lv09f3
v10  =   0.7123*f3     +   0.7019 e10
                lv10f3
v11  =   0.5419*f3     +   0.8404 e11
                lv11f3
v12  =   0.8455*f3     +   0.5340 e12
                lv12f3
```

FIGURE 5.22
Manifest variable equations with standardized estimates.

Variable	Parameter	Estimate	Standard Error	t Value
f1		1.00000		
f2		1.00000		
f3		1.00000		
e01	vare01	0.19699	0.01633	12.06
e02	vare02	0.35563	0.02878	12.36
e03	vare03	0.36203	0.03197	11.32
e04	vare04	0.45760	0.03090	14.81
e05	vare05	0.51755	0.03532	14.65
e06	vare06	0.69818	0.04834	14.44
e07	vare07	0.38384	0.03598	10.67
e08	vare08	0.51875	0.04709	11.02
e09	vare09	0.34880	0.02927	11.92
e10	vare10	0.73671	0.05471	13.46
e11	vare11	0.76976	0.05176	14.87
e12	vare12	0.34179	0.03409	10.03

FIGURE 5.23
Variances of exogenous variables.

```
Var1 Var2 Parameter Estimate

 f1   f2    cf1f2    0.72214
 f1   f3    cf1f3    0.73052
 f2   f3    cf2f3    0.80487
```

FIGURE 5.24
Correlations among exogenous variables.

```
    Data _items_9;
    Set  _items_;
    Keep v1-v9;
    Run;

Proc Calis COV data=_items_9 G4=1000 GCONV=1E-10 Method=ML ALL;

    LINEQS
       v1   = lv01f1 f1 + e01,
       v2   = lv02f1 f1 + e02,
       v3   = lv03f1 f1 + e03,
       v4   = lv04f1 f1 + e04,

       v5   = lv05f2 f2 + e05,
       v6   = lv06f2 f2 + e06,
       v7   = lv07f2 f2 + e07,
       v8   = lv08f2 f2 + e08
        ;

    STD
    f1=1, f2=1,
    v9=varv9,
    e01 =   vare01,
    e02 =   vare02,
    e03 =   vare03,
    e04 =   vare04,
    e05 =   vare05,
    e06 =   vare06,
    e07 =   vare07,
    e08 =   vare08
     ;

    COV
    f1  f2  =   cf1f2,
    f1  v9  =   cf1v9,
    f2  v9  =   cf2v9;
    Run;
```

FIGURE 5.25
Nonstandard confirmatory factor analysis model.

5.6 Real-Life Examples

5.6.1 Minnesota Nicotine Withdrawal Scale

Consider a version of the Minnesota Nicotine Withdrawal Scale (MNWS) for use in a smoking cessation trial. This version contains the following nine items: urge to smoke (Item 1); depressed mood (Item 2); irritability, frustration, or anger (Item 3); anxiety (Item 4); difficulty concentrating (Item 5); restlessness (Item 6); increased appetite (Item 7); difficulty going to sleep (Item 8); and difficulty staying asleep (Item 9). Each item is rated on a 0–4 ordinal response scale (0 = not at all, 1 = slight, 2 = moderate, 3 = quite a bit, and 4 = extreme). The objective was to identify the structure of this nine-item version of the MNWS and, in doing so, to refine and enhance its measurement properties of nicotine withdrawal symptoms.

EFA of the MNWS was conducted in a study (n = 626) across all available subjects at times when varying levels of withdrawal symptoms were expected (week 0 [baseline], week 2, week 4) (Cappelleri et al., 2005). This study was a phase 2, multicenter, randomized, double-blind, parallel-group, and placebo- and active-controlled study with a 7-week treatment phase (Nides et al., 2006). Subjects were randomized to one of three varenicline dose regimens (0.3 mg QD, 1.0 mg QD, or 1.0 mg BID); to the active control, sustained-release bupropion, 150 mg BID; or to a placebo. The baseline or initial survey of subjects (week 0, prequit) was 8 days before the target quit date (Week 1 + 1 day).

For the data on the MNWS questionnaire, the scree plot (Figure 5.26) depicted an abrupt break or discontinuity before eigenvalue 3, suggesting

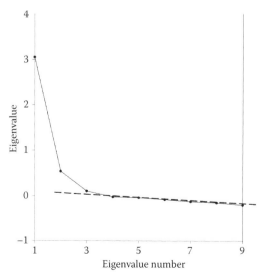

FIGURE 5.26
Scree plot using data at baseline on the MNWS.

```
Rotated Factor Pattern (Standardized Regression Coefficients)
(as produced by SAS)
Variable        Factor1            Factor2
Item 3          0.70973            0.00495
Item 4          0.70729            0.01137
Item 2          0.63702            0.08121
Item 5          0.61167            0.15788
Item 6          0.38553            0.38416
Item 1          0.12647           -0.05186
Item 8         -0.07937            0.73473
Item 9         -0.05459            0.69227
Item 7          0.09194            0.37309
```

FIGURE 5.27
Rotated factor pattern at baseline on the MNWS.

that only the first two factors were meaningful to be retained. An approximate straight line can be drawn from eigenvalue 3 to eigenvalue 9 throughout all points in between, but not from eigenvalue 1 or eigenvalue 2 to eigenvalue 9. The same pattern of eigenvalues was observed at week 2 and week 4.

Figure 5.27 represents the rotated factor pattern for data at baseline. Based on results at different time points (baseline, week 2, and week 4) the following two multi-item domains emerged: Negative Affect with four items (depressed mood; irritability, frustration, or anger; anxiety; difficulty concentrating) and Insomnia with two items (difficulty going to sleep, difficulty staying asleep). In addition, three single items (manifest variable: Urge to Smoke, Restlessness, Increased Appetite), each measuring a distinct element of withdrawal, completed the remaining part of the MNWS structure.

Consequently, a CFA using data from two phase 3 studies (Gonzales et al., 2006; Jorenby et al., 2006) confirmed the hypothesis that this MNWS scale should be structured as two multi-item domains and three manifest variables. Figure 5.28 represents the measurement model of MNWS, Table 5.1 represents its comparative fit indices, and Table 5.2 gives the standardized factor loadings for the two multi-domain domains. Values of the CFI exceeded 0.90 (Table 5.1), indicating that this model has acceptable fit to the data, and other goodness-of-fit statistics (not shown) were consistent with these findings. In addition to the fit indices, the standardized factor loadings of the individual items on their respective factors were acceptably high and consistent across measurement points (Table 5.2). In all instances, these (standardized) factor loadings were larger than 0.4, indicating that the items loaded solidly on their respective factors.

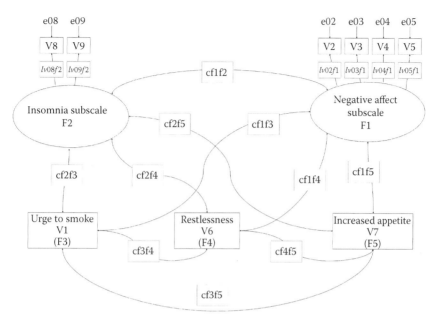

FIGURE 5.28
Hypothesized measurement model of Minnesota Nicotine Withdrawal Scale.

TABLE 5.1

Comparative Fit Indices for the Measurement Model
of the Minnesota Nicotine Withdrawal Scale

Week	Phase 3: Study 1	Phase 3: Study 2
	Comparative Fit Index	*Comparative Fit Index*
Baseline	0.97	0.98
Week 1	0.98	0.98
Week 4	0.98	0.99

In the simulated example in Section 5.5.2 and Figure 5.25, we showed how a nonstandard model with just one manifest variable should be implemented using the CALIS procedure. Let us expand upon that example. In Figure 5.29, we see that, with three manifest variables, the variance needs to be defined for all three of them (v1 = varf03, v6 = varf04, v7 = varf05). We also need to have all correlations among latent domains and manifest variables as part of the model (f1 f2 = cf1f2, f1 v1 = cf1f3, …, v1 v7 = cf3f5, v6 v7 = cf4f5).

5.6.2 Sexual Experience Questionnaire

The previous example illustrated one of the most used approaches in the development of scale construction. An EFA is used to form and quantify a hypothesis

TABLE 5.2

Standardized Factor Loadings for the Negative Affect and Insomnia Subscales
of the Minnesota Nicotine Withdrawal Scale

Study and Week	Factor Loadings for the Four Items of the Negative Affect Scale				Factor Loadings for the Two Items of the Insomnia Scale	
	Depressed Mood	Irritability, Frustration, or Anger	Anxiety	Difficulty Concentrating	Difficulty Going to Sleep	Difficulty Staying Asleep
Phase 3 Study 1						
Baseline	0.67	0.70	0.75	0.70	0.82	0.70
Week 1	0.59	0.79	0.81	0.70	0.86	0.78
Week 4	0.70	0.78	0.82	0.76	0.78	0.76
Phase 3 Study 2						
Baseline	0.65	0.72	0.74	0.68	0.87	0.76
Week 1	0.58	0.75	0.81	0.72	0.82	0.83
Week 4	0.74	0.78	0.85	0.72	0.86	0.79

of a scale's structure. This hypothesized structure is then tested using CFA using a new batch of data. The example now illustrated will showcase a different approach: if a strong initial conceptual framework (model) exists, then CFA can be used to develop a measurement model of a scale from the outset.

The absence of a single and brief measure that can assess functional, health-related quality of life, and satisfaction concepts prevents the rapid evaluation of the sexual experience in men. To address this unmet need, researchers sought to develop a new instrument—eventually called the Sexual Experience Questionnaire—to assess PROs regarding concepts that are most pertinent to men in connection with their sexual experience.

Much preparatory work was undertaken before the birth of the Sexual Experience Questionnaire. Contributions from an expert panel consisting of sexologists and urologists plus a systematic literature review of existing male sexual function instruments were used to identify seven key concepts of concern to men and to develop open-ended questions (Mulhall et al., 2008). These input streams were used to elicit qualitative information from 2 h focus groups and 1 h individual in-depth telephone interviews of sexually active men aged 35–69 years in Germany, Spain, the United Kingdom, and the United States. The moderators/interviewers were all native speakers and residents of their respective countries and were trained by the core research group, and the focus groups and interviews were recorded.

After review of the results, the expert panel proposed a qualitative approach using three domains, including a focus on partners, to define the sexual experience. Further input was elicited from a group of 10 physicians in clinical practice to develop the initial conceptual framework of the draft questionnaire and the pool of items.

```
Proc Calis COV data=_tmp_cfa_1 GCONV=1E-10 Method=ML All;

LINEQS
/* Domain #1 - "Negative Affect Subscale" */
v2 = lv02f1 f1 + e02,
v3 = lv03f1 f1 + e03,
v4 = lv04f1 f1 + e04,
v5 = lv05f1 f1 + e05,

/* Domain #2 - "Insomnia Subscale" */
v8  = lv08f2 f2 + e08,
v9  = lv09f2 f2 + e09;

STD
f1=1, f2=1,

v1=varf03,
v6=varf04,
v7=varf05,

e02 =    vare02,
e03 =    vare03,
e04 =    vare04,
e05 =    vare05,

e08 =    vare08,
e09 =    vare09;

COV
f1   f2  =    cf1f2,
f1   v1  =    cf1f3,
f1   v6  =    cf1f4,
f1   v7  =    cf1f5,

f2   v1  =    cf2f3,
f2   v6  =    cf2f4,
f2   v7  =    cf2f5,

v1   v6  =    cf3f4,
v1   v7  =    cf3f5,

v6   v7  =    cf4f5
;
Run;
```

FIGURE 5.29

Nonstandard confirmatory factor analysis model for Minnesota Nicotine Withdrawal Scale.

Based on this initial conceptual framework, preliminary elements of the Sexual Experience Questionnaire were considered that consisted of 15 items and 3 domains labeled Erection, Relationship, and Satisfaction (see Figure 5.30) (Mulhall et al., 2008). Two datasets were used for the development of the measurement model: (1) a clinical trial data on a sample of men enrolled in a double-blind, placebo-controlled trial of flexible-dose

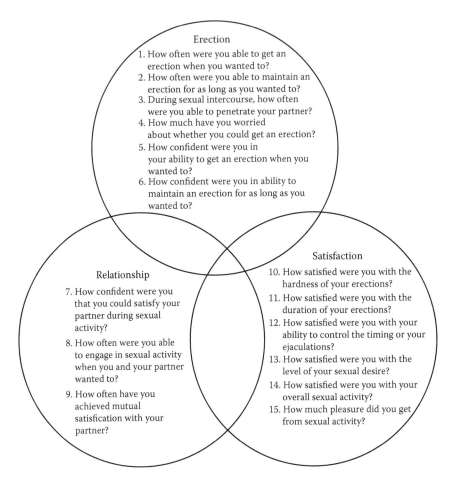

FIGURE 5.30
Initial conceptual framework of the Sexual Experience Questionnaire.

sildenafil citrate who thereafter became part of an open-label study with sildenafil and (2) a survey dataset on multiple samples of men who were to complete the draft questionnaire a single time as part of a consumer health survey on the Internet.

CFA was used to determine the factor structure in the context of the over-lapping three-factor conceptual model. This CFA methodology provides a relatively simple and straightforward algorithm to take the 15-item draft questionnaire structured as a three-factor conceptual model to a final model that satisfactorily fitted the data. Bentler's CFI was used to help determine fit (for the final model the CFI had to be >0.9 in order to be deemed acceptable; Hatcher, 1994).

In a stepwise iteration process, deletion or reassignment (or both) of individual items and factor paths (factor to item) was tested for improvement in model fit, targeting those items and paths with the largest Lagrange multiplier at each step. The Lagrange multiplier estimates the extent to which the model chi-square statistic would decrease (e.g., improve) if a given parameter were freed (e.g., if a given path were added to the model). If the deletion or reassignment of an item improved fit but weakened the other items or resulted in paths that were not statistically significant, the deletion or reassignment of the item was not incorporated into the model. A weak item was defined as having a standardized loading less than 0.4 or not being statistically significant. The clinical trial dataset at screening was used for development of the measurement model. The final measurement model was tested in both datasets (clinical trial and survey).

This preceding set of procedures reduced the number of items to 12, with some items reassigned to different domains than originally planned based on the qualitative research. As a result, names of the domains were also redefined (relative to the initial structure): Domain 1—Erection, Domain 2—Individual Satisfaction, and Domain 3—Couple Satisfaction.

The fit of the revised three-factor, 12-item model—which became the Sexual Experience Questionnaire—was confirmed by testing the clinical trial dataset at baseline (with 213 men who were first screened and subsequently enrolled in the trial; CFI = 0.91), at the interim stage in the double-blind, placebo-controlled trial (week 6; sample size, $n = 194$ men; CFI = 0.94), at the end-of-treatment part of the double-blind, placebo-controlled trial (week 10, $n = 177$ men; CFI = 0.93), and at the end-of-study assessment, which occurred at the end of the open-label phase (week 16, $n = 177$ men; CFI = 0.94), as well as in the survey dataset ($n = 904$ men, CFI = 0.95).

5.6.3 Power of Food Scale

This example combines all earlier discussed methods from EFA, including parallel analysis, to CFA. The example also introduces and highlights a second-order factor as the next level of generalization of latent factors in CFA.

The PFS was developed to assess the psychological impact of living in food-abundant environments, as reflected in feelings of being controlled by food, independent of food consumption itself (Cappelleri et al., 2009). The 21 items on the PFS were designed to reflect responsiveness to the food environment involving three levels of food proximity: (1) food readily available in the environment but not physically present, (2) food present but not tasted, and (3) food when first tasted but not consumed. Every item was measured on the following five-category scale: I do not agree (1), I agree a little (2), I agree somewhat (3), I agree quite a bit (4), and I strongly agree (5).

Data from obese adults in a clinical trial for a weight management drug ($n = 1741$) were used in EFAs to form a hypothesis about the structure of the scale. Data from overweight, obese, and normal weight adults, which came from a web-based survey ($n = 1275$), were used to perform a CFA.

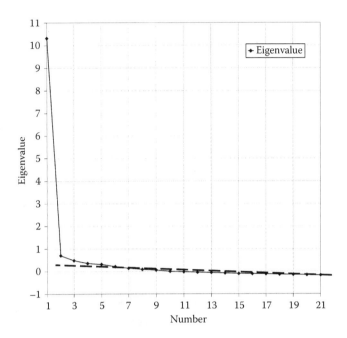

FIGURE 5.31
Scree plot using data from obese adults in a clinical trial.

While executing EFA, the researchers found that the initial analysis of the scree plot (Figure 5.31) indicated that probably only one factor should be considered. However, an attempt to fit the model in a CFA with just one latent factor for all 21 items (using the same dataset) failed; CFI was less than 0.9. This result motivated the researchers to consider parallel analysis in order to define the number of factors beyond chance. Based on the results of this analysis (Figure 5.32), it was concluded that at least eight eigenvalues were larger than the 95th percentile from random calculations (meaning that it is possible that there could be as many as eight factors in the model).

To resolve this issue the researchers decided to continually extract solutions (one-factor, two-factor, three-factor, and so on) using EFA and then immediately test these solutions using CFA. In addition to CFI, two indices were used to compare models: the Parsimonious Normed Fit Index (PNFI) (Cattell, 1966) and the Expected Cross Validation Index (ECVI) (Schumacker and Lomax, 2004). The PNFI simultaneously reflects both the fit and the parsimony of the model; the model with the largest PNFI is the most parsimonious one. The ECVI gauges the applicability or generalizability of results; the model with the smallest ECVI value is considered to be the most stable in the same population.

CFIs for one- and two-factor models were less than 0.90, indicating that these models did not adequately fit the data. CFIs for the three-, four-, and five-factor solutions were more than 0.90; therefore, these models fit the data (Table 5.3). Extracting a solution beyond five factors did not produce a new structure

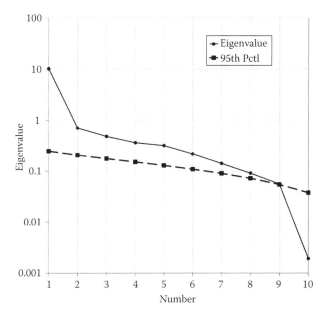

FIGURE 5.32
Original scree plot overlaid with results of the parallel analysis (showing only first 10 eigenvalues, with vertical axis on a logarithmic scale).

TABLE 5.3

Fit Indices of Confirmatory Factor Analysis Models
in the Power of Food Scale

Model	Comparative Fit Index	Parsimonious Normed Fit Index	Expected Cross Validation Index
Three factor	0.92	0.79	1.04
Four factor	0.93	0.77	0.81
Five factor	0.94	0.78	0.82

compared with the five-factor model. In this example, EFA and CFA were used sequentially to enlist (EFA) and confirm (CFA) the most plausible factor structures that resonant most with the empirical data.

From the three-, four-, and five-factor models, the three-factor model (with three weak items removed resulting in an 18-item model) was selected to represent the PFS measurement model as the most parsimonious solution (based on PNFI). This three-factor model with 18 items, though, also gave the largest ECVI. These findings indicate that, although this model was the most parsimonious one, it could be less generalizable than the four- and five-factor models. Additional calculations were performed to refine the three-factor model and achieve better generalizability and fit of the model. On the basis of obtaining a CFI and ECVI better

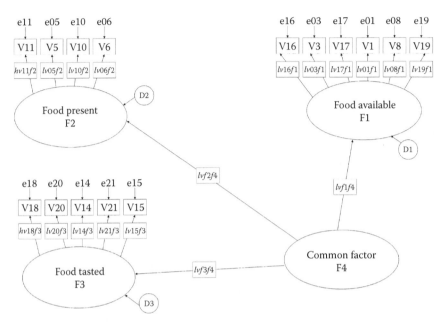

FIGURE 5.33
Second-order confirmatory factor analysis model with one second-order (common) factor and three single-order factors.

than those obtained for the existing three-, four-, and five-factor models, a three-factor model containing 15 items emerged.

For the 15-item questionnaire, the relatively high correlations among the three factors (factors 1 and 2: 0.73; factors 1 and 3: 0.72; factors 2 and 3: 0.69) suggested that a three-factor, second-order model is a well-suited and appropriate model. Figure 5.33 represents a second-order factor model with 15 final items that includes three first-order latent variables and one second-order factor, which represents the general and common concept of power of food that encompasses the more specific concepts defined in the three first-order factors (the second-order can be viewed as the *parent* and its first-order factors as the *children*). The CFI for this model was 0.95. All of the model's standardized path coefficients, including those from the aggregated factor, were statistically significant and exceeded 0.4. This second-order model also provided a good fit to the data from the web-based survey.

Figure 5.34 represents the implementation of the second-order model using the CALIS procedure. Comparing this implementation with previous examples, we can note that there are no correlations between the first-order latent factors, because now the second-order latent common factor affects all three first-order latent factors and *absorbs* their correlations. Earlier it was noted that the structural part of the standard first-order CFA is represented

```
Proc Calis COV data=_tmp_2 GCONV=1E-10 All;
LINEQS
  v1   = lv01f1 f1 + e01,
  v3   = lv03f1 f1 + e03,
  v8   = lv08f1 f1 + e08,
  v16  = lv16f1 f1 + e16,
  v17  = lv17f1 f1 + e17,
  v19  = lv19f1 f1 + e19,

  v5   = lv05f2 f2 + e05,
  v6   = lv06f2 f2 + e06,
  v10  = lv10f2 f2 + e10,
  v11  = lv11f2 f2 + e11,

  v14  = lv14f3 f3 + e14,
  v15  = lv15f3 f3 + e15,
  v18  = lv18f3 f3 + e18,
  v20  = lv20f3 f3 + e20,
  v21  = lv21f3 f3 + e21,
f1   = lvf1f4 f4 + d1,
f2   = lvf2f4 f4 + d2,
f3   = lvf3f4 f4 + d3
 ;
STD
f4=1,
d1=1,
d2=1,
d3=1,
 e01 =    vare01  ,
 e03 =    vare03  ,
 e05 =    vare05  ,
 e06 =    vare06  ,
 e08 =    vare08  ,
 e10 =    vare10  ,
 e11 =    vare11  ,
 e14 =    vare14  ,
 e15 =    vare15  ,
 e16 =    vare16  ,
 e17 =    vare17  ,
 e18 =    vare18  ,
 e19 =    vare19  ,
 e20 =    vare20  ,
 e21 =    vare21
 ;
Bounds
 vare01 >=0. ,
 vare03 >=0. ,
```

FIGURE 5.34
Implementation of the second-order model.

(*continued*)

```
        vare05  >=0. ,
        vare06  >=0. ,
        vare08  >=0. ,
        vare10  >=0. ,
        vare11  >=0. ,
        vare14  >=0. ,
        vare15  >=0. ,
        vare16  >=0. ,
        vare17  >=0. ,
        vare18  >=0. ,
        vare19  >=0. ,
        vare20  >=0. ,
        vare21  >=0.
     ;

   Run;
```

FIGURE 5.34 (continued)
Implementation of the second-order model.

by covariances between latent variables. In the second-order CFA model, the relationship between the first-order latent factors and the second-order latent common factor should be depicted in the same way as the relationship between the observed items and the first-order latent factors. Thus, in Figure 5.34, the last three equations in the LINEQS part (f1 = lvf1f4 f4 + d1, f2 = lvf2f4 f4 + d2, f3 = lvf3f4 f4 + d3) describe the structural part. Note that three additional disturbance terms (D1, D2, and D3) are introduced and there are no covariances in this model.

5.7 Summary

This chapter covers EFA and CFA for items on a scale that are effect indicators, homogeneous items that are influenced by the construct of interest. In general, factor analysis does not apply to causal indicators, heterogeneous items on an index that cause the construct and bear no intrinsic relationship among themselves with respect to the construct. EFA is discussed in terms of its role, model, number of factors, sample size, and assumptions.

Contrasted with EFA, CFA is described in terms of its measurement model, along with model types and depiction. Also described is identification of residual terms and estimated parameters in the model, along with assessment of model fit. Simulated examples using SAS on EFA and CFA are provided in order to delve deeper into both methodologies and to enrich the reader's understanding of the concepts (even for readers with not much exposure to SAS). These simulations are grounded in, and motivated by, real-life experiences and the material in the chapter. Finally, applications from the published literature on three questionnaires (Minnesota Nicotine Withdrawal Scale, Sexual Experience Questionnaire, and Power of Food Scale) are provided to illustrate key aspects and practical implementations of EFA and CFA.

References

Bollen, K.A. 1989. *Structural Equations with Latent Variables*. New York, NY: John Wiley & Sons Ltd.

Brown, T.A. 2006. *Confirmatory Factor Analysis for Applied Research*. New York, NY: The Guilford Press.

Cappelleri, J.C., Bushmakin, A.G., Baker, C.L., Merikle, E., Olufade, A.O., and D.G. Gilbert. 2005. Revealing the multidimensional framework of the Minnesota nicotine withdrawal scale. *Current Medical Research and Opinion* 21:749–760.

Cappelleri, J.C., Bushmakin, A.G., Gerber, R.A., Kline Leidy, N., Sexton, C.C., Karlsson, J., and M.R. Lowe. 2009. Evaluating the Power of Food Scale in obese subjects and a general sample of individuals: Development and measurement properties. *International Journal of Obesity* 33:913–922.

Cappelleri, J.C. and R.A. Gerber. 2010. Exploratory factor analysis. In: Chow, S.-C. (editor). *Encyclopedia of Biopharmaceutical Statistics*, 3rd edition, Revised and Expanded. New York, NY: Informa Healthcare, pp. 480–485.

Cattell, R.B. 1966. The scree test for the number of factors. *Multivariate Behavioral Research* 1:245–276.

Fayers, F.M. and D. Machin. 2007. *Quality of Life: The Assessment, Analysis and Interpretation of Patient-Reported Outcomes*, 2nd edition. Chichester, England: John Wiley & Sons Ltd.

Gonzales, D., Rennard, S.I., Nides, M., Oncken, C., Azoulay, S., Billing, C.B., Watsky, E.J., Gong, J., Williams, K.E., and K.R. Reeves. 2006. Varenicline, an alpha4beta2 nicotinic acetylcholine receptor partial agonist, vs sustained-release bupropion and placebo for smoking cessation: A randomized controlled trial. *JAMA* 296:47–55.

Hatcher, L. 1994. *A Step-by-Step Approach to Using the SAS® System for Factor Analysis and Structural Equation Modeling*. Cary, NC: SAS Institute Inc.

Hayton, J.C., Allen, D.G., and V. Scarpello. 2004. Factor retention decisions in exploratory factor analysis: A tutorial on parallel analysis. *Organizational Research Methods* 7:19.

Jorenby, D.E., Hays, J.T., Rigotti, N.A., Azoulay, S., Watsky, E.J., Williams, K.E., Billing, C.B., Gong, J., and K.R. Reeves. 2006. Efficacy of varenicline, an alpha-4beta2 nicotinic acetylcholine receptor partial agonist, vs placebo or sustained-release bupropion for smoking cessation: A randomized controlled trial. *JAMA* 296:56–63.

Kaplan, D. 2000. *Structural Equation Modeling: Foundations and Extensions*. Thousand Oaks, CA: Sage Publications.

Kline, R. 2010. *Principles and Practice of Structural Equation Modeling*, 3rd edition. New York, NY: The Guilford Press.

Mulhall, J.P., King, R., Kirby, M., Hvidsten, K., Symonds, T., Bushmakin, A.G., and J.C. Cappelleri. 2008. Evaluating the sexual experience in men: Validation of the Sexual Experience Questionnaire. *Journal of Sexual Medicine* 5:365–376.

Nides, M., Onchen, C., Gonzales, D., Rennard, S., Watsky, E.J., Anziano, R., and K.R. Reeves, for the Varenicline Study Group. 2006. Smoking cessation with varenicline, a selective 42 nicotine receptor partial agonist: Results from a 7-week, randomized, placebo-and bupropion-controlled trial with 1-year follow-up. *Archives of Internal Medicine* 166:1561–1568.

O'Connor, B.P. 2000. SPSS and SAS programs for determining the number of components using parallel analysis and Velicer's MAP test. *Behavior Research Methods, Instruments, & Computers* 32:396–402.

Pett, M.A., Lackey, N.R., and J.J. Sullivan. 2003. *Making Sense of Factor Analysis: The Use of Factor Analysis for Instrument Development in Health Care Research*. Thousand Oaks, CA: Sage Publications.

SAS Institute Inc. 2011. *SAS/STAT® 9.3 User's Guide*, 2nd edition. Cary, NC: SAS Institute Inc.

SAS Institute Inc. 2012. *Base SAS® 9.3 Procedure Guide*, 2nd edition. Cary, NC: SAS Institute Inc.

Schumacker, R.E. and R.G. Lomax. 2004. *A Beginner's Guide to Structural Equation Modeling*, 2nd edition. Mahwah, NJ: Lawrence Erlbaum.

Steiger, J.H. 1999. *EzPATH: Causal Modeling*. Evanston, IL: SYSTAT Inc.

Streiner, D.L. and G.R. Norman. 2008. *Health Measurement Scales: A Practical Guide to Their Development and Use*, 4th edition. New York, NY: Oxford University Press.

6

Item Response Theory

The analytic aspects of the previous chapters have implicitly relied on classical test theory (CTT) to evaluate the properties of a patient-reported outcome (PRO), especially when multiple items are intended to measure the same underlying concept. Alternative terms for the concept being measured include construct, attribute, trait, or ability. The most apt descriptor depends on what is being measured (e.g., trait or ability). In this chapter, the term *attribute* is used generally to describe the construct or latent characteristic that is being measured. CTT underpins the embodiment of traditional psychometric theory used to assess and improve the measurement properties of a scale. Having dominated the fields of health, psychological and educational measurement for nearly a century, CTT has made assumptions about measurement scales and their constituent items that are expected to be considered appropriate in most situations.

Over the last few decades, psychometricians have advanced another measurement model, one based on item response theory (IRT). IRT is a statistical theory consisting of mathematical models expressing the probability of a particular response to a scale item as a function of the (latent or unobserved) attribute of the person and of certain parameters or characteristics of the item. Rather than replacing CTT methodology, IRT methodology can be more constructively viewed as an important complement to CTT for scale development, evaluation, and refinement in certain circumstances. IRT assumes that patients at a particular level of an underlying attribute (e.g., with a particular level of physical functioning) will have a certain probability of responding positively to each question. This probability will depend, in part, on the difficulty of the particular item. For example, many patients with cancer might respond *Yes* to easy questions such as "Do you dress yourself?", but only patients with a high level of physical functioning are likely to reply *Yes* to the more difficult question "Do you engage in vigorous activities such as running, lifting heavy objects, or participating in strenuous sports?"

As with factor analyses and most other traditional psychometric paradigms, IRT may not be suited for certain symptoms and side effects whose interitem correlations do not arise as a consequence of a latent attribute that a scale was designed to measure. Instead, their interitem correlations (e.g., in a symptom cluster) arise solely through external considerations such as a consequence of treatment or disease; such correlations do not arise through items having a shared, inherent representation of a conceptually meaningful unidimensional attribute. Thus, if a patient does have severe nausea, this patient may or may not have severe diarrhea, vomiting, and other symptoms. Correlations may depend on the study population as well as the disease and treatment. A patient with poor symptomology does not necessarily imply that this patient is experiencing diarrhea or vomiting. Indeed, poor sympto-mology can be one symptom alone, such as severe nausea. In these types of situations, IRT (and factor analysis) should not be used.

This chapter revisits CTT, highlights several elements and fundamen-tal concepts of IRT methodology, motivates the rationale for using the IRT framework, and covers some relevant models of IRT. The chapter also pro-vides published and simulated examples intended to enrich the understand-ing of IRT methodology. Many additional resources, which can be used to complement and supplement this chapter, are available on IRT in general and in relation to PROs (Hambleton et al., 1991; Fischer and Molenaar, 1995; van der Linden and Hambleton, 1997; Embretson and Reise, 2000; Hays et al., 2000; Reeve, 2003; Baker and Kim, 2004; De Boeck and Wilson, 2004; Chang and Reeve, 2005; Reeve and Fayers, 2005; Wilson, 2005; Bond and Fox, 2007; Streiner and Norman, 2008; de Ayala, 2009; DeMars, 2010; Fayers and Machin, 2007; Massof, in press).

6.1 Classical Test Theory Revisited

6.1.1 Assumptions

CTT assumes that each person has a true score on a concept of interest that would be obtained if there were no errors in measurement (Crocker and Algina, 1986; Nunnally and Bernstein, 1994; Kline, 2005). A person's true score may be defined as the expected score over a hypothetically infinite number of independent administrations of the PRO measure. A person's true score is not observed, but inferences are made from an observed score. It is typically assumed that random errors are normally distributed and that the expected value of the error (i.e., mean of the distribution of errors over an infinite number of trials) is zero. In addition, those random errors are assumed to be uncorrelated with each other and with the true score. Practical solutions to some difficult measurement problems have been worked out within the CTT framework (Fan, 1998).

Advantages of CTT are its relatively weak assumptions (i.e., they are likely to be met or approximately met with most real data), well-known properties, and long track record. While CTT has centered on the overall test or scale score, item statistics (i.e., item difficulty and item discrimination) are a quite important, useful (and even underrated) aspect of CTT in scale develop-ment and validation (Crocker and Algina, 1986; Kline, 2005). The mean and standard deviations of items can provide clues about which items are useful and which ones are not. Generally, the higher the variability of the item and the closer its responses distribute evenly around the middle of the item's response options, the better the item will perform. Descriptive statistics at the item level, as well as at the scale level, can be valuable during not only later phases of psychometric testing but also earlier stages of scale development, including the content validity stage, where sample sizes are expected to be modest.

6.1.2 Item Difficulty, Discrimination, and Weighting

In the special case of dichotomous items, the proportion of respondents in a sample who endorse or respond to an item is equivalent to the mean item score. If a positive response to each item reflects an endorsement of a desirable indicator on the attribute or construct of interest (e.g., the ability to run or walk as indicators of the construct of physical functioning), an item with a lower proportion of endorsement suggests that it is more difficult to achieve than an item with a higher proportion. Items that have proportions of 0 or 1 are useless because they do not differentiate between individuals. In general, items with proportions of 0.50—that is, 50% of the group endorses the item—provide the highest levels of differentiation between individuals in a group. When response categories are ordinal rather than binary, they can be made so by appropriately collapsing adjacent categories (or left as stand-alone categories, depending on the objectives of the analysis).

The more the item discriminates among individuals with different amounts of the underlying concept of interest, the higher the item's discrimination index. The extreme group method can be used to calculate the discrimination index using three steps. Step 1 is to partition those who have the highest and lowest overall scores, aggregated across all items, into upper and lower groups. The upper group can be composed of the top $x\%$ who are the best performers (those with the most favorable overall PRO scores, say, those in the top 25th percentile); the lower group can be composed of the bottom $x\%$ who are the poorest performers (those with the least favorable PRO scores, say, those in the bottom 25th percentile). Step 2 is to examine each item and determine the proportion of individual respondents in the sample who endorse or respond to each item in the upper group and lower group. Step 3 is to subtract this pair of proportions from those two groups. The higher an item's discrimination index, the more the item will distinguish between individuals.

Another indicator of item discrimination is the corrected item-to-total correlation—how well an item correlates with the sum of the remaining items on the same scale or domain (*corrected* because the sum does not include that item). It is best to have moderate-to-high (corrected) item-to-total correlations (say, at least 0.40). Items with low correlations indicate that they do not correlate, or *go with*, the rest of the items in the dataset.

An item characteristic curve (ICC) can be produced by plotting the percentage of people choosing each response option (or each group of response options if adjacent categories are combined) on the vertical axis by the total score on the horizontal axis that can be expressed as percentiles (10th percentile, 20th percentile, and so on through the 100th percentile). A good response category displays a sigmoid or S-shaped curve, with the probability of endorsing an item increasing monotonically with increasing total score or amounts of the attribute (illustrations of such curves are given later in Figures 6.1 through 6.3). A particular category should also be centered or located as hypothesized relative to the other categories with respect to the total score or attribute.

Differential item weighting occurs when items are given more weight or less weight when being combined into a total score. This is in contrast to unit weighting items, where each item has a weight of 1.0 (i.e., effectively contributing equally to the total score). Different techniques are available to assign different weights to items. Three of them are mentioned here. One way is to estimate the test–retest reliability of each item and then assign the reliabilities as weights to their respective items. Another way is to run a factor analysis and use the factor loadings to assign weights to the items. A third way is to use the corrected item-to-total correlation coefficients to weight the items.

Unit (equal) weighting of items is generally preferred over differential weighting. Measures that assess a single concept will have items that are substantially intercorrelated. As a result, weights assigned to one item over

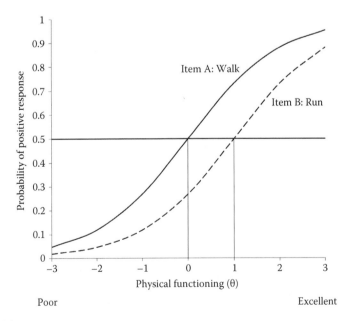

FIGURE 6.1
Item characteristic curves for two items of differing difficulty.

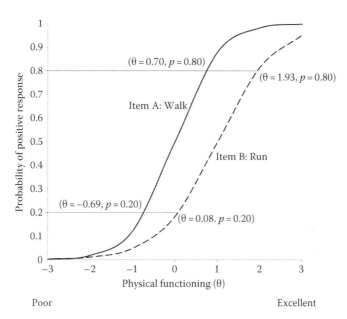

FIGURE 6.2
Item characteristic curves for two items of differing discrimination and difficulty.

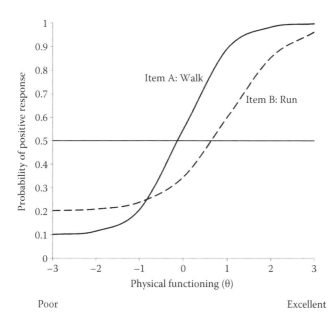

FIGURE 6.3
Item characteristic curves for two items of differing intercepts, difficulty, and discrimination.

another are likely to be relatively small and nonconsequential. That is, the correlation between differentially weighted and unit-weighted scores is expected to be high.

Items can be averaged together or summed to produce total scores. In addition, the raw score can be linearly transformed to a standardized Z score, computed as the difference between the individual's raw score and the mean of the chosen referent group, and then this difference is divided by the standard deviation of the referent group (so that the mean is 0 and standard deviation is 1 for the referent group). This difference would reflect the level of a person's attribute relative to other persons.

6.1.3 CTT and IRT

Certain aspects of CTT, such as item difficulty and discrimination, have their analogues in IRT, which will be the sole focus of subsequent sections in this chapter. While these two measurement paradigms have been perceived as being theoretically very different, documented research indicates that person and item statistics derived from the two measurement frameworks are quite comparable (Fan, 1998; Macdonald and Paunonen, 2002). Advocates of IRT highlight its distinctiveness with respect to sample independence, that the properties of the scale are separate and independent from the attributes of the people responding to it; differential item impact, that items can have varying influences on what is being measured; heterogeneity of errors in measurement, that more item information implies smaller errors of measurement and more precision (information) for patients in the middle range of scores and less precision for patients with more extreme scores; and equating scales, that scales with a different number or difficulty of items can be linked by responses to a common set of anchor items (Embretson and Reise, 2000).

6.2 Assumptions of IRT

Assumptions underlying the use of IRT models are more stringent that those required of CTT. IRT models also tend to be more complex, and the outputs are more difficult to understand, particularly for nontechnically oriented readers. IRT relies on three major assumptions, which need to be met: unidimensionality, local independence, and model fit.

6.2.1 Unidimensionality

The assumption of unidimensionality requires that a scale consists of items that tap into only one dimension. A person's level on this single continuous latent variable is what is taken to give rise to responses to the scale's questions.

The most common way of testing for unidimensionality is through exploratory factor analysis, including use of a scree plot, designed to evaluate the factor structure underlying the observed covariation among item responses. If the scale is unidimensional, then all of the items should be highly correlated with (or load on) the first factor (see Chapter 5 for a description of exploratory factor analysis).

If unidimensionality cannot be supported, one recommendation is to divide the scale into subscales based on both knowledge of the subject matter and a factor structure emanating from the factor analysis. Another recommendation is that, as long as these subscales or subdomains are sufficiently correlated with each other, the scale as a whole may still be considered unidimensional as when, for instance, the scale is a second-order factor and the subscales are first-order factors. Unidimensionality is not necessarily an all-or-nothing phenomenon; some judgment may be needed in order to determine whether a scale is unidimensional enough.

6.2.2 Local Independence

Local independence means that, once we remove the influence of the underlying attribute or factor being measured (i.e., the first factor in a factor analysis), there should be no association among the responses from any pair of items. In other words, for a subsample of individuals who have the same level on the attribute (which is one way to remove or control for the effect of the attribute), there should be no correlation among the items. Items are assumed to be correlated only because they are all affected, to varying degrees, by the latent attribute (factor); once the effect of the attribute is removed, the items should be uncorrelated. This rationale is another way of defining a strong first factor, so local independence and unidimensionality can be viewed as two different ways of saying the same thing.

If the item responses are not locally independent under a unidimensional model, another dimension must be causing the dependence. In this case, the scale is not unidimensional and is instead tapping two or more attributes, which can be revealed by a factor analysis. Redundant items can also lead to local dependence (lack of local independence) as when two items ask the same question in two different ways and share a very high correlation (say, above 0.80). Local dependence can also be caused by items that are linked, so that there is a carryover in answers from one item to the next. If, for example, two math problems are part of the measurement of cognitive ability, a person good in math may get both questions correct and a person not good in math may get both questions wrong. These highly correlated math problems may be measuring mathematics ability as a distinct attribute above and beyond that of cognitive ability.

A simple test, called Q_3, has been proposed to check pairs of items for local dependence (Yen, 1993; DeMars, 2010). An IRT model is fit to provide item parameter estimates and a residual (the difference between the observed value based on the actual data and the predicted value based on the model estimate) is calculated for each person's response to each item. After the calculation of the residuals, Q_3 is computed as the correlation between the residuals from one item and the residuals from another item. The correlation matrix of residuals is then examined to find pairs of items with *large enough* correlations between residuals. Correlations greater than 0.20 are suggestive of local dependence (Yen, 1993; DeMars, 2010).

6.2.3 Model Fit

The third assumption, which is not unique to IRT models, is correct model specification. Assessing fit in IRT models is performed at both the item level and the person level. The fit between the model and the data can be assessed to check for model misspecification. The goal of IRT modeling is to estimate a set of items and person parameters that reproduce the observed item responses as closely as possible. Graphical and empirical approaches are available for evaluating item fit, person fit, and overall model fit (van der Linden and Hambleton, 1997; Embretson and Reise, 2000; Baker and Kim, 2004; Bond and Fox, 2007; de Ayala, 2009; DeMars, 2010). These approaches are based on the concept of a residual: the difference between an observed response and a model-based response. Overall model fit might seem to be a reasonable consideration. While indices of overall model fit have been proposed to compare models, none of these indices has achieved widespread use and acceptance (DeMars, 2010). Instead, models are often selected based on the content and purpose of the instrument.

6.3 Item Characteristic Curves

As noted previously, IRT is a statistical theory consisting of mathematical models expressing the probability of a particular response to a scale item as a function of the true (but unknown) attribute of the person and of certain characteristics of the item. The mathematical description for the item response is often abbreviated as ICC (not to be mistaken for the intraclass correlation coefficient described in Chapter 4). An ICC is the fundamental unit in IRT and can be understood as the probability of endorsing an item (for a binary response) or responding to a particular category of an item (for a polytomous response) for individuals with a given level of the attribute.

Depending on the IRT model used, these curves can tell which items (or questions) are harder or more difficult and which items are better discriminators of the attribute. For example, if the attribute is mental health, the typical person would need better mental health to respond favorably in overcoming a harder or more difficult item. If an item is a

good discriminator of mental health, the proportion of people responding to this item would increase noticeably as the level of mental health
increases. The various IRT models (to be explained shortly in this section), which are variations of logistic models, are simply different mathematical functions for describing the ICCs as the relationship between
a person's level of an attribute and the probability of a specific response
on an item measuring that attribute.

6.3.1 Dichotomous Response Models

An ICC is based on the type of IRT model. Dichotomous models involve items
with two response options (e.g., yes/no, true/false). If a person endorses an
item, it is considered a positive response in agreeing with the content of the
question. The three most common IRT models for a dichotomous (binary)
response are the one-, two-, and three-parameter logistic models whose names
are associated with the number of item parameters that characterize an item's
functioning and hence need to be estimated (Table 6.1). These three models all
have an item difficulty parameter (b) and a latent attribute parameter (θ).

Difficulty is a suitable word for describing the ability to perform physical
functions, although it may be intuitively less clear for describing other aspects
of health status. *Difficulty* simply means that, for a given value of the latent
attribute θ, fewer patients are expected to answer positively (more favorably)
to a question related to a more advanced symptom or more demanding task
or endeavor. The latent person parameter θ is not a constant but a random
variable that varies from patient to patient. It should technically have a subscript to refer to a given patient but that subscript is omitted here to simplify
the notation. This parameter is merely a measure that quantifies the underlying characteristic of the attribute (construct) being measured for each individual. The parameter can represent an individual's underlying proficiency,
ability, trait, attribute, or disposition. Again, the most apt term depends on
the context.

TABLE 6.1

Dichotomous Item Response Models

Model	Mathematical Form	Item Parameter
One-parameter logistic	$P_{ij}(\theta_j) = \dfrac{1}{1+e^{-(\theta_j-b_i)}}$	Difficulty (b)
Two-parameter logistic	$P_{ij}(\theta_j) = \dfrac{1}{1+e^{-a_i(\theta_j-b_i)}}$	Difficulty (b), discrimination (a)
Three-parameter logistic	$P_{ij}(\theta_j) = c+(1-c)\left[\dfrac{1}{1+e^{-a_i(\theta_j-b_i)}}\right]$	Difficulty (b), discrimination (a), guessing (c)

Note: e is the mathematical constant and approximately equals 2.71828; i represents the
ith item; and j represents the jth subject.

The metric of the person and item parameters is somewhat arbitrary. The estimate mean of the respondent parameter θ, for instance, may be set to 0 (alternatively, the estimate mean of the item difficulty parameter b may be set to 0). Theoretically, θ can extend from positive to negative infinity. In practice, most values are between −3 and 3. The parameter θ is measured in log-odds units (called logits), which relates the level of the attribute to the probability of responding positively to an item (or to an item category).

As later formalized in Chapter 7 (cross-sectional analysis), the log odds is the natural log of the odds, with the odds being the probability of occurrence divided by the probability of no occurrence (Kleinbaum and Klein, 2010; Hosmer et al., 2013). In IRT models, the odds of responding positively to an item (or to an item category) are the probability of responding positively divided by the probability of not responding positively. Equations in IRT models look similar to equations in logistic regression models, except that in IRT models the log odds is expressed as a function of a predictor that is a latent variable (θ) that must be estimated (along with item characteristics like item difficulty) rather than an observable quantity (such as the number correct) (Hambleton et al., 1991; Embretson and Reise, 2000).

In IRT models, logits often get translated into a different unit before being communicated to stakeholders. Any linear transformation on θ preserves its probabilistic interpretation. Some researchers prefer to deal with mainly positive numbers. Hence, one possible translation of θ is to calibrate it to have a new mean of 100 and a new standard deviation of 10, which would keep most (if not all or almost all) values positive.

Item difficulty, or b parameter, is on the same metric as θ. Both parameters are measured on an interval scale. Like θ, item difficulty values have a theoretical range from negative to positive infinity. They tend in practice to be between −2 and 2, so that the items typically are not too easy or too difficult for the intended population. One of the distinguished features of IRT is that the difficulty parameter b, which reflects a property of an item, is expressed on the same scale as θ, which reflects the property of an individual. As Table 6.1 indicates, the difference between the respondent parameter and item difficulty parameter helps to determine the probability of responding positively to an item.

Consider the one-parameter logistic model, also known as the Rasch model, which requires only the single parameter b_i to describe an item i (Table 6.1, top panel). The probability of a positive response by a particular patient j to item i $[P_{ij}(\theta_j)]$ is a function of the difference between the amount of the patient's latent attribute θ_j and the item's difficulty b_i. The difficulty parameter (b_i) in relation to the attribute parameter (θ_j) indicates the extent of a positive response to a particular item.

For the Rasch model, the natural logarithm of the odds (i.e., a log odds or logit) is modeled by the simple difference between a person's attribute score, θ_j, and the difficulty for the *i*th item, b_i. That is, the ratio of the probability of a positive response for a person to the probability of a negative response is modeled as follows:

$$\ln\left[\frac{P_{ij}(\theta_j)}{1-P_{ij}(\theta_j)}\right] = (\theta_j - b_i), \tag{6.1}$$

where ln denotes the natural logarithm. If the attribute level equals item difficulty (e.g., $\theta_j = b_i$), then the log odds of a positive response (or logit) will be zero. Taking the antilog or exponentiating of zero yields an odds of $e^0 = 1$ (or 50:50 chance), which means that the patient is as likely to respond positively as to respond negatively; 50% of individuals would respond positively or endorse the item. If the attribute level exceeds item difficulty by one logit (e.g., $\theta_j - b_i = 2.5 - 1.5 = 1$), then the odds of a positive response increase by a factor of 2.718 (= e^1) and the probability of responding positively equals 73% [= $1/(1+e^{-1})$; see top panel or row of Table 6.1]. In general, when $\theta_j > b_i$, there is greater than a 50% chance that a subject would endorse the item. If the attribute level is less than item difficulty by one logit (e.g., $\theta_j - b_i = 1.5 - 2.5 = -1$), then the odds of a positive response decrease by a factor of 0.368 (= e^{-1}), or the odds of a negative response increase by a factor of 2.718 (= $1/0.368$), and the probability of responding positively equals 0.27 [= $1/(1+e^1)$]. In general, when $\theta_j < b_i$, there is less than a 50% chance that a subject would endorse the item.

For the one-parameter (Rasch) model, Figure 6.1 depicts the ICCs for two items of different difficulty (*b*), conditional on a person's level of physical functioning (θ). Without loss of generality, assume that higher levels of θ here indicate better (more favorable) levels of physical functioning and that each question inquires about an ability to perform a specific task. Values of θ range from −3 (the lowest level of physical functioning) to 3 (the highest level of physical functioning) with numbers in between representing, along the continuum, varying amounts of intermediate levels of physical functioning. Suppose patients were asked to regularly perform activities like walking and running. Item A could be the question "Were you able to walk several blocks without pain in the last 7 days?" (with a response of *Yes* or *No*) and Item B could be the question "Were you able to run several blocks without pain in the last 7 days?" (*Yes* or *No*).

In Figure 6.1, Item A (Walk) has a *b* value of 0 and Item B (Run) has a *b* value of 1. A horizontal line appears where the probability is 0.5; this line intersects the ICC for Item A at an attribute value of 0 ($\theta = 0$) and ICC for Item B at an attribute value of 1 ($\theta = 1$). This means that the difficulty value of 0 corresponds to the level of physical functioning ($\theta = 0$) needed to have a 50% probability for responding positively (*Yes*) to Item A on the ability to walk several blocks without pain. Similarly, the difficulty value of 1 corresponds to the level of physical functioning ($\theta = 1$) needed to have a 50% probability for responding positively (*Yes*) to Item B on the ability to run several blocks without pain. While patients with a true physical functioning score estimated to equal 0 ($\theta = 0$) will, on average, give a positive response to Item A on walking approximately half of the time, they have a smaller probability of 0.27 of responding positively to the more difficult Item B on running. Item A on walking is, as expected, an easier item to endorse than Item B on running for a majority of patients.

Now consider the two-parameter logistic model for a binary outcome (Table 6.1, middle panel or row). It keeps the difficulty item parameter and adds a second item parameter called the discrimination parameter for the *i*th item (a_i). Whereas the value of a_i was implicitly assumed to equal 1 for all items in the one-parameter model (i.e., all items have the same discrimination), the value of a is estimated for each item in the two-parameter model. Item discrimination concerns the ability of an item to separate patients into low and high levels on the *thing* being measured (θ). Discrimination corresponds to the steepness of the curve, the steeper the better (more discriminating).

The theoretical range of the a parameter is also negative to positive infinity but generally ranges from 0 to 3 and, more commonly, from 0 to 2. Items with negative discrimination would mean that respondents with higher θ are, contrary to expectation, less likely to answer the item correctly. Items with negative discrimination, therefore, may be screened out by some computer estimation programs, and these items should be removed from the questionnaire.

In Figure 6.2, Item A (Walk) and Item B (Run) have the same difficulty values as in Figure 6.1, with Item A ($b = 0$) being easier (or less difficult) to endorse than Item B ($b = 1$). However, Item A also generally discriminates ($a = 2$) between patients better than Item B ($a = 1.5$). For Item A ("Were you able to walk several blocks without pain in the last 7 days?") patients with a low score (low levels of physical functioning) of $\theta = -0.69$ have a 20% chance of responding positively to walking several blocks, while patients with a higher score (better physical functioning) of $\theta = 0.70$ have an 80% chance of responding positively. This increase in improved physical functioning of 1.39 [0.70 − (−0.69)] from 20% to 80% endorsement is less than what is needed than the larger increase of 1.85 (1.93 − 0.08) for the same 20%–80% increase in responding positively to Item B ("Were you able to run several blocks without pain, in the last 7 days?"), because Item A is more discriminating or sensitive than Item B for this particular range on physical functioning (where Item A has a steeper slope than Item B). On the other hand, Item B would be the better discriminator for higher levels of physical functioning, such as when $\theta = 2$, where Item B has a steeper slope than Item A. The point is that both items have merit as their levels of discrimination complement each other with respect to varying levels of physical functioning. Having items with psychometric properties that specialize in different levels across the spectrum of an attribute is a desirable feature.

The three-parameter logistic regression model for a binary outcome introduces a third parameter, c_i, to further characterize the ith item (Table 6.1, bottom panel or row). This parameter, which allows the baseline intercept to vary, is sometimes known as a guessing parameter because individuals with very low amounts of the attribute (θ) would be expected to endorse the item only by guessing. The parameter allows for persons, even those with low levels of the attribute, to have a minimal probability (c_i) of answering the ith item correctly.

In Figure 6.3, Item A has the same difficulty and discrimination as in Figure 6.2 ($b = 0$, $a = 2$), as does Item B ($b = 1$, $a = 1.5$). What has been added is the horizontal asymptote parameter, c, for Items A and B. In Figure 6.3, Item A (Walk) has a value of $c = 0.10$, while Item B (Run) has a value of $c = 0.20$. Although the guessing parameter may provide insightful information on understanding the behavior of persons with respect to items on a questionnaire and has a straightforward interpretation in educational measurement, the three-parameter model with its guessing parameter can be vague in health measurement and is not usually applied.

As Figures 6.1 through 6.3 show, a few important characteristics of ICCs are worth noting. One feature of ICCs is that they are S-shaped. They are also monotonic: the probability of answering the question in the positive direction consistently increases as the attribute (θ) increases. On the other hand, they can differ from each other in up to three ways—namely, in their location along the trait continuum (location, b), in the steepness of their slopes (discrimination, a), and where they flatten out at the bottom (guessing, c).

6.3.2 Polytomous Response Models

Items that have more than two response options (categories) are called polytomous items. Numerous PRO scales include items with ordered response categories (e.g., strongly disagree, disagree, neutral, agree, strongly agree). For ordinal responses, extra information about persons becomes available and polytomous IRT models capitalize on it to represent the nonlinear relationship of person attribute level and item characteristics on the probability of responding to a particular response category of an item. In these models, a function analogous to an ICC can be plotted for each category of an item. Although the term used to label such a curve is not universal, such a curve is referred to as a category characteristic curve in this chapter. For polytomous items, several models have been proposed. Among them are the partial credit model and the graded-response model for items in which the categories are ordered; they should not be used to determine the empirical ordering of the categories post hoc.

The partial credit model, which is a generalization of the one-parameter (Rasch) dichotomous IRT model, assumes that all items are equally good at discriminating among persons; therefore, item slopes are constrained to be equal (fixed to equal one) across items. The model depicts the probability of a person responding to a given category of an item as a function of the difference between a person's attribute level and a category intersection parameter. These category intersection parameters, also called category threshold parameters, are akin to the difficulty thresholds in the dichotomous IRT models and reflect the attribute level at which the response category of an item becomes as likely (50% chance) to be responded to as the previous category. Hence, this type of threshold is the point where the probability of a response in either one of two adjacent categories is 50%. A higher attribute level will make that particular response category more likely (more than 50%) to be chosen than the previous category.

The number of category intersection parameters is equal to one less than the number of response options. The set of intersection parameters can differ across different items; items do not have to have identical response options or even the same number of response options. The rating scale model is a special type of partial credit model that does require the same response format be used for all items and sets the category intersection parameters to be equal across items.

The graded response model, another type of two-parameter model, is intended for responses on an ordinal scale. As a direct extension of the two-parameter dichotomous model, the graded response model allows item discrimination to vary across items (unlike the partial credit model) and, in addition, allows spacing between each of the response categories to vary item by item (like the partial credit model). The mathematical function for the graded response model takes the following form:

$$P_{ik}^*(\theta) = \frac{1}{1 + e^{-a_i(\theta - b_{ik})}} \, , \tag{6.2}$$

where

$P_{ik}^*(\theta)$ is the probability of scoring in or above category k of item i (given θ and the item parameters), with the asterisk (*) added to P to indicate the probability of selecting a category k or higher (not only the probability of selecting that category k)

a_i as before is the item slope for item i

b_{ik} is the category boundary for category k of item i (and reflects the level of the attribute at which patients have an equal probability of scoring a category lower than k vs category k or higher)

Equation 6.2 can be used to arrive at the probability of scoring exactly in category k of item i (given θ and the item parameters) by subtracting adjacent probabilities:

$$P_{ik}(\theta) = \frac{1}{1+e^{-a_i(\theta-b_{ik})}} - \frac{1}{1+e^{-a_i(\theta-b_{i(k+1)})}},\qquad(6.3)$$

with this probability equal to the probability of selecting category k or higher minus the probability of selecting category $k + 1$ or higher. Because any subject should have responded to a category on an item, the probability of responding in or above the lowest category is 1, and the probability of responding above the highest category is 0.

For example, consider the question "During the last 7 days, how much of the time have you accomplished your daily activities as a result of your physical health?" with six response categories (0 = none of the time, 1 = little of the time, 2 = some of the time, 3 = a good bit of the time, 4 = most of the time, 5 = all of the time). The probability of responding in or above *none of the time* (category 0) is 1, and the probability of responding above the highest category (category 5) is 0. Figure 6.4 illustrates category characteristic curves, which gives the probability of responding to a particular category for a given level of θ; the sum of the probabilities across categories for a given θ adds up to one. For instance, given a value of $\theta = -1.5$, the probability of responding *none of the time* and, separately,

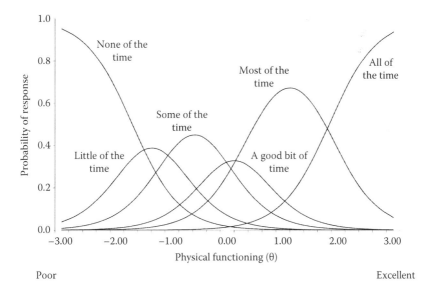

FIGURE 6.4
Category characteristic curves for graded-response model with a six-category item. (*Note:* The item reads "During the last 7 days, how much of the time have you accomplished your daily activities as a result of your physical health?")

little of the time is each approximately 0.40, with response to the category *some of the time* taking almost all of the remaining 0.20.

6.4 Item Information

Item information provides an assessment on the precision of measurement (i.e., reliability) of an item for distinguishing among patients across different levels of the underlying concept or attribute being measured (θ). Higher information implies more precision. Item information depends on the item parameters. For the two-parameter dichotomous logistic model, the item information function $I(\theta)_i$ for item i at a specific value of θ is defined as

$$I(\theta)_i = a_i^2 P_i (1 - P_i), \tag{6.4}$$

where P_i is the proportion of people with a specific amount of the attribute (a specific value of θ) who endorse or respond positively to item i. For a dichotomous item, item information reaches its highest value at $\theta = b$, specifically, when the proportion of people who endorse an item is $P_i = 0.5$. The amount of item information (precision) decreases as the amount of the attribute departs from item difficulty and approaches zero at the extremes of the attribute scale.

An item has more information and precision when the a parameter (the item discrimination parameter) is high than when it is low. If an item has a slope of $a = 1$, it has four times the information or discriminating ability than an item with $a = 0.5$ (per Equation 6.4). The value of the a parameter can be negative; however, this results in a monotonically *decreasing* item response function. People with high amounts of the attribute will then have a *lower* probability of responding correctly than people with lower amounts of the attribute. Such bad items are usually quickly weeded out of an item pool.

Figure 6.5 contains information functions for two items, "I feel calm and peaceful" (Item 1) and "I feel happy" (Item 2), with the same two response categories of yes or no. The latent attribute or construct of interest is mental health (θ). For each item, the item difficulty parameter (b) determines where the item information function is located and centered. More item information is contained around individuals whose mental health status is around b ($b_1 = 0.25$ for Item 1, $b_2 = -0.23$ for Item 2). Item 1 (discrimination parameter $a_1 = 2.83$) has more item information than Item 2 ($a_2 = 1.11$) and hence gives the taller and narrower curve. Good items like Item 1 provide a lot of information around its item difficulty, and less information further away, whereas items not as good like Item 2 provide less information that is more diluted and spread out over a larger range of the attribute.

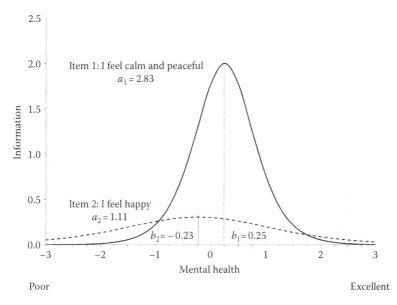

FIGURE 6.5
Item information function for a good item (Item 1) and a poorer item (Item 2).

With polytomous items, each category provides information. The item information function depends not only on the item slope (discrimination) but also on the distance it takes along the attribute (θ) to move from one category to the next. If categories within an item are close in their category threshold values (the point on θ where the probability of a response in either one of two adjacent categories is equal), the item information will be peaked for values of the latent construct or attribute near the center of the categorical threshold values. But if the categories are spread further apart in their category threshold values, varying amounts of information can be added at different locations of the attribute. Consequently, while the item information function for a dichotomous item resembles a normal curve, the item information function for a polytomous item may be broader, with information more spread over the range of the attribute, and may have multiple peaks. As a result of the greater number of response categories, polytomous items generally have more information than dichotomous items.

It should be noted that information functions for the items in the same scale sum to produce the information function for the entire scale. The reciprocal of the square root of the information function for a scale gives the standard error of measurement as a function of the underlying attribute; the lower the standard error of measurement, the more precise is the measure. Unlike reliability in classical test theory, IRT information functions for an item and for a scale of multiple items are not single coefficients but vary according to where the patient resides along the latent continuum of the attribute.

6.5 Item Fit and Person Fit

A desirable characteristic of a useful PRO scale is one that includes an efficient set of items that spans the entire range of the concept or attribute being measured. Consider when the metric is centered on persons, so that values of the person parameter are fixed to have a mean of zero ($\theta = 0$). Ideally, the amount of the attribute across persons should be stretched evenly and representatively across the continuum of attribute estimates. If the distribution of θ is approximately normal, most of the patients will be within 2 or 3 units of 0, with a larger proportion of individuals near 0 and fewer and fewer at the extremes. If the mean of the item difficulties is also near 0, the scale is well matched to the underlying levels of the attribute from patients. If the item difficulty parameters have a noticeably higher mean than 0, the scale is difficult on average; if they have a noticeably lower mean, the scale is easy on average.

Now consider the case when the metric is centered on item difficulty instead of person attribute, so that item difficulties (b) are constrained to have a mean of zero ($b = 0$). An ideal situation is to have a set of items in the range from about −3 to 3 units (or −4 to 4 units, depending on the data) below and above the mean, respectively. Estimates on the difficulty of items can be plotted along a continuum from −3 to 3 units, which is expected to cover all or almost all of the range (with most values being from −2 to 2 units, as noted in Section 6.3.1). If estimates of item difficulty tend to cluster together at the low end of the scale, these items are too easily endorsed and measure only low amounts of the underlying attribute. Conversely, if estimates of item difficulty tend to cluster at the other extreme, these items are too difficult to endorse and measure only high amounts of the underlying attribute. If estimates of item difficulty tend to cluster in the middle of the scale, these items cover only the middle portion of the attribute. Ideally, a questionnaire should have items covering the full range of difficulty to ensure complete assessment of the concept of interest.

6.5.1 Person-Item Maps

It is common in Rasch analysis to center the metric around item difficulty (instead of person attribute) so that the mean of the item difficulties is fixed to equal 0. If the PRO measure is easy for the sample of persons, the mean across person attributes will be greater than zero ($\theta > 0$); if the PRO measure is hard for the sample, the mean of θ will be less than zero. Rasch users produce person-item (or Wright) maps to show such relationships between item difficulty and person attribute.

Figure 6.6 portrays such a person-item map of a 10-item scale on physical functioning. Because of the scale content, person attribute here is referred as person ability. With a recall period of the past 4 weeks, each item is pegged to a different physical activity but raises the same question: "In the

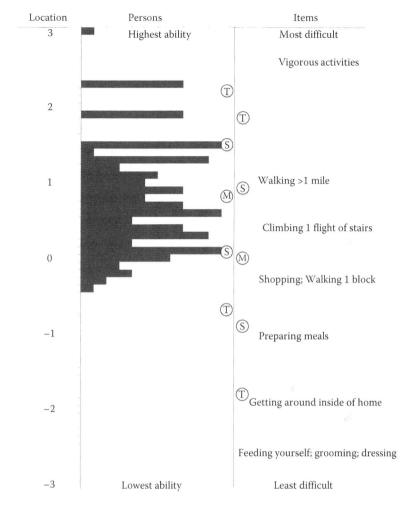

FIGURE 6.6

Illustration of person-item map on physical functioning. (*Note*: M = mean of person distribution or item distribution, S = single standard deviation from the person mean or the item mean, T = two standard deviations from the person mean or the item mean.)

past 4 weeks, how difficult was it to perform the following activity?" Each item also has the same set of five response options: 1 = extremely difficult, 2 = very difficult, 3 = moderately difficult, 4 = slightly difficult, 5 = not difficult. Assume that all activities were attempted by each respondent during the past 4 weeks. Also assume that item difficulty emanated from the rating scale model, a polytomous Rasch model, where each item has its own difficulty parameter separated from the common set of categorical threshold values across items (Bond and Fox, 2007). If the more general partial credit model was fit instead, the mean of the four category threshold parameters for each item can be used to represent an item's difficulty. If the response option was binary instead of ordinal, a one-parameter (Rasch) binary logistic model could have been fit to obtain the set of item difficulties and attribute values.

At least five points are noteworthy. First, the questionnaire contains more easy items than hard ones, as seven of the 10 items have location (logit) scores on item difficulty below 0. A consequence of this is that an attribute or ability score jumps from 1 (item on *Walking > 1 mile*) to slightly below 3 (*Vigorous activities*, such as running, lifting heavy objects, or participating in strenuous sports), which suggests that adding some moderately difficult items would be beneficial in order to measure and distinguish among individuals within this range.

Second, some items have the same difficulty scores: the dual items on shopping and walking one block and the triplet on feeding yourself, grooming, and dressing. Not much scale information would be sacrificed if one of the dual items and two of the triplet items were removed.

Third, if the items have been written based on a construct map (a structured and ordered definition of the underlying ability or attribute intended to be measured by the scale and conceived of in advance), the item map (e.g., right-hand side of Figure 6.6) that follows the construct map can be used as evidence of being congruent with content validity (Wilson, 2005). A construct map is informed by a strong theory of which characteristics or features of the attribute require higher levels of the attribute for endorsement.

Fourth, patients tend to cluster at the higher end of the scale (note that the mean location score is about 1 for the ability of persons and it exceeds the fixed mean location of 0 for difficulty of items), indicating that most of these patients would be likely to endorse (or respond favorably) to several of these items. Figure 6.6 shows which items fall toward the lower end (most persons would endorse or respond favorably to these items) and which items rose to the upper end (relatively few persons would endorse or respond favorably to these items). Thus, this group of patients had either a high degree of physical functioning or, consistent with the previous evaluation of the items, there are not enough challenging or more difficult items such as those on moderate activities (such as moving a table, pushing a vacuum cleaner, bowling, or playing golf). The ideal situation is to have a mean location score of around 0 ($\theta = 0$) across a representative sample of individuals.

Finally, it should be noted that ICCs, which cannot cross in the one-parameter Rasch model, can cross in the two-parameter and three-parameter models when the discrimination parameters among items vary, which can confound the item ordering. For two- and three-parameter models, a consequence of this is that Item 1 might be more difficult than Item 2 for low levels of the attribute, whereas Item 2 might be more difficult than Item 1 for high levels of the attribute. In such a case the item ordering will not correspond in the same way as the item difficulty parameters. The Rasch model, which assumes equal item discrimination, corresponds exactly to (and is defined by) the order of item difficulties and hence the order of the items is constant throughout levels of the attribute.

6.5.2 Fit Indices

As with any use of mathematical models, it is important to assess the fit of the data to the model. The fit of a model can be compared using indices of overall model fit. One straightforward procedure is to compare the observed total score distribution to the model-predicted score distribution. Their distributions could be visually compared or the difference between them could be assessed with a statistical test such as a chi-square test. Tests are also available for comparing the fit between different models (Hambleton et al., 1991; van der Linden and Hambleton, 1997; Embretson and Reise, 2000; Baker and Kim, 2004; De Boeck and Wilson, 2004; DeMars, 2010).

More commonly reported than model fit is item fit. Item fit indices can identify items that should be excluded, rewritten or replaced before rerunning the IRT analysis. For example, the question "Do you have any trouble going up stairs?" might have a high level of misfit since some patients who cannot go up stairs will reorganize their lifestyles accordingly by avoiding going up stairs. If they believe that the questionnaire concerns the degree to which they are inconvenienced or troubled, they might truthfully respond "no problem, because I no longer have any need to go upstairs."

For item fit, the key concept is the residual. The residual is the difference between an observed proportion and model-predicted (expected) proportion of a positive response for a binary item or in a response category for a polytomous item. The residual is calculated based on the same patient in Rasch models and conditional on groups of individuals with the same level on the attribute (θ) in non-Rasch models. Residual plots can prove helpful as well.

Rasch models offer two types of mean square statistics to assess item fit. The infit statistic is a weighted estimate that gives relatively more weight to responses close to an item's modeled estimates. Infit mean square statistic is more sensitive to the pattern of responses to items targeted on the person and vice versa. The infit statistic is usually influenced by response patterns, is hard to diagnose and remedy, and presents a threat to validity. In contrast, the outfit statistic is an unweighted estimate that is more likely to be influenced by unexpected responses, is easier to diagnose, and presents less of a threat to measurement. Outfit mean square statistic is more sensitive to responses to items with difficulty far from a person and vice-versa (imputed responses, lucky guesses, careless mistakes).

When a mean square value is greater than 1.0, the observed variance is more than expected (more haphazard than expected, with model underfit); when a mean square value is less than 1.0, the observed variance is less than expected (more orderly than expected, with model overfit). Therefore, a mean square of, say, 1.70 indicates 70% [i.e., 100% (1.7 − 1)] more variation in the observed data than the Rasch model predicted; a mean square of 0.4 indicates 60% [i.e., 100% (1 − 0.4)] less variation in the observed response pattern than was modeled. Both infit and outfit statistics have an expected value of 1 and an accepted range of fit is between 0.5 and 1.5 (Lincare, 2006).

A complementary way to assess item fit in IRT models in general is to examine the ordinal response categories of the items to determine whether the categories performed sufficiently well to create an interpretable measure. Average attribute estimates of patients are expected to increase as the category level increases (with each higher category reflecting more increments or amounts of the attribute). This monotonicity (a monotonic sequence being one in which successive values move in the same direction) of average attribute estimates is based on the assumption that patients with more of the attribute should endorse higher ladders or categories indicative of it, while those with less of the attribute should endorse lower ladders or categories reflective of it. Categories showing a violation of this pattern are considered disordered and suspect.

Person-fit indices identify individuals who fail to fit the model well. The stability of the model estimation may be greatly improved by excluding these patients from analyses. For example, some patients might state that they are unable to take a short walk, yet, inconsistently, also indicate that they can take long walks. Such conflicting responses cause problems when fitting models. In the Rasch model, *infit* and *outfit* mean square indices can also be calculated for each patient by summing, respectively, the squared weighted residuals (*infit*) and the square unweighted residuals (*outfit*) across items within a particular score.

In Rasch measurement, the person separation index is used as a reliability index, because reliability reflects how accurately or precisely the scores separate or discriminate among persons; it is a summary of the genuine person separation relative to such separation and also measurement error. Measurement error consists of both random error and systematic error and represents the discrepancy between scores obtained and their corresponding true scores. The person separation index is akin to Cronbach's alpha and is based on the basic definition of reliability from CTT, as the ratio of true score variance to observed variance (which equals the true score variance plus the error variance). As noted earlier, the level of measurement error in IRT models is not uniform across the range of a PRO scale and is generally larger for more extreme scores (low and high scores).

6.6 Differential Item Functioning

One of the assumptions necessary to compare patients on an attribute is that the item response functions are the same for all individuals. As part of the process of validating multi-item PRO scales, it may be desirable to know whether each item behaves in the same way for different subgroups of respondents. For example, do males and females respond differently to the statement "I feel like crying," even after controlling for depression levels of every subject? In other words, do males and females respond differently to "I feel like crying" even when these two subgroups are adjusted to have the same overall level of depression? Is an item about fatigue answered similarly by older and younger age groups, given that they have the same overall fatigue level? Are responses to an item about carrying heavy objects answered similarly between respondents who completed the original English version of a questionnaire and respondents who completed the Spanish-translated version, even when these English and Spanish subgroups are taken to have the same overall level of physical functioning?

Two types of differential item functioning (DIF) exist. Uniform DIF occurs when the item shows the same amount of DIF between groups whatever the level of the total scale score on the PRO measure. For example, uniform DIF might occur in an item on depression (an item on a multi-item PRO scale to assess the overall attribute of mental health) when males with lower levels of mental health are likely to score higher on the depression item compared to females with the same lower levels of mental health and, to the same extent, males with higher levels of mental health are also likely to score higher on the depression item compared to females with the same higher levels of mental health. Nonuniform DIF occurs when the magnitude of the group effect depends on the total scale score. For example, nonuniform DIF might occur in a fatigue item (another item that constitutes mental health) when males with lower levels of mental health are more likely to score higher on the fatigue item than do females with the same lower levels of mental health, whereas males with higher levels of mental health are less likely (instead of more likely) to score higher on the fatigue item than do females with the same higher levels of mental health.

A range of techniques on DIF exist for evaluating whether there are different subgroup responses to items within a scale, after controlling for group differences in the overall attribute being assessed (Fayers and Machin, 2007; Scott et al., 2010). One widely used approach for detecting DIF is logistic regression, which is commonly regarded as robust and efficient as well as simple and straightforward. For items with two response categories, binary logistic regression can be used to relate the probability of a positive response to the group membership variable, the total scale score, and the interaction between the group membership and the total scale score. The presence of nonuniform DIF can be evaluated by testing whether the interaction coefficient between group membership and (total) scale score is statistically significant from zero. If it is not statistically significant, the presence of uniform DIF can be evaluated by testing whether the regression coefficient of group membership is statistically significant from zero and, if so, would indicate a constant difference between the groups across the entire range of the attribute.

DIF may occur for varied reasons and does not necessarily imply item bias per se. DIF simply assesses whether items behave differently between subgroups of patients, whereas the term *item bias* suggests a judgment as to the consequence and impact of DIF. If differential responses are not expected between, say, males and females, then DIF may suggest that the item be deleted or modified. If a scale is being developed simultaneously between two or more languages, then DIF may indicate a problem with either the concept or the translation, which would require further investigation. If persons at or above age 65 respond differently from persons with the same level of physical functioning who are below age 65 with respect to the employment item "Do you have trouble working?", then DIF may have risen because individuals at or above 65 (who tend to be retired more than individuals below 65) tend to interpret this question differently, resulting in item bias that would confound the comparison of these two age groups. On the other hand, if differential responses on a well-validated scale are expected between two cultural groups, with one group being more likely than the other to use the extreme response categories, then DIF would confirm the expectation that the location of the threshold values for the response options would differ between the two groups and substantiate the anticipated cultural differences between the groups.

6.7 Sample Size

What sample size is needed for a reliable IRT analysis? IRT models require large samples to obtain accurate and stable parameter estimates, although Rasch models (for dichotomous items and polytomous items) can result in stable estimates with more moderate samples. Several factors are involved in sample size estimation and no definitive answer can be given. First, the choice of IRT model affects the required sample size. Rasch models involve the estimation of the fewest parameters and thus smaller sample sizes are needed, relative to two-parameter and three-parameter models, in order to obtain stable parameter estimates on item difficulty and person location.

Second, the type of response options influences the required sample size. In general, as the number of response categories increases, a larger sample size is warranted as more item parameters must be estimated. For non-Rasch models, it has been shown that the graded response IRT model can be estimated with 250 respondents but around 500 respondents are often recommended for accurate and stable parameter estimates (Embretson and Reise, 2000). In general, the ideal situation is to have adequate representation of respondents for each combination of all possible response patterns across a set of items, something that is rarely achieved. It is important, though, to have at least some people respond to each of the categories of every item to allow the IRT model to be fully estimated.

Third, study purpose can affect sample size. A large sample size is not needed to obtain an initial or descriptive picture of response behavior or trends, provided that a heterogeneous sample is obtained that reasonably reflects the range of population diversity inherent in item and person responses. But if the purpose is to obtain precise measurements on item characteristics and person scores, with stable item and person calibrations declared definitively, sample sizes of at least 250 and generally over a few hundred are required. Also, when a finer level of precision is desired to measure individuals, and distinguish among them, a larger sample is needed to achieve a more refined set of measurement properties.

Fourth, the sample distribution of respondents is another important consideration. Ideally, respondents should be spread fairly uniformly over the range of the attribute (construct) being measured. If fewer people are located at the ends of the attribute, items also positioned at the extreme end of that construct will have higher standard errors associated with their parameters.

Fifth, questionnaires with more items may require larger sample sizes. Additional items increase the possibility that the parameters of any one item need a larger sample in order to be adequately estimated. Finally, if the set of items in a questionnaire has a poor or merely a modest relationship with the attribute, a larger sample size would be needed as more information is needed to compensate for the lackluster relationship. If such a relationship is lackluster, though, the credibility of the scale should be called into question.

6.8 Example

The National Eye Institute sponsored the development of the Visual Function Questionnaire (NEI-VFQ) to assess the dimensions of vision-targeted functional health status that are most important to persons with chronic eye disease (Mangione et al., 1998, 2001). Items are grouped into several subscales, each dealing with a specific aspect of visual functioning. In this example, the focus is on the attribute of near vision using the near-vision subscale (six items) from the German version of the NEI-VFQ, using 200 patients with broad stages of age-related macular degeneration (Thompson et al., 2007).

Each of the six items in the near-vision subscale has five ordinal categories (Table 6.2). Each item has the same set of categorical responses, codes, and descriptions: 100—no difficulty at all, 75—a little difficulty, 50—moderate difficulty, 25—extreme difficulty, 0—stopped doing because of eyesight. Each domain score also ranges from 0 (worst) to 100 (best).

The data were analyzed in Winsteps® and reported using the (Andrich) rating scale model (Lincare, 2006; Thompson et al., 2007). Each of the six items has five categories and thus four (= 5 − 1) thresholds for moving from one category to the next higher functioning category. The probability of responding in the lowest ability category or higher is predefined as 1, while the probability of responding above the highest functioning category is predefined as 0. Given a specific level of true functional ability and an item's characteristics, the probability of responding in a specific category of an item is the probability of responding in that category or higher minus the probability of responding in the next category or higher.

Item difficulties ranged from –2.02 to 1.45 units (logits) for the near-vision subscale in which *shaving/hair styling/makeup* was the least difficult task and

TABLE 6.2

Items on the Near-Vision Subscale of the NEI-VFQ

1. How much difficulty do you have *reading ordinary print in newspapers*?
2. How much difficulty do you have doing work or hobbies that require you to *see well up close*, such as cooking, sewing, fixing things around the house, or using hand tools?
3. Because of your eyesight, how much difficulty do you have *finding something on a crowded shelf*?
4. Wearing glasses, how much difficulty do you have reading the small print in a telephone book, on a medicine bottle, or on legal forms?
5. Because of your eyesight, how much difficulty do you have *figuring out whether bills you receive are accurate*?
6. Because of your eyesight, how much difficulty do you have doing things like *shaving, styling your hair, or putting on makeup*?

Source: National Eye Institute Visual Functioning Questionnaire 25 (VFQ-25), with 14-item appendix, 1996. The NEI-VFQ was developed at RAND under the sponsorship of the National Eye Institute.

TABLE 6.3

Results of Rasch Model for the Near-Vision Subscale of the NEI-VFQ: Items Ranked from Most to Least Difficulty

Item	Item Difficulty	Infit Mean Square	Outfit Mean Square
Reading small print	1.45	1.03	1.00
Seeing close up	0.93	0.88	1.13
Reading newsprint	0.77	0.71	0.70
Reading bills/mail	−0.34	0.92	0.69
Finding objects on shelf	−0.78	1.28	1.34
Shaving/hair styling/makeup	−2.02	1.39	0.92
Mean across items	0.00	1.04	0.96

reading small print the most difficult (Table 6.3). Standard errors of the item difficulties ranged from 0.10 to 0.14. Infit mean squares of the items ranged from 0.71 to 1.39; outfit mean squares ranged from 0.69 to 1.34. Both sets of item fit indices were therefore in the acceptable range (between 0.5 and 1.5).

As defined here, in the rating scale model, a category threshold parameter for an item defines the attribute or ability level (in logit units) necessary to have a 50% probability of responding in the next higher category. The ability level to have an equal chance (50:50) of responding *stopped doing* or *extreme difficulty* was −2.06 (standard error = 0.15) units, *extreme difficulty* or *moderate difficulty* was −0.26 (0.11), *moderate difficulty* or *little difficulty* was 0.89 (0.10), and *little difficulty* or *no difficulty* was 1.43 (0.09). Notice that these threshold values increase according to the logical order principle required by the Rasch measurement model.

A content-based interpretation using ICCs can also be made in order to enrich interpretation and enhance meaning of scores on a PRO measure. An example with the NEI-VFQ is given in Chapter 11 on interpretation.

6.9 Example: Rasch Model Implementation

In this section, we illustrate the implementation of the Rasch model by creating a simulated dataset in SAS. Consider a scale with five binary items [no (0) and yes (1)] given to 1000 subjects. The outcome variable is represented by the variable U with a value of 1 if a subject responded *yes* and a value of 0 if a subject responded *no*. Figure 6.7 represents the implementation to simulate data. Note that the SAS line

```
prob = 1/(1 + exp(-1*(Theta - b[j])));
```

corresponds to the one-parameter logistic model in Table 6.1. Figure 6.7 creates a dataset with a simulated binary outcome U—a subject's response to an item—and indicator variables $Item1_i$, $Item2_i$, $Item3_i$, $Item4_i$, and $Item5_i$ (to be discussed shortly), as well as an ID variable to represent a subject.

Figure 6.8 represents a structure of the dataset for the analysis with the first 2 subjects shown. The first subject (ID = 1) responded 1 (*yes*) to Items 3 and 4 where $U = 1$, and 0 (*no*) to Items 1, 2, and 5 where $U = 0$. The second subject (ID = 2) responded 1 (*yes*) to Items 1 and 3 where $U = 1$, and 0 (*no*) to Items 2, 4, and 5 where $U = 0$.

Before illustrating the implementation of the Rasch analysis, we need to transform the first equation in Table 6.1 to an exactly equivalent equation as shown here:

$$p_{ij} = \frac{1}{1 + e^{-(\theta_j - b_1 \, Item1_i - b_2 \, Item2_i - b_3 \, Item3_i - b_4 \, Item4_i - b_5 \, Item5_i)}}, \qquad (6.5)$$

where
  p_{ij} is the probability of responding *yes* for subject j on item i ($j = 1, 2,..., 1000$;
    $i = 1, 2,..., 5$)
  θ_j is the value of the attribute θ for subject j (or ability of subject j)
  b_1, b_2, b_3, b_4, and b_5 are the five difficulty parameters for the five items
  $Item1_i$, $Item2_i$, $Item3_i$, $Item4_i$, and $Item5_i$ are the binary indicator variables for
    item i and each of these variables could have only a value of 0 or 1

Therefore, for every item, only one indicator variable corresponding to a particular item will be equal to 1, with all others to be equal to 0 (see Table 6.4 and Figure 6.8). After accounting for the values of the indicator variables,

```
/*
For this example we have 1000 subjects (NumberOfRows) and a
scale with five binary items.
*/
options nofmterr nocenter pagesize = 2000 linesize = 256;

%Let NumberOfRows = 1000;

%Let seed1 = 100;
%Let seed2 = 200;

Data _irt_;

Array b{1:5} (-2.5 -0.5 0.7 1.9 3.0); /*Difficulty parameters*/
Array Item{1:5} (0 0 0 0 0);

        Do i = 1 To &NumberOfRows;

        ID = i;
        Theta = rannor(&seed1);

            Do j = 1 to 5;

               prob = 1/(1 + exp(-1*(Theta - b[j])));

               U = ranbin(&seed2,1,prob);

                 Do k = 1 to 5;
                 Item[k] = 0;
                 End;

                 Item[j] = 1;

               output;
               End;
        End;

    Keep ID U Item1-Item5;
  Run;
```

FIGURE 6.7
SAS codes to create a simulated dataset for a Rasch model.

Item1	Item2	Item3	Item4	Item5	ID	U
1	0	0	0	0	1	0
0	1	0	0	0	1	0
0	0	1	0	0	1	1
0	0	0	1	0	1	1
0	0	0	0	1	1	0
1	0	0	0	0	2	1
0	1	0	0	0	2	0
0	0	1	0	0	2	1
0	0	0	1	0	2	0
0	0	0	0	1	2	0

FIGURE 6.8
Structure of the dataset for the Rasch modeling.

TABLE 6.4

Indicator Variable Values

i	Item1$_i$	Item2$_i$	Item3$_i$	Item4$_i$	Item5$_i$
1	1	0	0	0	0
2	0	1	0	0	0
3	0	0	1	0	0
4	0	0	0	1	0
5	0	0	0	0	1

we can see that Equation 6.5 reduces to an equation with only one difficulty parameter for every particular item. For example, for Item 2, Equation 6.5 reduces to the following:

$$p_{2j} = \frac{1}{1+e^{-(\theta_j - b_1 \times 0 - b_2 \times 1 - b_3 \times 0 - b_4 \times 0 - b_5 \times 0)}},$$

$$p_{2j} = \frac{1}{1+e^{-(\theta_j - b_2)}}.$$

Figure 6.9 represents the implementation of the Rasch model using the NLMIXED procedure in SAS. A detailed discussion of the NLMIXED procedure is beyond the scope of this book and can be found elsewhere (SAS, 2008). Here we highlight the most salient points of the implementation for the purpose at hand. First, note that the SAS code line

```
prob = 1/(1+exp(-1*(theta-b1*Item1-b2*Item2-b3*Item3-b4*Item4-
b5*Item5)));
```

corresponds exactly to Equation 6.5 and represents probability of response to a binary item. The MODEL statement specifies that the dependent variable *U* is from a binary distribution defined by the probability value *prob*. The RANDOM statement defines the random effects and their distribution (for more on the definition of random effects, see Chapter 8). In our particular case, the random effect is the ability (θ) of every subject. Note that the ability (θ) is normally distributed with a mean of 0 and a standard deviation of 1, which is consistent with how ability (θ) was simulated in Figure 6.7 (Theta = rannor(&seed1);). The *subject* statement (subject = ID) indicates that observations with the same ID come from the same subject, and, as a result, only one value of ability (θ) will be estimated for each subject (OUT = Theta_out in Figure 6.9).

Figure 6.10 represents partial output with estimates of the difficulty parameters. As expected, the estimated values (−2.5580, −0.4120, 0.6570, 1.8246, 2.9451) are close to the values used to simulate the data in Figure 6.7 (Array b{1:5} (−2.5 −0.5 0.7 1.9 3.0); /*Difficulty parameters*/).

```
Proc Nlmixed Data = _irt_ method = gauss technique = newrap
noadscale qpoints = 100;

Parms b1 = 0 b2 = 0 b3 = 0 b4 = 0 b5 = 0;

prob = 1/(1+exp(-1*(theta-b1*Item1-b2*Item2-b3*Item3-b4*Item4-
b5*Item5)));

   MODEL U~binary(prob);

   RANDOM theta~normal(0,1) subject = ID OUT = Theta_out;

Run;
```

FIGURE 6.9
Implementation of the Rasch model using the NLMIXED procedure in SAS.

Parameter Estimates

Parameter	Estimate	Standard Error	DF	Pr > |t|	Alpha	Lower	Upper
b1	-2.5580	0.1160	999	<.0001	0.05	-2.7856	-2.3304
b2	-0.4120	0.07729	999	<.0001	0.05	-0.5636	-0.2603
b3	0.6570	0.07857	999	<.0001	0.05	0.5028	0.8112
b4	1.8246	0.09473	999	<.0001	0.05	1.6388	2.0105
b5	2.9451	0.1318	999	<.0001	0.05	2.6865	3.2038

FIGURE 6.10
Partial output of NLMIXED procedure.

6.10 Summary

CTT underpins the traditional embodiment of psychometric theory used to assess and improve the measurement properties of a scale. Assumptions of CTT about measurement scales and their constituent items are expected to be considered appropriate in most situations. IRT, the topic of this chapter, offers a complementary or alternative measurement framework and provides additional insight into the measurement and validation of PRO instruments. IRT is a statistical framework consisting of mathematical models expressing the probability of a particular response to a scale item as a function of the (latent or unobserved) attribute of the person and of certain parameters or characteristics of the item. IRT assumes that patients at a particular level of an underlying attribute (e.g., with a particular level of physical functioning) will have a certain probability of responding positively to a binary question or to a category of a polytomous question. This probability will depend on the item characteristics and their relation to the person's level on the attribute.

This chapter describes the assumptions of IRT, ICCs, the different types of IRT models, item information, item fit and person fit, DIF, and sample size consideration. In addition, the chapter provides a published example and an instructive simulated example.

References

Baker, F.B. and S.-H. Kim. 2004. *Item Response Theory: Parameter Estimation Techniques*, 2nd edition, revised and expanded. New York, NY: Marcel Dekker.

Bond, T.G. and C.M. Fox. 2007. *Applying the Rasch Model: Fundamental Measurement in the Human Sciences*, 2nd edition. Mahwah, NJ: Lawrence Erlbaum Associates.

Chang, C.H. and B.B. Reeve. 2005. Item response theory and its applications to patient-reported outcomes measurement. *Evaluation in the Health Professions* 28:264–282.

Crocker, L. and J. Algina. 1986. *Introduction to Classical and Modern Test Theory*. Belmont, CA: Wadsworth Publishing.

de Ayala, R.J. 2009. *The Theory and Practice of Item Response Theory*. New York, NY: The Guilford Press.

De Boeck, P. and M. Wilson (editors). 2004. *Explanatory Item Response Models: A Generalized Linear and Nonlinear Approach*. New York, NY: Springer-Verlag.

DeMars, C. 2010. *Item Response Theory*. New York, NY: Oxford University Press.

Embretson, S.E. and S.P. Reise. 2000. *Item Response Theory for Psychologists*. Mahwah, NJ: Lawrence Erlbaum Associates.

Fan, X. 1998. Item response theory and classical test theory: An empirical comparison of their item/person statistics. *Educational and Psychological Measurement* 58:357–381.

Fayers, F.M. and D. Machin. 2007. *Quality of Life: The Assessment, Analysis and Interpretation of Patient-Reported Outcomes*, 2nd edition. Chichester, England: John Wiley & Sons Ltd.

Fischer, G.H. and I.W. Molenaar (editors). 1995. *Rasch Models: Foundations, Recent Developments, and Applications*. New York, NY: Springer-Verlag.

Hambleton, R.K., Swaninathan, H.J., and H.J. Rogers. 1991. *Fundamentals of Item Response Theory*. Newbury Park, CA: Sage Publications.

Hays, R.D., Morales, L.S., and S.P. Reise. 2000. Item response theory and health outcomes measurement in the 21st century. *Medical Care* 38:9 (Suppl. II):II-28–II-43.

Hosmer, D.W., Jr., Lemeshow, S., and R.X. Sturdivant. 2013. *Applied Logistic Regression*, 3rd edition. Hoboken, NJ: John Wiley & Sons.

Kleinbaum, D.G. and M. Klein. 2010. *Logistic Regression: A Self-Learning Text*, 3rd edition. New York, NY: Springer.

Kline, T. 2005. *Psychological Testing: A Practical Approach to Design and Evaluation*. Thousand Oaks, CA: Sage Publications.

Lincare, J.M. 2006. *A User's Guide to WINSTEPS® MINISTEP: Rasch-Model Computer Programs*. Chicago, IL: MESA Press.

Macdonald, P. and S.V. Paunonen. 2002. A Monte Carlo comparison of item and person statistics based on item response theory versus classical test theory. *Educational and Psychological Measurement* 62:921–943.

Mangione, C.M., Lee, P.P., Gutierrez, P.R., Spritzer, K., Berry, S., and R.D. Hays, for the National Eye Institute Visual Function Questionnaire Field Test Investigators. 2001. Development of the 25-item National Eye Institute Visual Function Questionnaire. *Archives of Ophthalmology* 119:1050–1058.

Mangione, C.M., Lee, P.P., Pitts, J., Gutierrez, P., Berry, S., and R.D. Hays, for the NEI-VFQ Field Test Investigators. 1998. Psychometric properties of the National Eye Institute Visual Function Questionnaire (NEI-VFQ). *Archives of Ophthalmology* 116:1496–1504.

Massof, R.W. In press. A general theoretical framework of interpreting patient-reported outcomes estimated from ordinally scaled item responses. *Statistical Methods in Medical Research*. Published online 19 February 2013. E-pub ahead of print. DOI: 10.1177/0962280213476380.

Nunnally, J.C. and I.H. Bernstein. 1994. *Psychometric Theory*, 3rd edition. New York, NY: McGraw-Hill.

Reeve, B.B. 2003. Item response theory modeling in health outcomes measurement. *Expert Review of Pharmacoeconomics & Outcomes Research* 3:131–145.

Reeve, B.B. and P. Fayers. 2005. Applying item response theory modelling for evaluating questionnaire item and scale properties. In: Fayers, P. and Hays, H. (editors). *Assessing Quality of Life in Clinical Trials*, 2nd edition. New York, NY: Oxford University Press, pp. 55–73.

SAS Institute Inc. 2008. *SAS/STAT® 9.2 User's Guide*. Cary, NC: SAS Institute Inc.

Scott, N.W., Fayers, P.M., Aaronson, N.K., Bottomley, A., de Graeff, A., Groenvold, M., Gundy, C., Koller, M., Petersen, M.A., and M.A.G. Sprangers. 2010. Differential item functioning (DIF) analyses of health-related quality of life instruments using logistic regression. *Health and Quality of Life Outcomes* 8:81. Open access.

Streiner, D.L. and G.R. Norman. 2008. *Health Measurement Scales: A Practical Guide to Their Development and Use*, 4th edition. New York, NY: Oxford University Press.

Thompson, J.R., Cappelleri, J.C., Getter, C., Pleil, A., Reichel, M., and S. Wolf. 2007. Enhanced interpretation of instrument scales using the Rasch model. *Drug Information Journal* 41:541–550.

van der Linden, W.J. and R.K. Hambleton (editors). 1997. *Handbook of Modern Item Response Theory*. New York, NY: Springer-Verlag.

Wilson, M. 2005. *Constructing Measures: An Item Response Modeling Approach*. Mahwah, NJ: Lawrence Erlbaum Associates.

Yen, W.M. 1993. Scaling performance measures: Strategies for managing local item dependence. *Journal of Educational Measurement* 30:187–213.

7

Cross-Sectional Analysis

Thus far, we have covered major concepts and analytic methods on the use of either a single- or multi-item patient-reported outcome (PRO) instrument. In this chapter, both nonparametric and parametric statistical methods for analyzing the PRO data cross-sectionally (e.g., at a certain time point) will be examined and exemplified. This chapter also covers a single measurement of change from baseline, which, although not strictly cross-sectional, reflects longitudinal data in its most basic form and involves the same type of cross-sectional analytic methods.

7.1 Types of PRO Data and Exploratory Methods

7.1.1 Types of PRO Data

PRO instruments may employ binary, ordinal, or continuous scales defined by their specific types of response formats. A *rating scale* may be defined differently by different researchers. Here, a rating scale is defined generally as a method to elicit a direct quantitative estimate of the magnitude on attribute. A rating scale has many variations.

For example, a visual analog scale (VAS) is a line of fixed length, usually 100 mm, with words that anchor the scale at the extreme ends and no words describing intermediate positions. The VAS, as the term *analog* in the name implies, is a continuous scale. Patients are instructed to indicate the place on the line corresponding to their perceived state. The mark's position is measured as the score (Figure 7.1).

The VAS approach has merit for its simplicity and its potential to detect differences within patients and between patients. In addition, when used repeatedly over time, the use of the VAS makes it difficult or impossible for patients to recall precisely where a mark was previously made along a featureless line (unless one of its two endpoints was chosen), and thereby facilitating the targeting of response to the current assessment rather than confounding the current response with a previous response. On the other hand, the VAS approach has potential limitations that may include the wording of its endpoints (what is the "The worst pain imaginable" if an individual has never experienced it?), their meaning (different individuals may have experienced different levels of "worst pain imaginable"), and the evaluation being made in different dimensions by different individuals (e.g., frequency,

How severe is your pain right now? Place a vertical mark on the line below to indicate the severity of your pain.

No pain |‾‾‾‾‾‾‾‾‾‾‾‾‾‾‾‾‾‾‾‾‾‾‾‾‾‾‾‾‾‾‾‾‾‾| Worst pain
at all |_____| imaginable

FIGURE 7.1
An example of a VAS for pain.

intensity, and duration). Another consideration is that, because the VAS is based on only one item, test–retest reliability of this single measurement is not expected to be high and internal consistency reliability cannot be calculated. An anchored or categorized VAS has the addition of one or more intermediate marks positioned along the line with reference terms assigned to each mark to help patients identify the locations between the scale's two extremes. For example, the 0–10 numeric rating scale (NRS) has discrete numbers that patients can choose between to indicate their level of pain (or whatever concept is being measured). This feature has an advantage over the VAS because it allows easier scoring but is still on a 0–10 metric.

Unlike the typical VAS or NRS, which labels only the endpoints, an adjectival scale has descriptors along a continuum. An example for the question "How anxious do you feel right now?" would be response categories of none, mild, moderate, and severe.

A Likert scale is widely used in measuring opinions, beliefs, and attitudes. A Likert scale is a type of adjectival scale with one notable exception: While adjectival scales are unipolar, with responses on an attribute that range from none or little of the attribute to much or the maximal amount, a Likert scale is (strictly speaking) bipolar. Response options may tap agreement (strongly agree to strongly disagree), acceptance (most agreeable to least agreeable), similarity (most like me to least like me), or probability (most likely to least likely), among other characteristics (and their descriptors). For the item "Exercise is an essential component of a healthy lifestyle," an example of a Likert scale is 1 = strongly agree, 2 = moderately agree, 3 = slightly agree, 4 = neither agree nor disagree, 5 = slightly disagree, 6 = moderately disagree, and 7 = strongly disagree.

Two major considerations should be kept in mind for a Likert format. One consideration is that the question should be appropriate and align with its adjectival response categories. A useful criterion is "How are patients with different amounts of strengths of the attribute in question likely to respond?" For instance, a very mild statement such as "My health is important" may elicit too much agreement so that a person could strongly agree with the statement (i.e., choose an extreme response option on agreement) without really holding such an extreme opinion. Changing the statement to be fairly strong (though not extremely strong), "My health is a top priority," may be more suitable. The second consideration with Likert scales is how to label the middle position, if there is to be one, which should reflect a middle amount of the attribute and not an inability to answer the question. Good choices for a midpoint include *neither agree nor disagree, agree and disagree equally,* and *no preference.*

The following types of response scales among others, may also be found in practice (FDA, 2009):

1. Recording of events as they occur by using an event log that can be included in a patient diary or other reporting system (e.g., interactive voice response system).

2. Pictorial scale uses a set of pictures applied to any of the other response option types. Pictorial scales are often used in pediatric questionnaires but also have been used for patients with cognitive impairments and for patients who are otherwise unable to speak or write.

3. Checklist provides a simple choice between a limited set of options, such as *Yes*, *No*, and *Do not know*. Some checklists ask patients to place a mark in a space if the statement in the item is true. Checklists should be reviewed for completeness and nonredundancy.

Other sources are available for a detailed or informed description of rating scales (McDowell, 2006; Streiner and Norman, 2008; DeVellis, 2012).

Because of the various types of data—some having continuous responses and others having binary or ordinal categorical responses—suitable statistical methods should be employed and many references are available for consultation (e.g., Fleiss et al., 2002; Zou 2003a,b; van Belle et al., 2004; Rosner, 2010). In the following sections, we will review some commonly used descriptive and inferential methods for analyzing binary and continuous data on PRO variables. Implementation of the main concepts is shown using a two-group treatment comparison.

7.1.2 Exploratory Methods and Descriptive Statistics

Exploratory data analysis and visualization methods including boxplots, histograms, and bar diagrams are generally useful to visually compare between treatment groups at a fixed time point such as at baseline or postbaseline.

Descriptive statistics for PRO scores are an essential element of data summarization. For quantitative PRO scores (be it at the domain level or item level), descriptive statistics typically include sample size, mean score, standard deviation (SD) or standard error (SE, which is the SD divided by the square root of the sample size), median, first and third quartiles (their difference being the interquartile range, used as a measure of dispersion), and minimum and maximum (their difference being the range). For PRO scores measured as discrete or qualitative variables, the proportion (or percentage), counts, and sample size are typically reported as descriptive statistics. Descriptive statistics for PRO scores are typically stratified by treatment group.

In addition to summarizing the data numerically, it is often useful to explore the distribution of the data. A normal quantile–quantile (Q–Q) plot is one way to graph whether the data are normally distributed, which is (strictly speaking) an assumption of parametric statistical tests. (A quantile is the point below which a given fraction (or percent) of points lies: for example, if the value of 2 is associated with the 0.90 (or 90%) quantile, then 90% of the data fall at or below the value of 2 and 10% fall above that value.)

Both axes of normal Q–Q plot can be portrayed in units of their respective datasets, with the observed sample data ordered typically on the vertical axis and the quantiles of the corresponding theoretical (normal) distribution on the horizontal axis. If the sample observations follow the theoretical distribution, an approximately straight line with a positive slope will be formed.

A probability plot is a specific type of Q–Q plot with the ordered observations from a sample (vertical axis) plotted against the corresponding percentiles from the postulated distribution (horizontal axis). It is this latter metric of normal percentiles that gives the normal probability plot its distinction. (Essentially the same as a quantile, a percentile is the value or score below which a certain percent of observations fall; for example, the 20th percentile is the value or score below which 20% of the observations may be found.)

In addition to graphical techniques like Q–Q and probability plots, formal statistical tests are available to examine whether the scores follow a normal distribution. The null hypothesis is that the sample comes from a population with a normal distribution of scores and the alternative is that the samples come from a population with non-normal distribution of scores. To test these hypotheses, the Shapiro–Wilk test uses the normal probability plot. Other tests of normality in common use are the Anderson–Darling, Cramér–von Mises, and Kolmogorov–Smirnov tests. These tests compare the sample (empirical) cumulative distribution functions to the normal cumulative distribution functions with the same sample mean and variance. (A cumulative distribution function describes the probability that scores will be less than or equal to a particular value.) The Kolmogorov–Smironov test is based on the maximum absolute difference between the sample cumulative distribution function and the normal cumulative distribution function. The Anderson–Darling and the Cramér–von Mises tests are based on weighted integral of the squared difference between the sample and normal cumulative distribution functions. For all of these tests, small p-values (say, less than 0.05) are evidence that the sample is not from a normal distribution.

7.1.3 Simulated Examples Using SAS: Q–Q Plot, Probability Plot, and Normality Test

A simulated dataset is used to illustrate the construction of the normal Q–Q plot, a normal probability plot, and tests for normality. Consider a hypothetical example of a clinical study with two treatment arms, where each subject is randomly assigned to an active treatment or a placebo treatment. Two outcomes for 1000 subjects are simulated. The outcome variables are Y as a normally distributed variable and $Y1$ as a log-normally distributed variable. The SAS code in Figure 7.2 generated the simulated dataset with 1000 observations (subjects) and two random values Y and $Y1$ representing the two outcomes. The SAS code line

```
Y = rannor(&seed2)*sqrt(1.2*1.2);
```

```
options nocenter;

%Let NumberOfRows = 1000;
%Let seed1 = 2;
%Let seed2 = 2;
%Let seed3 = 3;

Data _response_;

    b1 = 1.5;         /* Treatment effect */

        Do i=1 To &NumberOfRows;

            If rannor(&seed1)>0 Then
              Do;
              Treatment=0;
              Y = rannor(&seed2)*sqrt(1.2*1.2);
              Y1= exp(Y);
              End;
            Else
              Do;
              Treatment=1;
              Y = b1+rannor(&seed3)*sqrt(1.3*1.3);
              Y1= exp(Y);
              End;

            output;

          End;

        Keep Y Y1 Treatment;
Run;
```

FIGURE 7.2
Simulating a dataset.

defines Y as a normally distributed outcome with mean of 0 and standard deviation of 1.2. The SAS code line

$Y1 = \exp(Y);$

generates a log-normally distributed outcome.

Figure 7.3 represents implementation of the Q–Q plot using the UNIVARIATE procedure for Y. Figure 7.5 depicts the Q–Q plot, with the data points joining pairs of Y values (vertical axis) and standardized normal values (the theoretical distribution on the horizontal axis) associated with a given quantile. Note that, as expected, the observations form a straight line.

```
proc univariate data=_response_ NORMAL ;

qqplot Y/normal (mu=est sigma=est);

run;
```

FIGURE 7.3
SAS implementation of the Q–Q plot using the UNIVARIATE procedure.

```
proc univariate data=_response_ NORMAL ;
probplot Y/normal(mu=est sigma=est) pctlminor;
run;
```

FIGURE 7.4
SAS implementation of the probability plot using the UNIVARIATE procedure.

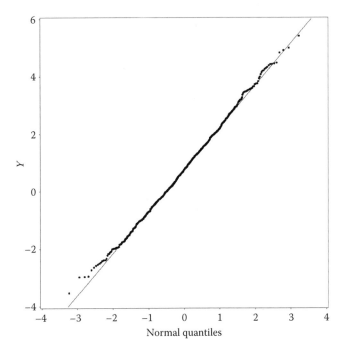

FIGURE 7.5
Q–Q plot for a normally distributed variable.

A normal probability plot, which uses percentiles on the horizontal axis and essentially represents the same information as the normal quantile plot, can enrich interpretation. Figure 7.4 shows the UNIVARIATE procedure to produce a probability plot. From it, Figure 7.6 shows that the vast majority of the data starting from the 3rd percentile to 95th percentile is arranged in a line, meaning that at least 92% of the data can clearly be represented by normal distribution; the rest of the data is close enough to a line and is also consistent with data coming from a normal distribution.

Figure 7.7 is based on the same code represented by Figure 7.4 but has the variable Y1 in the "probplot" statement. Being very different from Figure 7.6, as it should be, Figure 7.7 clearly gives a probability plot that is not linear and indicates that the data represented by variable Y1 is extremely different from that emanating from a normal distribution.

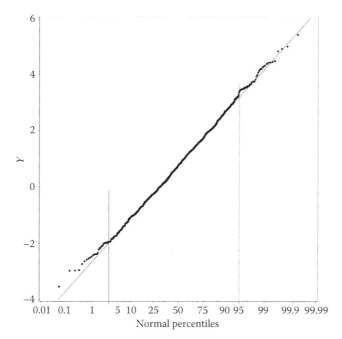

FIGURE 7.6
Probability plot for a normally distributed variable.

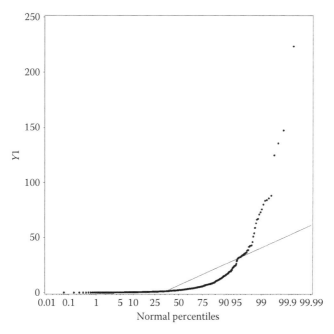

FIGURE 7.7
Probability plot for a log-normally distributed variable.

```
proc univariate data=_response_ NORMAL ;

Class Treatment;

run;
```

FIGURE 7.8
The UNIVARIATE procedure to produce normality tests by treatment.

The same dataset "_response_" described previously (see Figure 7.2) is used to illustrate tests of normality. Figure 7.8 shows the SAS implementation of the UNIVARIATE procedure to perform normality tests separately for each treatment cohort. Figure 7.9 includes descriptive statistics and displays the goodness-of-fit test results on normality for variable Y (normally distributed) in the cohort with *Treatment* = 0. All p-values for the tests of normality are above 0.05 and, therefore, provide evidence that normality cannot be rejected for variable Y.

Figure 7.10 displays the goodness-of-fit test results for normality for variables $Y1$ (not normally distributed) for the same cohort with *Treatment* = 0. Here, all p-values are below 0.05 and provides evidence to reject the hypothesis that $Y1$ comes from a population normal distribution.

```
The UNIVARIATE Procedure
Variable: Y
Treatment = 0
                              Moments
N                         486    Sum Weights               486
Mean               0.03459659    Sum Observations    16.8139429
Std Deviation      1.18430234    Variance            1.40257203
Skewness          -0.0726295     Kurtosis            -0.4183164
Uncorrected SS       680.82914   Corrected SS        680.247435
Coeff Variation     3423.17648   Std Error Mean      0.05372105
                  Basic Statistical Measures

      Location                        Variability

Mean       0.034597    Std Deviation           1.18430
Median     0.057941    Variance                1.40257
Mode         .         Range                   6.17128
                       Interquartile Range     1.64727

                  Tests for Normality

Test                    --Statistic---    -----p Value------

Shapiro-Wilk         W     0.995607    Pr < W        0.1904
Kolmogorov-Smirnov   D     0.020793    Pr > D       >0.1500
Cramer-von Mises     W-Sq  0.041573    Pr > W-Sq    >0.2500
Anderson-Darling     A-Sq  0.364193    Pr > A-Sq    >0.2500
```

FIGURE 7.9
The UNIVARIATE procedure: partial output for variable Y.

```
The UNIVARIATE Procedure
Variable: Y1
Treatment = 0

                  Tests for Normality

Test                    --Statistic---      -----p Value------

Shapiro-Wilk            W      0.643165      Pr < W      <0.0001
Kolmogorov-Smirnov      D      0.234846      Pr > D      <0.0100
Cramer-von Mises        W-Sq   8.59438       Pr > W-Sq   <0.0050
Anderson-Darling        A-Sq   45.82249      Pr > A-Sq   <0.0050
```

FIGURE 7.10
The UNIVARIATE procedure: partial output for variable Y1.

7.2 Comparing Two or More Samples

7.2.1 Nonparametric Methods

Consider PRO scores measured cross-sectionally (i.e., at a single time point) or as a single change from baseline between two treatment groups. A common practice is to assign the ordered categories of the scale with consecutive integer values as if the responses were measured on a continuous scale. Ordinal data are generally bounded and may have skewed distributions, for which nonparametric methods in principle may be considered more appropriate than parametric methods. In addition, inclusion and exclusion criteria may engender a truncation of the scores at baseline, with the observed data being restricted because subjects before treatment intervention are more likely to share more similar or homogeneous set of responses than they would after treatment intervention (assuming it is beneficial on average), which would lead to an increased range of responses.

Nonparametric methods do not rely on the assumption that data are drawn from a specified distribution. Nonparametric methods, such as the Wilcoxon rank-sum test for two independent groups and Kruskal–Wallis test for more than two independent groups, may be conducted to compare the distributions of different treatment groups on a quantitative outcome. The Wilcoxon signed-rank test can be used to compare two quantitative measurements from the same individual. Spearman's rank correlation can be used to estimate the degree of association between two quantitative variables. For binary outcomes, appropriate procedures include the chi-square test for the difference between two proportions from two independent groups and the McNemar test for the difference between two proportions from two related samples.

7.2.2 Parametric Methods

Although nonparametric tests have the desirable property of not requiring that the individual data values come from a normal distribution, they have two main drawbacks. The first is that they are generally less powerful than parametric procedures when the data are approximately normally distributed and hence less likely to show a significant difference when in fact one exists. The second drawback of nonparametric tests is that their results are often less easy to interpret than the results of parametric tests. Nonparametric tests involve tests of distributions, which may differ between groups because of differences in their medians, variances, or both, while parametric tests involve tests of means, which is generally what is desired.

Parametric methods, such as the two-sample Student's t-test for two independent groups and analysis of variance (ANOVA) for more than two independent groups, may be conducted for quantitative measurements to compare the underlying means between different treatment groups. The 95% confidence interval for the population mean PRO score at a particular visit or the population mean change score from baseline to a particular visit may be constructed. Hypothesis tests are based on using the t-test or the F-test. The paired t-test can be used to compare two quantitative measurements from the same individual. Pearson's rank correlation can be used to estimate the degree of linear association between two quantitative variables.

Conventional parametric statistical methods are generally robust enough to approximate correct inference on quantitative data. Although there may be concern that the assignment of integers to the categories is somewhat arbitrary and that the distances between adjacent scores do not represent equal gradations, moderate differences among various scoring systems seldom produce marked changes in conclusions (Baker et al., 1966; Snedecor and Cochran, 1980). For example, it has been recommended to assign integer scores to ordinal categories and conduct parametric methods when the data have an underlying continuous scale (Snedecor and Cochran, 1980).

The central limit theorem for means, one of the most celebrated results in statistics, makes the assumption of normality appropriate on the sampling distribution of the mean even if the individual data are not normally distributed, provided that the sample size is large enough. Therefore, parametric statistical tests for means are generally appropriate for quantitative data because of the central limit theorem (whether or not the individual data are normally distributed). Further support for parametric methods is based on the assignment of consecutive integers being viewed as just a monotonic transformation that is analogous to other types of transformations such as log and square root transformations, which are commonly employed to help correct departures from the usual assumptions. Thus, from a pragmatic perspective, under most circumstances (unless the distribution of scores is severely skewed), data from ordinal rating scales can be analyzed as if they were based on interval-level measurements without introducing severe bias.

7.2.3 Simulated Examples Using SAS: *t*-Test

In Section 7.1.3, the dataset "_response_" was generated (see Figure 7.2). All simulated subjects were assigned into one of two cohorts defined by the variable "Treatment": This dataset "_response_" is used in the current example (see Figure 7.11) to compare the means between two treatment groups via a two-sample *t*-test. Note that simulated data for *Treatment* = 0 were normally distributed values with mean of 0 and standard deviation of 1.2 (see Figure 7.2: Y = rannor(&seed2) * sqrt(1.2*1.2);), and for *Treatment* = 1 data were also normally distributed, but with mean of 1.5 and standard deviation of 1.3 (see Figure 7.2: Y = b1 + rannor(&seed3) * sqrt(1.3*1.3);).

Figure 7.12 represents the corresponding output. The difference in the sample means is −1.4385, which is close to the value of 1.5 specified in the simulation. The standard deviations for both distributions are estimated as 1.1843 and 1.3599 (vs 1.2 and 1.3 respectively in the simulation). It is important to first check "Equality of Variances." Here a *p*-value of 0.0021 would indicate rejection of the null hypothesis that the two populations, which gave rise to the two samples, have the same variance. Therefore, the Satterthwaite version of the two-sample Student's *t*-test should be used, as the Satterthwaite test assumes that these populations have unequal variances. With a *t*-value of −17.86 (whose absolute value is greater than 1.96, the critical *t*-value for a two-tailed test using a 0.05 level of significance) and corresponding *p*-value of $<.0001$, evidence exists to conclude that the underlying population means are statistically significantly different. Note that if the line from Figure 7.1 were changed from

```
Y = b1 + rannor(&seed3) * sqrt(1.3*1.3);
```

to

```
Y = b1 + rannor(&seed3) * sqrt(1.21*1.21);
```

then the "Equality of Variances" would not have been statistically significant (*p*-value of $0.1381 > 0.05$). In this case, the two-sample *t*-test that uses the pooled sample variance should be used.

```
Proc TTest data=_response_;
    Class Treatment;
    Var Y;
Run;
```

FIGURE 7.11
SAS codes for conducting a two-sample *t*-test to compare means.

```
The TTEST Procedure

Variable: Y

Treatment        N       Mean    Std Dev    Std Err    Minimum    Maximum

0              486     0.0346     1.1843     0.0537    -2.9685     3.2028
1              514     1.4731     1.3599     0.0600    -3.5290     5.4097
Diff (1-2)            -1.4385     1.2776     0.0808
```

Treatment		Mean	95% CL Mean		Std Dev	95% CL	Std Dev
0		0.0346	-0.0710	0.1402	1.1843	1.1142	1.2638
1		1.4731	1.3552	1.5909	1.3599	1.2816	1.4486
Diff (1-2)	Pooled	-1.4385	-1.5971	-1.2799	1.2776	1.2239	1.3362
Diff (1-2)	Satterthwaite	-1.4385	-1.5965	-1.2805			

Method	Variances	DF	t Value	Pr > |t|
Pooled	Equal	998	-17.80	<.0001
Satterthwaite	Unequal	991.36	-17.86	<.0001

```
Equality of Variances
```

Method	Num DF	Den DF	F Value	Pr > F
Folded F	513	485	1.32	0.0021

FIGURE 7.12
Two-sample *t*-test output.

7.3 Regression Analysis

PRO scores at a particular postbaseline time, or changes in PRO scores from baseline to a particular postbaseline time, may be modeled by adjusting or controlling for the baseline PRO value and other covariates in a multivariable model. The type of model depends in part on the type of outcome data. The treatment variable is generally considered as the main predictor (covariate) of interest, while the ancillary predictors (i.e., those to be adjusted for) are covariates such as baseline patient characteristics.

Provided the sample size is large enough, randomization in randomized trials is expected to make the distribution of both known confounders and unknown confounders similar between the treatment groups, so that any treatment effect is due to the treatment itself and not due to other variables. In randomized studies, covariates expected to be related to the outcome (e.g., a baseline PRO score is often used as a covariate because it is expected to be associated with a postbaseline PRO score) are often included in models in order to increase the precision of the treatment effect estimate, making it more efficient by decreasing its standard error. For instance, a PRO measure at baseline is frequently used as a covariate when the outcome or dependent variable is the corresponding PRO measure at postbaseline. In nonrandomized studies, covariates are included in models primarily to address the potential bias for the treatment effect estimate when these covariates, as confounders, are associated with not only the outcomes but also the treatment variable. This section covers two common types of multivariable models: logistic regression for a binary outcome and linear regression for a continuous outcome.

7.3.1 Binary Outcome Variable

Logistic regression models, which allow for the inclusion of covariates, are versatile enough for the analysis of nominal (including binary) and ordinal outcomes. The logistic model is popular because the logistic function, on which the model is based, provides two attractions: (1) estimates for the response categories of an outcome which lie in the range between 0 and 1 (thereby giving probability estimates to foster interpretation) and (2) an appealing S-shaped description of the combined effect of several covariates on the probability of response, which is discussed in more details in Section 7.3.3. A binary logistic regression analysis can be performed for a binary outcome.

As an extension of binary logistic regression, ordinal logistic regression can be performed for an ordinal outcome (i.e., ordered levels with more than two categories). The proportional odds model (also known as the cumulative logit model) is an example of an ordinal logistic regression model and assumes the same odds ratio regardless of where the response categories are dichotomized (i.e., the odds ratio is invariant to where the outcome categories are dichotomized) (Ananth and Kleinbaum, 1997; O'Connell, 2005; Cappelleri et al., 2007; Arostegui et al., 2012).

A detailed exposition on logistic regression models is found elsewhere (Kleinbaum and Klein, 2010; Hosmer et al., 2013). In this section, the focus is on binary logistic regression for a PRO measure with a dichotomous response.

Consider a PRO measure with only two response categories, such as yes or no, success or failure, present or absent, and improved or not improved (deterioration or stay the same). For instance, a PRO measure may require the choice of improved (*responder*) vs not improved (*nonresponder*) reported by patients from baseline to the end of the treatment. In this case, a binary logistic regression can be conducted with the following logit form:

$$\text{logit}(p) = \ln\left[\frac{p}{1-p}\right],$$

where
   p denotes the probability of response (success)
   ln denotes the natural logarithm (to base $e = 2.718281828...$)

The log odds of the probability of success may be modeled as a linear combination of the predictor variables.

Consider, for illustration, a two-arm study with 1000 subjects and each subject is given an active drug or a placebo. The outcome variable is represented by Y with a value of 1 given to a patient considered a responder and a value of 0 given to a patient not considered a responder. In addition to the treatment variable (0 = placebo, 1 = active drug), the main predictor or covariate of interest, age, is taken as a covariate in the model. Then the multivariable binary logistic regression model for subject i on treatment k can be written as

$$\ln\left[\frac{p_{ik}}{1-p_{ik}}\right] = a + b_i + r_k, \tag{7.1}$$

where
   p_{ik} is the probability to be a responder for subject i on treatment k ($i = 1, 2, ...,$
      1000; $k = 1, 2$)
   a is the model intercept
   b_i is the effect of age for subject i
   r_k is the effect of treatment k

For this model configuration, the corresponding simulated dataset is represented by Figure 7.13. This figure creates a dataset with a simulated binary outcome *Y*, *Treatment* assignment as the predictor of interest, and *Age* at baseline as an additional covariate. In order to understand how the simulation is created, some transformations are needed starting with Equation 7.1. An exponentiation of Equation 7.1 (to base *e*) gives

$$\exp\left[\ln\left[\frac{p_{ik}}{1-p_{ik}}\right]\right] = \exp[a + b_i + r_k].$$

```
/*
This example has 1000 subjects (NumberOfRows) and two covariates,
namely, Treatment (0 or 1) and Age (with values from 20 to 30).
*/

options nofmterr nocenter pagesize=2000 linesize=256;

%Let NumberOfRows = 1000;

%Let seed1 = 1;
%Let seed2 = 2;
%Let seed3 = 3;

Data binary_response;
    b0 = -1;                /* Intercept     */
    b1 = 1;                 /* Treatment effect */
    b2 = 0.07;              /* Age effect */

        Do i=1 To &NumberOfRows;

            Age= 20 + 10*ranuni(&seed1);

            If ranuni(&seed2)>=0.5 Then
              Do;
              Treatment=1;
              End;
            Else
              Do;
              Treatment=0;
              End;

            eta = b0 + b1*Treatment + b2*Age;
            prob = exp(eta) / (1 + exp(eta));

            Y= ranbin(&seed3,1,prob);
            output;

        End;

    Keep Y Treatment Age;
  Run;
```

FIGURE 7.13
SAS codes to create simulated dataset for logistic regression.

Then, through a series of algebraic transformations, the following set of equations unfolds and results in Equation 7.2:

$$\frac{p_{ik}}{1-p_{ik}} = \exp[a+b_i+r_k]$$

$$p_{ik} = (1-p_{ik}) \times \exp[a+b_i+r_k]$$

$$p_{ik} + p_{ik} \times \exp[a+b_i+r_k] = \exp[a+b_i+r_k]$$

$$p_{ik}(1+\exp[a+b_i+r_k]) = \exp[a+b_i+r_k]$$

$$p_{ik} = \frac{\exp[a+b_i+r_k]}{1+\exp[a+b_i+r_k]}. \tag{7.2}$$

Note that the following two lines of SAS code (from Figure 7.13) directly correspond to Equation 7.2:

```
eta = b0 + b1*Treatment + b2*Age;

prob = exp(eta)/(1 + exp(eta));
```

Figure 7.14 represents the implementation of the logistic regression using the SAS LOGISTIC procedure and Figure 7.15 represents its partial output. The p-values from this logistic regression analysis show that the effects of *Treatment* and *Age* are estimated, respectively, as 0.9206 and 0.0698 (which were defined, respectively, as 1 and 0.07 in the simulated dataset). The estimated intercept value of -0.9944 also corresponds well to the value of -1 assigned to the intercept parameter in the simulation.

To understand and interpret the odds ratio, let us consider an equation where the function g depends on treatment and age. This particular equation is based on our example and corresponds to the general Equation 7.1:

$$g(Treatment, Age) = \ln\left[\frac{p_1}{1-p_1}\right] = b_0 + b_1 Treatment + b_2 Age.$$

```
Proc Logistic data=binary_response;
       Model Y (event='1') = Treatment Age / CLODDS=WALD;
       Unit Treatment=1 Age=10;
   Run;
```

FIGURE 7.14
SAS implementation of logistic regression.

```
                Analysis of Maximum Likelihood Estimates

                              Standard         Wald
     Parameter   DF    Estimate    Error    Chi-Square    Pr > ChiSq

     Intercept    1    -0.9944     0.6655      2.2328        0.1351
     Treatment    1     0.9206     0.1557     34.9463       <.0001
     Age          1     0.0698     0.0264      6.9925        0.0082

                Odds Ratio Estimates

                    Point             95% Wald
     Effect        Estimate       Confidence Limits

     Treatment      2.511          1.850         3.407
     Age            1.072          1.018         1.129

     Association of Predicted Probabilities and Observed Responses

     c              0.637

                Wald Confidence Interval for Odds Ratios

     Effect            Unit      Estimate    95% Confidence Limits

     Treatment        1.0000      2.511        1.850         3.407
     Age             10.0000      2.010        1.198         3.372
```

FIGURE 7.15
Partial output from the binary logistic regression analysis.

Now consider two subjects. The first subject is on active treatment (*Treatment* = 1) and has Age_1:

$$g(1, Age_1) = \ln\left[\frac{p_1}{1-p_1}\right] = b_0 + b_1 1 + b_2 Age_1.$$

The second subject is on placebo (*Treatment* = 0) and has Age_2:

$$g(0, Age_2) = \ln\left[\frac{p_2}{1-p_2}\right] = b_0 + b_1 0 + b_2 Age_2.$$

The odds ratio (OR) to be a responder is defined as the ratio of the odds of being a responder in one group relative to another group. Then the (natural) logarithm of the odds ratio can be formulated as

$$\ln(OR) = g(1, Age_1) - g(2, Age_2)$$

$$\ln(OR) = (a + b_1 1 + b_2 Age_1) - (a + b_1 0 + b_2 Age_2)$$

$$\ln(OR) = b_1 + b_2 (Age_1 - Age_2).$$

If $Age_1 = Age_2$ (i.e., the two subjects have the same age), then

$$\ln(\text{OR}) = b_1.$$

The parameter b_1 associated with *Treatment* represents the change in the logarithm of the odds from *Treatment* = 0 to *Treatment* = 1. As such, the odds ratio is calculated by exponentiating the value of the parameter associated with *Treatment*. In Figure 7.15, the value of b_1 is 0.9206 and hence OR = $e^{0.9206}$ = 2.511. This odds ratio estimate may be interpreted as follows: the odds of being a responder for a patient who received active treatment (*Treatment* = 1) is two and a half (2.511) times that for a patient who received placebo treatment. Note that this simple interpretation of the OR is appropriate only if both subjects have the same age and there is no age-by-treatment interaction (as noted previously). Hence, the odds ratio of 2.51 for treatment effect is adjusted (or controlled) for age.

Consider next the covariate *Age*. For two subjects with a 1-year age difference, the odds of being a responder for the *older* subject is 1.07 (1.072) times that for the *younger* subject. Note that for this interpretation to be correct both patients need to have received the same treatment, which follows the same logic given for the interpretation of the treatment effect odds ratio for subjects of the same age. Hence, the odds ratio of 1.07 for the age effect is adjusted for treatment.

A difference of only 1 year may be viewed as too small for practical interest. If so, the "Unit" statement in the LOGISTIC procedure provides the solution. For example, the statement (from Figure 7.14)

```
Unit Treatment = 1 Age = 10;
```

will trigger a set of additional estimated odds ratios (see the last two lines in Figure 7.15). A 10-year difference leads to an odds ratio of two (2.010). The treatment effect (odds ratio of 2.511) does not change as the difference between treatment codes was already based on one unit (0 = placebo, 1 = active).

It is important to verify the association of predicted probabilities and observed responses (see "Association of Predicted Probabilities and Observed Responses" in Figure 7.15). In particular, the *c*-statistic is a commonly used measure of how well the model can be used to discriminate subjects having the event (e.g., responder) from those not having the event (e.g., nonresponder). This *c*-statistic is the same as the area under curve for the receiver operating characteristic curve discussed in Sections 3.2.3, 7.2.1, and elsewhere (Zou et al., 2011; Alemayehu and Zou, 2012). In the current chapter, the *c*-statistic addresses how often a randomly chosen (true) responder will have a higher probability of being predicted to be a responder (based on a model that includes treatment and age) than a randomly true nonresponder. As a measure of discrimination and a goodness of fit to compare different logistic regression models, the *c*-statistic has values that cover perfect discrimination (*c*-statistic = 1), positive discrimination ($0.5 < c \leq 1$), negative discrimination

$(0.0 \leq c < 0.5)$, and no discrimination $(c = 0.5)$. Thus, a c-statistic value of 0.5 indicates that the model is no better than chance (no better than a coin toss) at making a prediction of membership in a group. A value of 1.0, on the other hand, indicates that the model perfectly identifies true group membership.

In the simulation, the c-statistic is 0.637. As a gauge for interpretation, values of c-statistic greater than 0.7 but less than 0.8 indicate acceptable discrimination and values greater than 0.8 but less than 0.9 indicate excellent discrimination (Hosmer et al., 2013). While useful, these ranges should be taken as a rough guideline. For example, if only 100 observations (instead of 1000 observations) were generated in our simulated example, by assigning a value of 100 to NumberOfRows (Figure 7.13: %Let NumberOfRows = 1000;), then the c-statistic will be 0.731. Although the guideline would suggest that the corresponding model has *acceptable discrimination*, estimations for the effects of treatment and age, as well as intercept, turned out to be well off the population values assigned to them in the simulations.

7.3.2 Continuous Outcome Variable

For a dependent variable taken as a single continuous outcome, such as many PRO measures, specialized regression models are commonly employed (Kleinbaum et al., 2007; Chatterjee and Hadi, 2012). Such a regression analysis is a standard approach to model the relationship between a dependent variable taken as a continuous outcome and one or more explanatory variables, which may be continuous, categorical, or both. The case of one explanatory variable (covariate or predictor) can be referred to as simple regression and more than one explanatory variable (multiple covariates or predictors) can be referred to as multiple regression. These regression models are often referred to as ordinary linear regression models (ordinary simple linear regression and multiple linear regression) because the continuous outcome depends linearly on the unknown parameters (regression coefficients) associated with the set of covariates.

As with logistic regression (for a categorical outcome), regression for a continuous outcome involves the modeling of data using a predictor function and the unknown model parameters are estimated from the data. Like logistic regression, regression for a continuous outcome is popular because of its rich and abundant applications that generally involve characterization or prediction: (1) characterizing the relationship—the extent, direction, and strength—between outcome and explanatory variables and (2) predicting the outcome as a function of predictors via a quantitative formula or equation.

Methods for simple and multiple regression analyses are general enough to encompass predictors taken as continuous, categorical, or both types. When the dependent variable is considered as a continuous outcome, models with specialized names and techniques have been applied frequently. When all predictors are nominal categories, an analysis of variance model can be used. If at least one predictor is continuous while at least another is categorical, an analysis of covariance model can be implemented.

More complicated models, including those involving an interaction effect of two covariates on the outcome and those with a covariate requiring a transformation (e.g., a continuous covariate with both a quadratic term and linear term) to satisfy a model assumption, also fall under the same rubric of multiple linear regression analysis. Even more generally, all models mentioned in this chapter, as well as several others not mentioned in this book, belong to a family of statistical models called generalized linear models because these models share a number of properties such as linearity, where some function of the expected value of the response variable is based on a linear equation with respect to the covariates (McCullagh and Nelder, 1989).

Regression models for continuous outcomes are expected to perform well even when the outcomes are ordinal and therefore not strictly continuous. For example, the analysis of covariance on differences between groups applied to ordinal data arising in randomized controlled trials has been shown to be *robust* and have good *power* even in small samples (Sullivan and D'Agostino, 2003). *Robust* here means that the observed type I error rates (i.e., the probability of rejecting the null hypothesis of no difference in adjusted treatment means between two groups when it should not be rejected) are close to the preselected (or nominal) type I error rates in the presence of violations of assumptions. *Power* here means the probability of rejecting the null hypothesis when it should be rejected and is equal to one minus the observed type II error rates (i.e., one minus the probability of not rejecting the null hypothesis of no difference in adjusted treatment means between two groups when it should be rejected).

To illustrate linear regression analysis, we borrow from the simulated example described in Section 7.3.1. The difference will be in the outcome variable, now taken as a continuous outcome Y instead of a binary outcome. A linear regression model for subject i on treatment k can then be written as a sum of four terms:

$$Y_{ik} = a + b_i + r_k + e_{ik}, \tag{7.3}$$

where
  Y_{ik} is the PRO response for subject i on treatment k ($i = 1, 2, \ldots, 1000; k = 1, 2$)
  a is the model intercept
  b_i is the effect of age for subject i
  r_k is the effect of treatment k
  e_{ik} is the error term associated with the outcome measurement Y_{ik}

It is assumed that errors e_{ik} are independent between subjects. The error term is assumed to be from a normal distribution with mean 0 and variance σ^2—that is, for any subject i on treatment k, $e_{jk} \sim N(0, \sigma^2)$.

A simulated dataset corresponding to the aforementioned example is represented by Figure 7.16. The following SAS code line (from Figure 7.16)

```
Y = b0 + b1*Treatment + b2*Age + rannor(&seed3)*sqrt(0.4*0.4);
```

directly corresponds to Equation 7.3. Figure 7.17 represents the implementation of the regression analysis using the SAS REG procedure, and Figure 7.18 represents its partial output. The output shows that estimations of the *Treatment* effect and *Age* effect (respectively, 1.02461 and 0.08290) are close to values used in the simulation (respectively, 1 and 0.07). At the same time, even with 1000 subjects, the REG procedure was a bit off in

```
/*
This example has 1000 subjects (NumberOfRows) and two covariates
called Treatment (0 or 1) and Age (with values from 20 to 30).
*/

options nofmterr nocenter pagesize=2000 linesize=256;

%Let NumberOfRows = 1000;

%Let seed1 = 1;
%Let seed2 = 2;
%Let seed3 = 3;

Data cont_response;

    b0 = -1;                /* Intercept     */
    b1 = 1;                 /* Treatment effect */
    b2 = 0.07;              /* Age effect */

        Do i=1 To &NumberOfRows;

          Age= 20 + 10*ranuni(&seed1);

          If ranuni(&seed2)>=0.5 Then
            Do;
            Treatment=1;
            End;
          Else
            Do;
            Treatment=0;
            End;

          Y = b0 + b1*Treatment + b2*Age + rannor(&seed3) *sqrt(0.4*0.4);
          output;

        End;

    Keep Y Treatment Age;
  Run;
```

FIGURE 7.16
SAS code to create simulated dataset for linear regression analysis.

```
Proc Reg data=cont_response ;

          Model Y = Treatment Age ;

Run;
```

FIGURE 7.17
SAS implementation of linear regression analysis.

Analysis of Variance					
Root MSE	0.40640		R-Square	0.6596	
Parameter Estimates					
Variable	DF	Parameter Estimate	Standard Error	t Value	Pr > |t|
Intercept	1	-1.34656	0.11196	-12.03	<.0001
Treatment	1	1.02461	0.02570	39.86	<.0001
Age	1	0.08290	0.00439	18.88	<.0001

FIGURE 7.18
Partial output from the linear regression analysis.

estimating the intercept well enough (the estimated value of −1.34656 was noticeably different from the simulated value of −1). The estimation of the variance of the error term was 0.41 (Figure 7.18: Root MSE = 0.40640), close to the value of 0.4 used in simulations. For linear regression, the estimated R^2 is often reported (here R-square = 0.6596). Hence, about 70% of variability in Y can be explained by the regression model (Equation 7.3) used to model the data.

7.3.3 Advanced Example: Logistic Regression versus Ordinary Linear Regression

In the prior sections, two models, represented by Equations 7.1 and 7.3, were discussed. Although generally looking the same, they are quite different and they have very important distinctions. First, Equation 7.1 has no error term but Equation 7.3 has. Second, in case of the ordinary linear regression (Equation 7.3), the outcome is the *observed* value. But in logistic regression (Equation 7.1), the outcome is the logit of the *predicted* probability. In the case of ordinary linear regression, *if* we already estimated parameters of the model, the error term also would not and should not be present. The reason is that now this is the exact formula for relationships between variables, and Equation 7.3 can be expressed as

$$YPRED_{ik} = a + b_i + r_k, \qquad (7.4)$$

where
   $YPRED_{ik}$ is the predicted value of PRO response for subject i on treatment
      k ($i = 1, 2,..., 1000; k = 1, 2$)
   a, b_i, r_k are the same as in Equation 7.3

It is important to stress that in Equation 7.1 the probabilities p_{ik} are, in fact, estimated (predicted) probabilities and, as a result, Equation 7.1 can be considered to represent exact relationships between variables, and the error term is not needed and should not be there. This leads us to ask how the observed binary outcomes (*responder* vs *nonresponder*) are related to the predicted probabilities p_{ik}.

To understand this, we can first consider a linear probability model in the following form:

$$Y_{ik} = a + b_i + r_k + e_{ik}, \qquad (7.5)$$

where
   Y_{ik} is 1 if a subject is a *responder* and 0 if *nonresponder* ($i = 1, 2,...,1000; k = 1,2$)
   a is the model intercept
   b_i is the effect of age for subject i
   r_k is the effect of treatment k
   e_{ik} is the error term associated with the outcome measurement Y_{ik}

Two points need to be addressed here. First, the observed outcome is binary (either 0 or 1), but, after fitting the model, the predicted values of the outcome can be not only between 0 and 1 (which are required of probabilities) but also outside this range, taking values more than 1 or even less than 0. Second, error terms for responders ($Y_{ik} = 1$) can be expressed as

$$e_{ik} = 1 - YPED_{ik}, \qquad (7.6)$$

and error terms for nonresponders ($Y_{ik} = 0$) can be expressed as

$$e_{ik} = 0 - YPED_{ik}. \qquad (7.7)$$

From Equations 7.6 and 7.7, the following two conclusions can be drawn: first, the error term is not normally distributed and, second, the values of the errors are dependent on the predicted values of the outcomes, in contrast to ordinary linear regression where the error term is independent with mean of zero and constant variance (see Equation 7.3).

To resolve these issues found with the linear probability model, the logistic regression was proposed. The most important part in this approach is that we do not model directly the binary outcome Y_{ik} but rather model it through the *logit* function. The *logit* function has the advantages of being continuous and constraining the values of probabilities to be between 0 and 1 (see Figure 7.19).

To further understand the inner workings of logistic regression, we can consider the following example. Suppose there are 34 subjects with effect X (e.g., age) and binary outcome Y (responder vs nonresponder):

$$Y_i(1 \text{ if a responder, 0 if nonresponder}) \tag{7.8}$$

$$\ln\left[\frac{p_1}{(1-p_1)}\right] = a + b \times X_i, \tag{7.9}$$

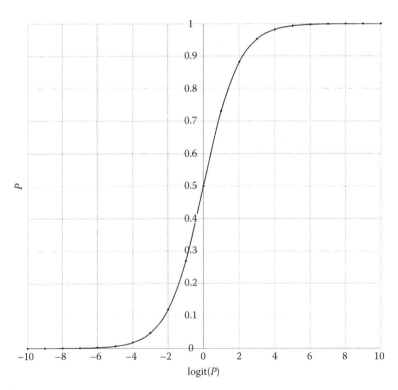

FIGURE 7.19
Relationship between probability P and logit(P).

TABLE 7.1

Data for Logistic Modeling

ID	X	Y
1	12	1
2	16	1
3	4	0
4	8	0
...		
30	18	1
31	14	1
32	18	1
33	6	0
34	4	0

where

Y_i is the observed binary outcome (1 if a responder, 0 if nonresponder) ($i = 1, 2,...,34$; see Table 7.1)

p_i is the probability to be a responder for subject i ($i = 1, 2,...,34$)

a is the model intercept

b is the slope coefficient for the effect of X_i on response Y_i for subject i

The question of interest is how Equation 7.8 can be linked to Equation 7.9. To do this, a maximum likelihood (ML) algorithm needs to be introduced. The idea behind the ML algorithm is to maximize the probability of success associated with the observed results. To estimate these probabilities, Equation 7.2 can be rewritten as

$$p_i = \frac{\exp[a + b \times X_i]}{1 + \exp[a + b \times X_i]},$$

which can be further transformed into

$$p_i = \frac{1}{1 + \exp[-a - b \times X_i]}. \tag{7.10}$$

The first subject (ID = 1) has covariate $X = 12$ and outcome $Y = 1$. By using Equation 7.10, the probability of this result can be estimated as

$$p_1 = \frac{1}{1 + \exp[-a - b \times 12]}.$$

It is important to note that this is the probability of success (e.g., being a responder). But for the third subject (ID = 3), $X = 4$ and $Y = 0$. Because this subject was a nonresponder, this means that the probability of this outcome should be calculated as

$$1 - (\text{probability of success}),$$

which means that probability of this result can be estimated as

$$p_3 = 1 - \frac{1}{1 + \exp[-a - b \times 4]}.$$

Now the likelihood (L) can be estimated to observe all 34 outcomes (from the 34 subjects) simultaneously. Under the assumption that all 34 observations are independent, the probability to observe them together is simply the product of those probabilities:

$$L = p_1 \times p_2 \times p_3 \times \cdots \times p_{34}.$$

To simplify calculations without loss in generality, the LOG transformation (to base 10) is typically applied:

$$\log(L) = \log(p_1) + \log(p_2) + \log(p_3) + \cdots + \log(p_{34}). \tag{7.11}$$

What is now needed is to find values of the parameters a and b that will maximize the value of $\log(L)$. For this, we can use any general algorithm that can minimize or maximize a function. In SAS, the general NLP procedure can be used (see Figure 7.20; SAS, 2012). Traditionally, instead of maximizing $\log(L)$, minimizing $-2 \log(L)$ is used instead (the negative sign makes the result positive and the "2" is used in the event that the fits of two models are to be compared using a chi-square distribution).

Figure 7.20 illustrates the ML estimation algorithm to estimate parameters of the logistic regression using the NLP procedure. Note that the SAS code

```
LogL = -2* (

Log(1/(1+exp(-a-b*12))) +

Log(1/(1+exp(-a-b*16))) +

Log(1-1/(1+exp(-a-b*4)))+

...

Log(1-1/(1+exp(-a-b*4)))));
```

```
Data binary_response;
Input ID X Y;
Datalines;
1   12  1
2   16  1
3    4  0
4    8  0
5   18  1
6    6  0
7   10  0
8    8  1
9   14  1
10  10  1
11  16  1
12   6  0
13  12  1
14   8  0
15  10  1
16   8  0
17  18  1
18  12  1
19   6  1
20   4  0
21   6  0
22  14  1
23   4  0
24   8  0
25  10  1
26   6  0
27  16  1
28  12  1
29  12  0
30  18  1
31  14  1
32  18  1
33   6  0
34   4  0
;
Run;

Proc NLP data=_null_;
min LogL;
parms a=1, b=1; /*initial values to get procedure started */

LogL= -2*(
Log(1/(1+exp(-a-b*12))) +
Log(1/(1+exp(-a-b*16))) +
```

FIGURE 7.20
Example of the implementation of the logistic regression through *hand-written* maximum likelihood.

(*continued*)

```
Log(1-1/(1+exp(-a-b*4)))+
Log(1-1/(1+exp(-a-b*8)))+
Log(1/(1+exp(-a-b*18)))  +
Log(1-1/(1+exp(-a-b*6)))+
Log(1-1/(1+exp(-a-b*10)))+
Log(1/(1+exp(-a-b*8)))  +
Log(1/(1+exp(-a-b*14)))  +
Log(1/(1+exp(-a-b*10)))  +
Log(1/(1+exp(-a-b*16)))  +
Log(1-1/(1+exp(-a-b*6)))+
Log(1/(1+exp(-a-b*12)))  +
Log(1-1/(1+exp(-a-b*8)))+
Log(1/(1+exp(-a-b*10)))  +
Log(1-1/(1+exp(-a-b*8)))+
Log(1/(1+exp(-a-b*18)))  +
Log(1/(1+exp(-a-b*12)))  +
Log(1/(1+exp(-a-b*6)))  +
Log(1-1/(1+exp(-a-b*4)))+
Log(1-1/(1+exp(-a-b*6)))+
Log(1/(1+exp(-a-b*14)))  +
Log(1-1/(1+exp(-a-b*4)))+
Log(1-1/(1+exp(-a-b*8)))+
Log(1/(1+exp(-a-b*10)))  +
Log(1-1/(1+exp(-a-b*6)))+
Log(1/(1+exp(-a-b*16)))  +
Log(1/(1+exp(-a-b*12)))  +
Log(1-1/(1+exp(-a-b*12)))+
Log(1/(1+exp(-a-b*18)))  +
Log(1/(1+exp(-a-b*14)))  +
Log(1/(1+exp(-a-b*18)))  +
Log(1-1/(1+exp(-a-b*6)))  +
Log(1-1/(1+exp(-a-b*4)))));
Run;

Proc Logistic data=binary_response ;
      model Y ( EVENT='1') = X ;
Run;
```

FIGURE 7.20 (continued)
Example of the implementation of the logistic regression through *hand-written* maximum likelihood.

corresponds to Equation 7.11 (multiplied by −2). Figure 7.20 also involves an assessment of the model's parameters using the LOGISTIC procedure. Figure 7.21 demonstrates that *a* and *b* estimated by the *hand-written* ML (using NLP procedure) are the same as those produced by LOGISTIC procedure estimates for *a* (Intercept = −6.3441) and *b* (the slope parameter; X = 0.6900). Also note that the "Value of Objective Function" in the NPL results is exactly the same as the value of "−2 Log L" in the LOGISTIC results.

The LOGISTIC Procedure				PROC NLP: Nonlinear Minimization			
Model Fit Statistics							
	Intercept and						
Criterion	Covariates						
AIC	25.414						
SC	28.466			Value of Objective Function =			
-2 Log L	21.414			21.413516299			
Analysis of Maximum Likelihood Estimates				Optimization Results Parameter Estimates			
							Gradient Objective
Parameter DF	Estimate	Pr > ChiSq		N Parameter		Estimate	Function
Intercept 1	−6.3441	0.0031		1 a		−6.344269	−9.93897E−13
X 1	0.6900	0.0026		2 b		0.690055	−5.20331E−11

FIGURE 7.21
Results of the estimations using NLP and LOGISTIC procedures.

7.4 Summary

This chapter focuses on an outcome at a particular time point within a study or a single measurement of change from baseline to a later time point. We have confined our attention to methods for a single postbaseline time point or a single change from baseline to a postbaseline time point, with the postbaseline assessment typically made at either the end of the study or at a clinically relevant time point. Two major regression models—logistic regression and linear regression—are described and simulated. The estimation of the parameters of the logistic regression is illustrated via the use of the ML algorithm. For cross-sectional multivariable regression analysis of PRO data, it is generally recommended to prespecify the statistical model, including the covariates of interest, in the protocol and analysis plan. In Chapter 8, the longitudinal analysis of PRO data simultaneously across all time points will be discussed in detail.

References

Alemayehu, D. and K.H. Zou. 2012. Applications of ROC analysis in medical research: Recent developments and future directions. *Academic Radiology* 19:1457–1464.

Ananth, C.V. and D.G. Kleinbaum. 1997. Regression models for ordinal responses: A review of methods and applications. *International Journal of Epidemiology* 26:1323–1333.

Arostegui, I., Núñez-Antón, V., and J.M. Quintana. 2012. Statistical approaches to analyse patient-reported outcomes as response variables: An application to health-related quality of life. *Statistical Methods in Medical Research* 21:189–214.

Baker, B.O., Hardyck, C.D., and L.F. Petrinovich. 1966. Weak measurements vs. strong statistics: An empirical critique of S. S. Steven's proscriptions on statistics. *Educational and Psychological Measurement* 26:291–309.

Cappelleri, J.C., Bell, S.S., and R.L. Siegel. 2007. Interpretation of a self-esteem subscale for erectile dysfunction by cumulative logit model. *Drug Information Journal* 41:723–732.

Chatterjee, S. and A.S. Hadi. 2012. *Regression by Example*, 5th edition. Hoboken, NJ: John Wiley & Sons.

DeVellis, R.F. 2012. *Scale Development: Theory and Applications*. Thousand Oaks, CA: Sage Publications.

Fleiss, J.L., Levin, B., and M. Cho Paik. 2002. *Statistical Methods for Rates & Proportion*, 3rd edition. Hoboken, NJ: Wiley-Interscience.

Food and Drug Administration (FDA). 2009. Guidance for industry on patient-reported outcome measures: Use in medical product development to support labeling claims. *Federal Register* 74(235):65132–65133. Also available at : http://www.fda.gov/Drugs/DevelopmentApprovalProcess/DrugDevelopmentToolsQualificationProgram/ucm284399.htm. (Accessed on August 31, 2013).

Hosmer, D.W., Jr., Lemeshow, S. and R.X. Sturdivant. 2013. *Applied Logistic Regression*, 3rd edition. Hoboken, NJ: John Wiley & Sons.

Kleinbaum, D.G. and M. Klein. 2010. *Logistic Regression: A Self-Learning Text*, 3rd edition. New York, NY: Springer.

Kleinbaum, D.G., Kupper, L.L., Mizam, A., and K.E. Muller. 2007. *Applied Regression Analysis and Other Multivariable Methods*, 4th edition. Belmont, CA: Duxbury Press.

McCullagh, P. and J.A. Nelder. 1989. *Generalized Linear Models*, 2nd edition. Boca Raton, FL: Chapman & Hall/CRC Press.

McDowell, I. 2006. *Measuring Health: A Guide to Rating Scales and Questionnaires*, 3rd edition. New York, NY: Oxford University Press.

O'Connell, A.A. 2005. *Logistic Regression Models for Ordinal Response Variables*. Thousand Oaks, CA: Sage Publications.

Rosner, B. 2010. *Fundamentals of Biostatistics*, 7th edition. Boston, MA: Duxbury Resource Center.

SAS Institute Inc. 2012. *SAS/OR® 9.3 User's Guide: Mathematical Programming*. Cary, NC: SAS Institute Inc.

Snedecor, G.W. and W.G. Cochran. 1980. *Statistical Methods*, 7th edition. Ames, IA: The Iowa State University Press.

Streiner, D.L. and G.R. Norman. 2008. *Health Measurement Scales: A Practical Guide to Their Development and Use*, 4th edition. New York, NY: Oxford University Press.

Sullivan, L.M. and R.B. D'Agostino Sr. 2003. Robustness and power of analysis of covariance applied to ordinal scaled data as arising in randomized controlled trials. *Statistics in Medicine* 22:1317–1334.

van Belle, G., Heagerty, P.J., Fisher, L.D., and T.S. Lumley. 2004. *Biostatistics: A Methodology for the Health Sciences*, 2nd edition. Hoboken, NJ: John Wiley & Sons.

Zou, K.H., Fielding J.R., Silverman S.G., and C.M. Tempany. 2003a. Hypothesis testing I: Proportions. *Radiology* 226:609–613.

Zou, K.H., Liu, A., Bandos, A., Ohno-Machado, L., and H.E. Rockette. 2011. *Statistical Evaluation of Diagnostic Performance: Topics in ROC Analysis*. Boca Raton, FL: Chapman & Hall/CRC Press.

Zou, K.H., Tuncali, K., and S.G. Silverman. 2003b. Correlation and simple linear regression. *Radiology* 227:617–622.

8

Longitudinal Analysis

Patient-reported outcomes (PROs) measures are often incorporated into a study by administering questionnaires at multiple time points with the goal of characterizing the outcome over time (Fairclough, 2004, 2005, 2010). These measurements are provided by the same individual repeatedly over time, allowing for the direct study of change. Such longitudinal data arise in most PRO investigations because interest centers on how a disease or intervention affects an individual's functioning and well-being over time. Longitudinal analysis also considers how groups change over time and how between-group factors like treatment affect different intervention groups over time. Longitudinal analysis has become central in drawing inferences about PRO measures.

The design of a longitudinal study is an important prerequisite in the analysis of longitudinal data (Fairclough, 2010). The number and timing of PRO assessments are influenced by the study objectives, such as when meaningful change is expected, and practical considerations, such as patient burden and when investigators have access to the subjects for clinical assessments.

Longitudinal data can appear in different forms for different purposes, for example in the estimation of clinical important differences (Chapter 11). This chapter focuses on longitudinal models for examining effects in the context of a single-group design or parallel multiple-group design. The conceptual and practical importance of PRO instruments assessed longitudinally is featured by a detailed description on the implementation of the two approaches generally referred to as random coefficient models and repeated measures models. These models are mainstream approaches for the analysis of longitudinal data.

Methodology is illustrated with applications to the data from clinical studies on renal cell carcinoma and smoking cessation. Simulated SAS examples also highlight and illustrate the methods discussed. In this chapter PRO measures are considered and analyzed as continuous variables. For modeling discrete outcomes, generalized estimating equations and generalized linear mixed-effects models are available, which are not discussed in this chapter and can be found elsewhere (see, for example, Fitzmaurice et al., 2011).

8.1 Analytic Considerations

Descriptive statistics on means (and their variability) at each time point can be analyzed cross-sectionally (at one particular time point, without considering the other time points) for a useful preliminary examination of the data. But, unlike cross-sectional data analysis, longitudinal data analysis acknowledges and accounts for the repeated nature of PRO responses on the same subject over time rather than isolating the data at a given time points.

In doing so, longitudinal analysis allows for inferences on within-individual changes that cannot be made from cross-sectional analysis. A simple observed mean within treatment group and between treatment groups (as well as mean change from baseline), along with their corresponding sample sizes and 95% confidence intervals, at each follow-up assessment can provide valuable descriptive insights. Even more informative, however, is the coalescing of responses of temporal trajectories from two or more follow-up (correlated) measurements within a single integrated and cohesive model that encompasses all available data simultaneously (i.e., all available observations from all available participants).

The main objective of longitudinal analysis is to account for systematic patterns in within-individual changes in the response variable (e.g., a PRO measure) and to relate these changes to interindividual differences in selected covariates (e.g., treatment group). A single statistical model for longitudinal data, which incorporates all available data, can be used to capture both how individuals change over time and how to relate within-individual changes to selected covariates. Several models can be considered for different types of analyses; the specific type of longitudinal model depends on the nature of the data and the objective of the study.

Because the analysis of PRO measures is similar to that of other quantitative outcomes, no special allowances are described here for PRO measures. For more detail on longitudinal analysis, especially on the topics covered in this chapter, several books can be consulted (Singer and Willett, 2003; Weiss, 2005; Brown and Prescott, 2006; Hedeker and Gibbons, 2006; Littell et al., 2006; Fairclough, 2010; Fitzmaurice et al., 2011; Newsom et al., 2012; Vonesh, 2012).

8.2 Repeated Measures Model

The most common example of the repeated measures experiment is the randomized clinical study to investigate benefits of a new drug compared with another drug or placebo. Frequently, outcomes of interest are collected at prespecified time points at the same set of times for every subject, such as every week. It does not mean that all measurements should be collected exactly every 7 days, but the time points should be generalizable to be considered as if they were collected at the same time. For weekly measurements, for example, data collected at day 7 plus or minus 3 days can be considered simply as data collected at "Week 1," data collected at day 14 plus or minus 3 days can be considered as data collected at "Week 2," and so on. It is not necessary that data be collected at equal time intervals; for instance, data could be collected daily during the first week of the study and weekly afterward.

One of the most important advantages of modeling data using repeated measures analysis is the ability to model relationships between error or disturbance terms (unexplained or random variation not accounted for by the model, and quantified by the difference between the observed response and the predicted response) at different time points for a subject—that is, the ability to approximate the variance–covariance matrix of error (or residual) terms. It is not necessarily assumed that the variance of error terms should be the same at every time point for a given subject. Errors between time points are also allowed to covary for a subject.

8.2.1 Repeated Measures with Time as a Categorical Covariate

Consider a hypothetical example of a clinical two-arm study for a new treatment. Six hundred subjects are selected from the population of interest. Each subject is given an active drug or placebo during the 4-week study. The outcome variable is a PRO measure (Y) and the covariates are time and treatment. Generally, treatment is referred to as a within-subject fixed effect (again, common or shared by all individuals) and time is referred to as a within-subject fixed effect (again, common or shared by all individuals). One simple form of a regression model for subject i at measurement occasion j on treatment k can be denoted as a sum of four terms:

$$Y_{ijk} = a + b_j + r_k + e_{ijk}, \tag{8.1}$$

where
  Y_{ijk} is the PRO response for subject i at the measurement occasion j on treatment k ($i = 1, 2,\ldots,600; j = 1, 2, 3, 4; k = 1, 2$)
  a is the overall mean
  b_j is the fixed time effect at week j
  r_k is the fixed effect of the treatment k
  e_{ijk} is the error term associated with outcome measurement Y_{ijk}

It is assumed that errors e_{ijk} are independent between subjects but covary within a subject. For example, for any subject at week j, the error term is assumed to be from a normal distribution with mean 0 and variance σ_j^2, that is, for any subject i at week j on treatment k, $e_{ijk} \sim N(0, \sigma_j^2)$. As mentioned previously, it is also generally presumed that error terms covary over time within a subject. For example, the error term at week n will covary with the error term at week m ($n = 1, 2, 3, 4; m = 1, 2, 3, 4; n \neq m$) with covariance $cov(e_{ink}, e_{imk}) = \sigma_{nm}$ for any subject i and treatment k.

8.2.2 Implementation of the Repeated Measures Model Using the SAS MIXED Procedure

8.2.2.1 Simulated Dataset

A simulated dataset is used to illustrate the implementation of a repeated measures model, with time taken as a categorical (discrete) covariate. As described previously in Section 8.2.1, consideration is given to a hypothetical clinical study with 600 subjects and two treatment arms. Each subject is randomized to an active drug or placebo during the 4-week study. The outcome variable is a weekly PRO measure (Y) and covariates represent time (variable Visit represents study week) and treatment (variable *Treatment* = 1 for the active treatment arm and *Treatment* = 2 for the placebo arm). The weekly outcome variable Y is simulated based on Equation 8.1.

The SAS code in Figure 8.1 generates the dataset with 2400 observations (300 subjects per treatment arm and four measurements for every subject). The SAS code line

```
a = 10;/* the overall mean */
```

defines the overall mean and corresponds to the term a in Equation 8.1. The SAS code line

```
Array b{1:4} (1.5 2.5 4 3);/*the time effect at week j =
1,2,3,4*/
```

defines the array of fixed time effects and corresponds to the term b_j in Equation 8.1. The SAS code line

```
Array r{1:2} (3 1);/*the effect of the treatment k = 1,2*/
```

defines the array of fixed treatment effects and corresponds to the term r_k in Equation 8.1. And the SAS code line

```
Array e{1:4};/*simulated error term at week j = 1,2,3,4*/
```

defines the array of errors to be simulated during the calculations. The SAS code line

```
Y = a + b[j] + r[k] + e[j];
```

represents Equation 8.1.

The value of the error term (Keep Y Error ID Visit Treatment;) is kept as a part of the dataset only to highlight later the relationship between those error term values and the estimated variance–covariance matrix. In this example, the outcome error term is modeled so that it has a different variance at every week. For example, at week 1 the variance is 3.5 (Call rannor(seed1,X); e[1] = sqrt(3.5)*X;). The simplest model for pedagogical purposes was defined here with only three fixed effects: overall mean, week, and treatment. The SAS code in Figure 8.2 outputs the variance–covariance matrix for the variable Error, which characterizes the error term in Equation 8.1 (see Figure 8.3 for output).

```
/*
This example has 600 subjects (NumberOfSubjectsPerTreatment *
NumberOfTreatments).
For every subject there are 4 visits (NumberOfVisits = 4;).
There are 2 treatments arms (NumberOfTreatments = 2;).
*/

options nofmterr nocenter pagesize=2000 linesize=256;

%Let NumberOfSubjectsPerTreatment    = 300;
%Let NumberOfVisits       = 4;
%Let NumberOfTreatments = 2;

data mixed_ds;

Retain seed1 1 seed2 2 seed3 3 seed4 4 ;

a=10;    /* the overall mean  */

Array b{1:4} (1.5 2.5 4 3); /*the time effect at week j=1,2,3,4 */
Array r{1:2} (3 1); /*the effect of the treatment k=1,2 */
Array e{1:4} ; /*simulated error term at week j=1,2,3,4*/

        ID=0;

        Do k=1 to &NumberOfTreatments;
        Do i=1 To &NumberOfSubjectsPerTreatment;

        Call rannor(seed1,X); e[1]=sqrt(3.5)*X;
        Call rannor(seed2,X); e[2]=sqrt(2.5)*X;
        Call rannor(seed3,X); e[3]=sqrt(4)*X;
        Call rannor(seed4,X); e[4]=sqrt(5)*X;

        ID=ID+1;

        Do j=1 To &NumberOfVisits;

            Y      = a + b[j] + r[k] + e[j];
            Error = e[j]   ;
            Visit = j      ;
            Treatment = k ;
            Output;

        End;
        End;
        End;

Keep Y Error ID Visit Treatment;

run;
```

FIGURE 8.1
Generating dataset for the analysis.

```
Proc Transpose data=mixed_ds out=mixed_ds_tr;
Var Error;
By ID;
Run;

Proc Corr data=mixed_ds_tr COV;
Var Col1-Col14;
Run;
```

FIGURE 8.2
Generating variance–covariance matrix for error term.

	COL1	COL2	COL3	COL4
		Covariance Matrix, DF = 599		
COL1	3.417866921	0.030607355	0.084758122	0.148561233
COL2	0.030607355	2.487089319	-0.013618685	0.019986091
COL3	0.084758122	-0.013618685	3.995026967	0.063440883
COL4	0.148561233	0.019986091	0.063440883	4.565678753

FIGURE 8.3
Variance–covariance matrix for error term (results of the CORR procedure).

```
Data mixed_ds_1;
Set mixed_ds;
Keep ID Y Visit Treatment;
Run;
```

FIGURE 8.4
SAS data step to create final simulated dataset for the analysis.

Here only four columns (see Figure 8.4; "Keep ID Y Visit Treatment;") were kept in the final dataset. Only those data are needed to model the data. Figure 8.5 shows an example of a final simulated dataset.

8.2.2.2 Implementation

Figure 8.6 represents implementation of the repeated measures model using the MIXED procedure (SAS, 2011). To model repeated measures data with the MIXED procedure, the MODEL and REPEATED statements should be specified. The understanding of how those two statements work together to describe a repeated measures model is essential. As described earlier, Equation 8.1 includes three fixed effects $a + b_j + r_k$ and the error term e_{ijk}. In the MIXED procedure, the MODEL statement always describes only fixed effects, so the statement "Model Y = Visit Treatment" corresponds to "$Y_{ijk} = a + b_j + r_k$" from Equation 8.1. The statement "Repeated Visit / Subject=ID Type=UN"

	ID	Y	Visit	Treatment
1	1	17.87651456	1	1
2	1	17.57418471	2	1
3	1	18.83472073	3	1
4	1	17.26800528	4	1
5	2	14.35049269	1	1
6	2	14.45005108	2	1
7	2	17.6328927	3	1
8	2	18.19990252	4	1
9	3	15.24192736	1	1
10	3	16.35546213	2	1
11	3	18.22579649	3	1
12	3	17.3896992	4	1

FIGURE 8.5
Simulated dataset (data for the first three subjects are shown).

```
Proc Mixed data=mixed_ds_1;
    Class Visit Treatment ID ;
    Model Y = Visit Treatment  / Solution ddfm=kr;
    Repeated Visit / Subject=ID Type=UN R rcorr;
Run;
```

FIGURE 8.6
Implementation of the repeated measures model.

describes the error term "e_{ijk}" from Equation 8.1. Note that in the MODEL statement we do not need to include the intercept (which represents overall mean a) because it is computed by default. Figure 8.7 summarizes the relationship between Equation 8.1 and the MODEL and REPEATED statements.

The option "Subject = ID" in the REPEATED statement defines the variable which will serve to identify subjects, that is, to inform the model that certain portions of data belong to the same subject. Note that "ID" should be the part of the CLASS statement. The option "Type = UN" defines the unstructured covariance structure, that will be used to define relationships

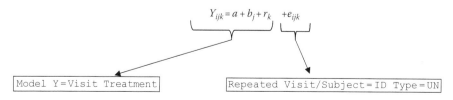

FIGURE 8.7
Relationship between Equation 8.1 and the MODEL and REPEATED statements.

between error terms in a subject. In this example, the variance–covariance structure takes the following form:

$$\begin{bmatrix} \sigma_1^2 & \sigma_{21} & \sigma_{31} & \sigma_{41} \\ \sigma_{21} & \sigma_2^2 & \sigma_{32} & \sigma_{42} \\ \sigma_{31} & \sigma_{32} & \sigma_3^2 & \sigma_{43} \\ \sigma_{41} & \sigma_{42} & \sigma_{43} & \sigma_4^2 \end{bmatrix}.$$

The option "ddfm = kr" performs the degrees-of-freedom calculations using the Kenward and Roger algorithm (Kenward and Roger, 1997), which is the preferable method for most longitudinal data. Option "Solution" requests the output for the fixed effects.

Figure 8.8 shows results of modeling for estimations of covariance parameters and fixed effects. With these simulated data, a determination can be made as to how close the estimated parameters are to the values assigned to those parameters when data were simulated. For instance, the modeled variance σ_1^2 for the error term at week 1 is 3.4192 (Figure 8.8), while in the simulations the value is 3.417866921 (Figure 8.3). Further, comparing the rest of the covariance parameter estimates from Figure 8.8 with results of CORR

```
Covariance Parameter Estimates

Cov Parm     Subject      Estimate

UN(1,1)      ID            3.4192
UN(2,1)      ID            0.03207
UN(2,2)      ID            2.4887
UN(3,1)      ID            0.08599
UN(3,2)      ID           -0.01222
UN(3,3)      ID            3.9962
UN(4,1)      ID            0.1501
UN(4,2)      ID            0.02173
UN(4,3)      ID            0.06495
UN(4,4)      ID            4.5675
```

Solution for Fixed Effects

Effect	Visit	Treatment	Estimate	Standard Error	DF	t Value	Pr > |t|
Intercept			14.0102	0.09549	767	146.72	<.0001
Visit	1		-1.4979	0.1132	599	-13.23	<.0001
Visit	2		-0.5233	0.1081	599	-4.84	<.0001
Visit	3		1.0694	0.1186	599	9.02	<.0001
Visit	4		0	.	.	.	.
Treatment		1	1.997	0.07760	598	25.74	<.0001
Treatment		2	0	.	.	.	.

FIGURE 8.8
Covariance parameter and fixed effect estimates.

procedure from Figure 8.3, we can see that the estimates are very close to the values used in the simulation.

The comparison of the estimated fixed effects with the values we used to simulate the dataset needs additional explanation. Recall that the values of 3 and 1 were assigned for effects of the active drug and placebo (Figure 8.1), respectively, but from Figure 8.8 the corresponding values are 1.99750 and 0. The reason for this is that the MIXED procedure uses an overparameterized model. The treatment variable here is a class (categorical or discrete) variable and has two levels, meaning that it is enough to have only one variable with values of 0 and 1 to describe this covariate. But the MIXED procedure will create two variables for treatment (according to the number of levels). The same applies for the time effects with four levels; the MIXED procedure will create the vector of four variables with values 0 or 1. As a result, the last level for every CLASS variable is used as a reference, meaning that the fixed effect for the last level is assigned the reference value of zero and effects for all other levels are defined relative to this last level. The effect of the active treatment was estimated as 1.9975, and, to be consistent with MIXED procedure, we need to subtract 1 (the simulated value for placebo) from value of 3 (simulated value for the active treatment) to obtain virtually the same value of 2 as the effect of active treatment over placebo.

For time effects, the estimated values are –1.4979 (Visit 1), –0.5233 (Visit 2), 1.0694 (Visit 3), and 0 (Visit 4) (Figure 8.8). Note that simulated values for time effects are represented by 1.5, 2.5, 4, and 3 at weeks 1, 2, 3, and 4, respectively (Figure 8.1). Subtracting the reference value of 3 from these numbers, we get the respective values of –1.5, –0.5, 1.0, and 0, which match well to the corresponding recalculated values used in the simulations.

Recall that in the simulation the value of 10 is assigned to the overall mean (or intercept) in the model. But in the SAS output the estimated value of the intercept is 14.0102 (Figure 8.8). This result is also attributed to over-parameterization from the MIXED procedure. The outcome variable Y is equal to the intercept (a), when all the covariates in the model are equal to zero. In the MIXED procedure, though, zero values of covariates correspond to the last levels of the covariates. But, originally in the data simulation, values for those reference levels are different from zero. Based on Equation 8.1 the estimated values for PRO response when covariates are equal to the reference levels can be written as

$$Y = a + b_4 + r_2.$$

Replacing a, b_4, and r_2 by 10 (the overall mean), 3 (the time effect at week 4), and 1 (the effect of the treatment for placebo), respectively, we obtain the same value of 14, as estimated by the MIXED procedure.

8.2.3 Covariance Structures

There are several predefined forms of variance–covariance structures available in the MIXED procedure. The unstructured covariance structure (Type=UN) used in the previous simulated example is the most general and does not assume any predefined pattern among errors over time. The unstructured covariance structure does not require equally spaced time intervals. It is the most flexible one and can be recommended as the variance–covariance structure of first choice for most repeated measures models, provided that the number of time points is not too large relative to the number of patients in the study.

Another possible structure is TYPE = CS (compound symmetry), which assumes the same covariance between any pair of error terms. For our simulated example (Section 8.2.2) this means that, for any subject i at any week j and any treatment k, the error term is assumed to be from a normal distribution with mean 0 and variance σ^2 [$e_{ijk} \sim N(0, \sigma^2)$]. An error term at any week n will covary with an error term at any other week m ($n = 1, 2, 3, 4; m = 1, 2, 3, 4; n \neq m$) with the covariance $cov(e_{ink}, e_{imk}) = \sigma_1$ for any subject i and treatment k. The compound symmetry variance–covariance structure can be represented as follows:

$$\begin{bmatrix} \sigma^2 & \sigma_1 & \sigma_1 & \sigma_1 \\ \sigma_1 & \sigma^2 & \sigma_1 & \sigma_1 \\ \sigma_1 & \sigma_1 & \sigma^2 & \sigma_1 \\ \sigma_1 & \sigma_1 & \sigma_1 & \sigma^2 \end{bmatrix}. \tag{8.2}$$

For any two random variables x and y,

$$cov(x, y) = corr(x, y) \times \sigma_x \times \sigma_y.$$

In our case, this formula can be rewritten as

$$cov(e_{ink}, e_{imk}) = corr(e_{ink}, e_{imk}) \times \sigma \times \sigma.$$

Replacing $corr(e_{ink}, e_{imk})$ by ρ allows the Matrix 8.2 to be expressed as

$$\sigma^2 \begin{bmatrix} 1 & \rho & \rho & \rho \\ \rho & 1 & \rho & \rho \\ \rho & \rho & 1 & \rho \\ \rho & \rho & \rho & 1 \end{bmatrix}.$$

A frequently used structure is TYPE = AR(1), first-order autoregressive. It models the same variance σ^2 component for any error term and assumes the same correlation ρ between any pair of error terms separated by one interval. The correlation between error terms separated by two intervals is ρ^2, correlation between error terms separated by three intervals is ρ^3, and so on. The first-order autoregressive variance–covariance structure can be presented as

$$\sigma^2 \begin{bmatrix} 1 & \rho & \rho^2 & \rho^3 \\ \rho & 1 & \rho & \rho^2 \\ \rho^2 & \rho & 1 & \rho \\ \rho^3 & \rho^2 & \rho & 1 \end{bmatrix}.$$

Note that the first-order autoregressive structure [AR(1)], unlike the unstructured covariance structure, should only be used in analysis of data when outcomes were collected at equal intervals in time. For instance, if data are collected daily during the first week of the study and weekly thereafter, the first-order autoregressive structure should not be applied to these data.

In addition to compound symmetry and first-order autoregressive, other types of covariance structures exist, some more widely recognized than others (Singer and Willett, 2003; Fitzmaurice et al., 2011). The Toeplitz covariance pattern, of which the first-order autoregressive pattern is a special case, assumes that the variance of the error term is constant across occasions and the correlation is the same between any pair of error terms that are equally separated in time. Another covariance pattern is heterogeneous compound symmetry in which the main diagonal elements represent the variance of error terms at different times and, unlike the regular compound symmetry model, these variances are allowed to be different. In addition, all pairs of error terms have their own covariances, obtained by multiplying a constant correlation parameter (between time points) by the product of a pair of standard deviations (of error terms) at the corresponding times.

8.2.4 Repeated Measures with Time as a Continuous Covariate

Sections 8.2.1 through 8.2.3 discussed and illustrated a repeated measured model using time as a categorical predictor. This approach has an important advantage: it does not impose any functional relationship between outcome and time. But if there is strong evidence (theoretical or empirical) that the relationship between time and outcome can be described by a particular function, the MIXED procedure is flexible enough to implement this as well. This approach to model repeated measures data is also known as growth curve modeling.

Consider a case that the simulated effect of time is increasing during the first 3 weeks and then drops down. Based on this information, a quadratic model can be considered for a time effect. Figure 8.9 shows the SAS code that adds into the dataset (created in Figure 8.4) two additional variables, representing a linear time term and a quadratic time term. Note that it is generally recommended to center such variables representing time in order to reduce

```
Data mixed_ds_1;
Set mixed_ds_1;
Time = Visit-2.5;
Time2 = Time*Time;
Run;
```

FIGURE 8.9
Adding linear time term and quadratic time term into the dataset.

```
Proc Mixed data=mixed_ds_1;

   Class Visit Treatment ID;

   Model Y = Time Time2 Treatment / Solution ddfm=kr;

Repeated Visit / Subject=ID Type=UN R rcorr;

Run;
```

FIGURE 8.10
Implementation of a growth curve model.

collinearity between time and time squared, which is intended to provide more precise estimations of the model parameters. In our example, values for time range from 1 to 4, meaning that 2.5 will be the center value for the entire time interval.

Figure 8.10 shows the implementation of the growth curve model. It is important to note that the new variables "Time" and "Time2" work in concert with the variable "Visit". The REPEATED statement can only accept the class (categorical) variable, and, because of this, two variables are always needed to represent time for a growth curve model. One will be used by the REPEATED statement to describe time points for the variance–covariance matrix and another one—which should be a continuous variable—will represent time in the MODEL statement.

8.3 Random Coefficient Model

Consider the case of time as a continuous covariate. Random coefficient models allow a set or subset of regression coefficients to vary randomly from one individual to another. For example, each individual has a slope that measures a rate of change over time on the PRO measure, and each individual has an intercept that represents a baseline or natural level on the PRO measure. In doing so, these models account for natural sources of heterogeneity in the population.

A distinctive feature of random coefficient models is the modeling of mean response as a combination of population characteristics. Population characteristics are captured through population regression parameters, such as a common slope and intercept, that are assumed to be shared by all individuals (fixed effects) and also the estimation of subject-specific effects, such as a subject's unique slope and intercept, that are unique to a particular individual (random effects). Random coefficient models lead to a marginal mean response across individuals overall (averaged over the distribution of the subject-specific random effects) and a subject-specific or individual mean response profile for a given individual over time. Both types of mean responses, which are conditional on covariates (like treatment) in the model, can be combined to enable the modeling of individual growth trajectories over time and inferences specifically to each individual.

The model can be often described with relatively few parameters, regardless of the number and timing of measurement occasions. Another appealing aspect of random coefficient models is their flexibility: measurement occasions can vary among subjects, making this model well suited for unbalanced longitudinal data, as data need not be collected at the same time points. This section covers the most common random coefficient model: the random intercept–slope model. This model can be easily modified into the simplest model with just one random parameter (typically the intercept) or into more complex models with more than two random parameters.

8.3.1 Random Intercept–Slope Model

Now consider a simulated example based on a clinical one-arm study for a new treatment. Two hundred subjects are randomly selected from the population of interest. Each subject was given the same drug during the 10-week study. The outcome variable is a PRO measure (Y) and the covariate is a measure of time (t; representing study week). Data are collected weekly and every subject has up to 10 observations.

The regression model for the subject i at the measurement occasion j can be denoted as

$$Y_{ij} = \alpha_i + \beta_i \times t_{ij} + e_{ij}, \tag{8.3}$$

where
- Y_{ij} is the PRO response for subject i at the measurement occasion j ($i = 1, 2,..., 200; j = 1, 2,..., n_i$; n_i represents the number of observations for subject i, which could be from only one observation to a maximum of 10 observations)
- α_i is the individual-specific intercept for subject i (assumed to be from a normal distribution with mean a and variance σ_a^2, that is, $\alpha_i \sim N(a, \sigma_a^2)$)
- β_i is the individual-specific slope for subject i (assumed to be from a normal distribution with mean b and variance σ_b^2), that is, $\beta_i \sim N(b, \sigma_b^2)$)
- t_{ij} is the time of the assessment (taken as a continuous variable)
- e_{ij} is the error term (assumed to be from a normal distribution with mean 0 and variance σ^2, i.e., $e_{ij} \sim N(0, \sigma^2)$)

It is also generally assumed that random intercepts α_i and random slopes β_i covary, with covariance $\text{cov}(\alpha_i, \beta_i) = \sigma_{ab}$.

Figure 8.11 graphically illustrates Equation 8.3 with varying intercepts and slopes. The population regression line over time (depicted by the thick solid line in Figure 8.11) changes linearly and increases longitudinally. Random regression lines (thin lines) represent several individual subjects (from 200 subjects).

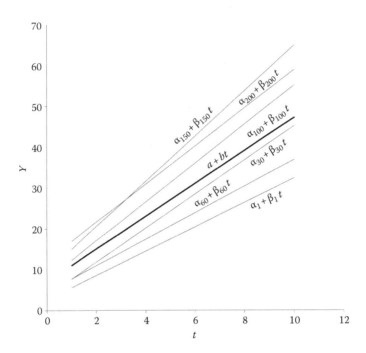

FIGURE 8.11
Depiction of the random intercept–slope model.

To transform Equation 8.3 into random coefficient mixed model, we need to represent it as a combination of fixed effects and random effects (mixed models are after all models that *mix* together fixed effects and random effects). In Equation 8.3, the subject-specific intercept α_i and the subject-specific slope β_i can be represented as

$$\alpha_i = a + \alpha_i', \tag{8.4}$$

$$\beta_i = b + \beta_i'. \tag{8.5}$$

The random effect for intercept α_i' for subject i represents the difference between the overall intercept a and the subject-specific intercept α_i; the random effect for slope β_i' for subject i represents the difference between the overall slope b and the subject-specific slope β_i. Because variables α_i' and β_i' were created by subtractions of constant values (a and b, respectively), they will have the same variances and covariances as the original variables α_i and β_i, but the means of the random effects α_i' and β_i' will be zero as follows:

$$\alpha_i' \sim N\left(0, \sigma_a^2\right), \tag{8.6}$$

$$\beta_i' \sim N\left(0, \sigma_b^2\right), \tag{8.7}$$

$$\text{cov}(\alpha_i', \beta_i') = \sigma_{ab}. \tag{8.8}$$

Appling the transformations in Equations 8.4 and 8.5 to Equation 8.3, we get

$$Y_{ij} = (a + \alpha_i') + (b + \beta_i') \times t_{ij} + e_{ij}$$

$$Y_{ij} = a + b \times t_{ij} + \alpha_i' + \beta_i' \times t_{ij} + e_{ij}. \tag{8.9}$$

In Equation 8.9, the portion $(a + b \times t_{ij})$ represents the fixed effects part of the model, where a and b correspond to the overall intercept and slope, respectively. The portion $(\alpha_i' + \beta_i' \times t_{ij} + e_{ij})$ of the same Equation 8.9 represents the random effects part of the model.

Like the repeated measures model, the random coefficient model can be further generalized to incorporate other factors like the effect of treatment. Covariates such as treatment group can be included, as can their interaction with time (e.g., time-by-treatment interaction). For example, the estimated means of intercepts and slopes across individuals can depend on treatment group. Section 8.4.2 discusses in detail a real-life application of the random intercept–slope model, which includes other covariates such as baseline, treatment, time-by-treatment interaction, as well as the detailed description of the implementation using SAS.

In general, random coefficient models can be expanded by including additional randomly varying regression coefficients, extending the structure for the residual errors, and allowing the means of the random effects to depend on covariates. These features enhance the flexibility and range of these models. In addition to including additional covariates, the models allow for transformations on time (e.g., the square root of time) and on outcome (e.g., PRO measure). These models incorporate all available data, including information from individuals who have less than a complete set of responses.

8.3.2 Implementation of Random Intercepts and Slopes Model Using SAS MIXED Procedure

8.3.2.1 Simulated Dataset

A simulated dataset is used to illustrate the implementation of the random intercept–slope model. As described in Section 8.3.1, consider a clinical one-arm study for a new treatment with 200 subjects. Each subject is given a drug during this 10-week study. The outcome variable is a PRO measure (variable Y) and the covariate is time (the variable Week represents study week). Weekly outcome variable Y is simulated and every subject could have up to 10 observations.

The first step is to simulate values of the individual intercepts and slopes. The SAS code in Figure 8.12 generated the dataset with 200 observations (200 subjects) and two random but correlated variables representing subject-specific intercepts and slopes, one pair for each individual. Results of the

```
Data _tmp_1;

Retain seed1 1 seed2 2;

NumberOfSubjects    = 200;

Do ID=1 To NumberOfSubjects;

Call rannor(seed1,X1);
sIntercept = 2+ID*0.025 + sqrt(.1)*X1;

Call rannor(seed2,X2);
sSlope = 3+ID*0.005 + sqrt(.2)*X2;

Output;
End;
Run;
```

FIGURE 8.12
Simulating values of the individual intercepts and slopes.

```
The MEANS Procedure

Variable      N      Mean      Std Dev      Minimum      Maximum
-----------------------------------------------------------------------
sIntercept   200   4.5259084   1.5039643   1.7574249   7.6259697
sSlope       200   3.4661792   0.5556389   2.1666971   5.2649625
-----------------------------------------------------------------------
```

FIGURE 8.13
Mean values for intercepts and slopes.

MEANS procedure show the mean values for the overall intercept and slope (see Figure 8.13). Note that at this stage our intercepts and slopes correspond to the values of the variables α_i and β_i in Equation 8.3.

The next step is to simulate fixed effects and random effects in the same way we had them depicted in Equations 8.4 and 8.5. The SAS code in Figure 8.14 adds new variables in the dataset, which would be used to generate fixed effects and random effects. Results of the CORR procedure show the variance–covariance matrix of the random effects for intercept and slope (represented by variables Random_Intercept and Random_Slope; see Figure 8.15). Note that the output from Figure 8.15 is directly related to Equations 8.6 through 8.8. Thus variable α_i' corresponds to the variable Random_Intercept and variable β_i' corresponds to the variable Random_Slope. From Figure 8.15 it is evident that the means for those variables are practically zeros and $\sigma_a^2 = 2.261908752$ and $\sigma_b^2 = 0.308734595$, and the covariance $cov(\alpha_i', \beta_i') = \sigma_{ab}$ is equal to 0.449230796.

Next a dataset is generated that will be used by SAS MIXED procedure to perform the analysis. The SAS code (see Figure 8.16) creates, based on values

```
Data _tmp_1;
Set   _tmp_1;

Fixed_Intercept =    4.5259084;
Fixed_Slope     =    3.4661792;
Random_Intercept=    sIntercept -   4.5259084;
Random_Slope    =    sSlope     -   3.4661792;

Run;

Proc Corr data=_tmp_1 COV;
Var Random_Intercept   Random_Slope;
Run;
```

FIGURE 8.14
Simulating values of the intercepts and slopes in terms of fixed and random effects.

```
             Covariance Matrix, DF = 199

                        Random_
                        Intercept      Random_Slope

Random_Intercept        2.261908752      0.449230796
Random_Slope            0.449230796      0.308734595

                     Simple Statistics

Variable          N      Mean    Std Dev     Sum    Minimum Maximum

Random_Intercept 200 4.56582E-9 1.50396 9.13164E-7 -2.76848 3.10006
Random_Slope     200 9.88818E-9 0.55564 1.97764E-6 -1.29948 1.79878

   Pearson Correlation Coefficients, N = 200
          Prob > |r| under H0: Rho=0

                        Random_          Random_
                        Intercept         Slope

Random_Intercept        1.00000          0.53758
                                         <.0001

Random_Slope            0.53758          1.00000
                        <.0001
```

FIGURE 8.15
Means, variances, and covariances for random intercepts and slopes.

of `Fixed_Intercept`, `Fixed_Slope`, `Random_Intercept`, and `Random_Slope`, up to 10 observations for every subject to simulate attrition that mimics a real clinical study.

Note that the SAS code line

Y = Fixed_Intercept + Fixed_Slope* Week + Random_Intercept + Random_Slope * Week + sqrt(0.15)*X4;

```
Data _tmp_2;
Set _tmp_1;

Retain seed3 3 seed4 4 ;

NumberOfVisits=10;

Call ranuni(seed3,X3);

Do Week=1 To (1+Int(NumberOfVisits * X3));

Call rannor(seed4, X4);
Y= Fixed_Intercept + Fixed_Slope* Week +
Random_Intercept + Random_Slope * Week + sqrt(0.15)*X4;
Output;
End;

Keep ID Y Week;

Run;
```

FIGURE 8.16
Generating dataset for the analysis.

represents Equation 8.9. So as to mimic a real clinical trial, only three columns (Keep ID Y Week;) are kept in the final dataset, which are the variables needed to model the data. Figure 8.17 shows how a final simulated dataset will look like. In the example, the first subject is in the study for 6 weeks and the second subject has data for all 10 weeks.

	ID	Week	Y
1	1	1	6.4070281153
2	1	2	10.160105482
3	1	3	13.611442179
4	1	4	17.470588405
5	1	5	20.483090734
6	1	6	24.657757745
7	2	1	4.6773041875
8	2	2	7.540056806
9	2	3	10.21563141
10	2	4	13.018953242
11	2	5	15.419948971
12	2	6	18.694451328
13	2	7	20.888545983
14	2	8	23.451088342
15	2	9	25.866276067
16	2	10	29.317560751

FIGURE 8.17
Final simulated dataset (data for the first two subjects are shown).

8.3.2.2 Implementation

Figure 8.18 represents the implementation of the random intercept–slope mixed-effects model using the SAS MIXED procedure. When the random coefficient model is used to model data using MIXED procedure, the MODEL and RANDOM statements should be specified. It is important to understand the way the two statements work together to describe the random intercept–slope mixed model. As noted previously, Equation 8.9 represents two types of effects—the fixed effects portion ($a + b \times t_{ij}$) and the random effects portion ($\alpha'_i + \beta'_i \times t_{ij} + e_{ij}$). The MODEL statement, as mentioned earlier, describes only fixed effects. Thus, the statement "Model Y = Week" corresponds to "$Y_{ij} = a + b \times t_{ij}$" in Equation 8.9. The statement "Random INTERCEPT Week" corresponds to "$\alpha'_i + \beta'_i \times t_{ij} + e_{ij}$" in Equation 8.9. Note that in the MODEL statement the intercept (as a fixed effect) does not need to be included as it is included by default. But in the RANDOM statement, all random effects including intercept should be spelled out exactly.

Figure 8.19 summarizes the relationship between Equation 8.9 and the MODEL and RANDOM statements. Another relevant point is that, although in both MODEL and RANDOM statements the same variable "Week" is used to identify the slope, in the MODEL statement it would denote (in this example) the overall population slope (represented by variable b in Equation 8.9), whereas in the RANDOM statement it denotes individual random slopes (represented by variables β'_i in Equation 8.9).

Option "Subject = ID" in the RANDOM statement defines the variable that will serve to identify subjects and hence to inform the model that certain portions of data belong to the same subject. Note that "ID" should be part of the

```
Proc Mixed data=_tmp_2;
    Class ID;

    Model Y = Week / Solution ddfm=kr;

    Random INTERCEPT Week / Subject=ID Type=UN Solution;
Run;
```

FIGURE 8.18
Implementation of the random intercept–slope mixed model.

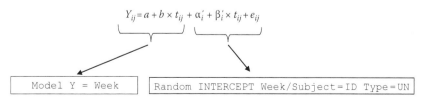

$$Y_{ij} = a + b \times t_{ij} + \alpha'_i + \beta'_i \times t_{ij} + e_{ij}$$

```
Model Y = Week        Random INTERCEPT Week/Subject=ID Type=UN
```

FIGURE 8.19
Relationship between Equation 8.9 and the MODEL and RANDOM statements.

CLASS statement. Option "Type=UN" defines that the unstructured covariance structure will be used to describe the relationship between the random effects for intercepts and slopes in the model. In this example, this variance–covariance structure will have the following form (see also Equations 8.6 through 8.8):

$$\begin{bmatrix} \sigma_a^2 & \sigma_{ab} \\ \sigma_{ab} & \sigma_b^2 \end{bmatrix}.$$

As discussed previously, there are several forms of variance–covariance structures available in MIXED procedure, but for the majority of random coefficient models, the unstructured covariance structure is recommended.

Option "Solution" requests output of the fixed effects (in the MODEL statement) and random effects (in the RANDOM statement). Figure 8.20 shows the results of modeling for estimations of covariance parameters and fixed effects. For example, the modeled variance for the random intercepts is 2.3409, which compares well with the simulated value of 2.261908752 (Figure 8.15). Similarly, the modeled variance for the random slopes is 0.3016, which corresponds to the simulated value of 0.308734595 (Figure 8.15). Moreover, the modeled covariance between the two random effects is 0.4574 (Figure 8.20), which is close to the simulated value of 0.449230796 (Figure 8.15).

The last parameter in this part of the output is the Residual. This parameter corresponds to e_{ij} in Equation 8.9 and to the last portion "...+sqrt(**0.15**)*X4" of the SAS code line to simulate outcome Y (see Figure 8.16). From this snippet of SAS code, it is known that the variance for this residual term is defined as 0.15; the model variance of the residual term is close to 0.15 (Residual 0.1475; Figure 8.20). Similarly, for the overall population means (fixed effects) for intercept and slope, the modeled values of 4.5425 and 3.4626 (Figure 8.20) are close to the values in the simulations (4.5259084 and 3.4661792, respectively; Figure 8.13).

```
Covariance Parameter Estimates

Cov Parm      Subject     Estimate

UN(1,1)       ID            2.3409
UN(2,1)       ID            0.4574
UN(2,2)       ID            0.3016
Residual                    0.1475

             Solution for Fixed Effects

                          Standard
Effect       Estimate       Error       DF      t Value     Pr > |t|

Intercept     4.5425        0.1124       199      40.41      <.0001
Week          3.4626        0.04165      182      83.13
```

FIGURE 8.20
Covariance parameter and fixed effect estimates.

```
                       Solution for Random Effects

                              Std Err
      Effect       ID    Estimate     Pred     DF    t Value    Pr > |t|

      Intercept    1     -1.5038     0.3493    986    -4.31      <.0001
      Week         1      0.09484    0.09473   993     1.00      0.3170

      Intercept    2     -2.3690     0.2768    970    -8.56      <.0001
      Week         2     -0.7815     0.05831   573   -13.40      <.0001
      . . . .
```

FIGURE 8.21
Partial output of modeled random effects.

When applying the random intercept–slope mixed model, we can also estimate individual intercept and slope for every subject. As noted earlier, the option "Solution" in the RANDOM statement requests output of the random effects. Figure 8.21 represents the modeled results for two subjects. Dataset "_tmp_1", created during the preparation of the simulated data, has variables Random_Intercept and Random_Slope that represent values used in the simulations for those subjects. Running the PRINT procedure (see Figure 8.22) against dataset "_tmp_1" for the first 2 subjects (with ID = 1 and ID = 2) allows for the comparison of random effects for intercepts and slopes known from the simulations vs those produced by the model.

Comparison of Figures 8.21 and 8.23 shows that, for the subject with ID = 2, modeled values of intercept and slope (Figure 8.21) are each statistically significant and close to their respective values from the simulate dataset (Figure 8.23). For subject with ID = 1, modeled and simulated

```
Proc Print data=_tmp_1 NOOBS;
Var ID Random_Intercept Random_Slope;
Where ID In (1 2);
Run;
```

FIGURE 8.22
SAS code to output values of random effects used in simulations.

```
      ID     Random_Intercept     Random_Slope

      1      -1.93017              0.12549
      2      -2.50118             -0.75315
```

FIGURE 8.23
Values of random effects used in simulations.

random effects for slope are 0.09484 and 0.12549, respectively, and the modeled slope is not statistically different from zero (p-value = 0.317). This pattern of individual results is based on the availability of information. In this simulation, 10 observations are available for subject 2 and only 6 observations are available for subject 1 (see Figure 8.17). For subject 1, the modeled and simulated random effects for intercept are –1.5038 and –1.93017, respectively.

8.4 Real-Life Examples

8.4.1 Repeated Measures Model

A randomized, double-blind, parallel-group, placebo- and active-treatment-controlled, phase 3 clinical trial was conducted on 1025 generally healthy smokers (at least 10 cigarettes per day) with less than 3 months of smoking cessation in the past year (Gonzales et al., 2006). Participants were randomly assigned in a 1:1:1 ratio to receive brief counseling and varenicline titrated to 1 mg twice per day (n = 352), bupropion sustained release (SR) titrated to 150 mg twice per day (n = 329), or placebo (n = 244) orally for 12 weeks.

One of the PROs measured in the trial was the Minnesota Nicotine Withdrawal Scale (MNWS), which assesses urge to smoke, depressed mood, irritability, anxiety, difficulty concentrating, restlessness, increased appetite, and sleep. In this section, attention is placed on the single-item question on urge to smoke. Higher scores on the MNWS urge to smoke (range of possible scores, 0–4) indicate greater intensity of symptoms.

Urge to smoke was analyzed as a continuous variable from data collected at each weekly study visit through the first 7 weeks of treatment. This analysis was based on a repeated-measures model with treatment, baseline urge to smoke, center, visit, and treatment-by-visit interaction as explanatory factors (fixed effects), with the visit time taken as a categorical (discrete) covariate. Given its flexibility, an unstructured variance–covariance structure was used to characterize the error terms over time within each individual. As no particular weekly time point was isolated as being most important, model estimates for each treatment gave the overall effect, averaged over week 1 through week 7.

The effects of varenicline and bupropion SR were compared with placebo on MNWS urge to smoke (Gonzales et al., 2006). Both varenicline and bupropion SR significantly reduced urge to smoke compared with placebo based on the least square means, which adjusted for the covariates in the model (Table 8.1). The standardized effect size (measured by the least-square mean difference between an active treatment and a placebo treatment on the urge-to-smoke outcome, divided by the pooled baseline standard deviation of that

TABLE 8.1

Urge to Smoke: Repeated Measures Analysis for Week 1 through Week 7

Treatment	Number[a]	Least Squares Mean (SE)	Comparison vs Placebo				
			Difference (SE)	95% CI	P-Value		Effect Size
Varenicline	341	1.11 (0.04)	−0.54 (0.06)	(−0.66; −0.42)	.001		−0.67
Bupropion SR	318	1.41 (0.05)	−0.24 (0.06)	(−0.36; −0.12)	.001		−0.30
Placebo	337	1.65 (0.05)	—	—	—		—

Abbreviations: SE, standard error; bupropion SR, sustained-release bupropion; CI, confidence interval.

[a] Sample size that includes data for all participants who had an assessment on urge to smoke both at baseline and at least one of the visits for weeks 1 through 7.

measure across all three treatment groups) showed that, relative to placebo, varenicline gave an (standardized) effect size of −0.67 and bupropion SR gave an effect size of −0.30 (Table 8.1).

To simulate the aforementioned example, we use the same approach described in Section 8.2.2. In addition to time and treatment, baseline PRO (urge-to-smoke) score, treatment-by-time interaction, and center are added in Equation 8.1 as fixed effects:

$$Y_{ijkz} = a + d \times x_i + b_j + r_k + g_{jk} + c_z + e_{ijkz},$$ (8.10)

where

Y_{ijkz} is the urge-to-smoke score for subject i at measurement occasion j on treatment k and at center z ($i = 1, 2, \ldots, 1050$; $j = 1, 2, 3, 4, 5, 6, 7$; $k = 1, 2, 3$; $z = 1, 2, 3, 4, 5$)

a is the overall mean (can be considered as an unknown fixed effect)

x_i is baseline score on urge to smoke for subject i and d is the corresponding regression coefficient (slope) for this covariate

b_j is the fixed time effect at week j

r_k is the fixed effect of the treatment k

g_{jk} is the interaction effect between drug k and time point j

c_z is the fixed effect of the center z

e_{ijkz} is the error term associated with outcome measurement Y_{ijkz}

Figure 8.24 represents the same technique used to generate the simulated dataset described in Section 8.2.2. The current example stimulates 1050 subjects. Each subject has 7 observations. There are three treatments and five centers. Figure 8.24 generates outcome values according to Equation 8.10 but without the error term.

In Section 8.2.2, the values from a simple normal distribution are taken to simulate error terms. These error terms are, in fact, independent between observations and any observed covariance is obtained just by chance. In the repeated measures modeling, however, the error term is considered to be from a multivariate normal distribution. In this example, the objective is to generate error terms so that they correlate more for adjacent observations and less for observations far from each other in time, a common and realistic scenario.

```
options nofmterr nocenter pagesize=2000 linesize=256;

%Let NumberOfSubjects  = 70;
%Let NumberOfVisits    = 7;
%Let NumberOfTreatments = 3;
%Let NumberOfCenters   = 5;

data mixed_ds;

Retain seed1 1 ;

a=3;    /* the overall mean */

d=0.07; /* baseline slope */

Array b{1:7} (-0.25 -0.50 -0.75 -1.00 -1.00 -1.00 -1.00);
/*the time effect at week j=1,2,3,...,7 */

Array r{1:3} (-1.00 -0.5 -0.25); /*the effect of the
treatments k=1,2,3 */

Array g{1:3,1:7}
(-0.10 -0.20 -0.30 -0.30 -0.30 -0.30 -0.30 /*interaction
effect between drug 1 and week j(j=1,2,...,7)*/
-0.02 -0.04 -0.06 -0.06 -0.06 -0.06 -0.06 /*interaction
effect between drug 2 and week j(j=1,2,...,7)*/
-0.01 -0.02 -0.03 -0.03 -0.03 -0.03 -0.03)/*interaction
effect between drug 3 and week j(j=1,2,...,7)*/
;

Array c{1:5} (0.01 0.02 -0.025 -0.01 0.02); /*the effect of
the center z=1,2,3,4,5 */

        ID=0;

        Do z=1 to &NumberOfCenters;
        Do k=1 to &NumberOfTreatments;
        Do i=1 To &NumberOfSubjects;

        ID=ID+1;

        Call rannor(seed1,e);
        x = 3 + sqrt(0.1)*e;

                Do j=1 To &NumberOfVisits;
```

FIGURE 8.24
Simulating *true* (without error term) outcomes for subjects.

```
                Y1 = a + d*x + b[j] + r[k] + g[k,j] + c[z];
                Visit = j ;
                Treatment = k ;
                Center = z;
                Baseline = x;
                Output;
                End;
        End;
        End;
        End;
Keep Y1 Baseline ID Visit Treatment Center;

run;
```

FIGURE 8.24 (continued)
Simulating *true* (without error term) outcomes for subjects.

Figure 8.25 generates seven error terms for each of the 1050 subjects. First, a dataset with type CORR is created in order to define correlations between error terms. More specifically, error terms adjacent in time are defined to correlate with a value of 0.5, error terms separated in time by 2 weeks should correlate with a value of 0.4, and so on. Error terms for the first and last

```
data _cov_ (type=corr);
input
_TYPE_ $ _NAME_ $  COL1   COL2   COL3   COL4   COL5   COL6   COL7;
datalines;
 CORR    COL1    1      0.5    0.4    0.3    0.2    0.1    0.05
 CORR    COL2    0.5    1      0.5    0.4    0.3    0.2    0.1
 CORR    COL3    0.4    0.5    1      0.5    0.4    0.3    0.2
 CORR    COL4    0.3    0.4    0.5    1      0.5    0.4    0.3
 CORR    COL5    0.2    0.3    0.4    0.5    1      0.5    0.4
 CORR    COL6    0.1    0.2    0.3    0.4    0.5    1      0.5
 CORR    COL7    0.05   0.1    0.2    0.3    0.4    0.5    1
 MEAN       .    0      0      0      0      0      0      0
 STD        .    0.5    0.7    0.6    0.4    0.8    0.3    0.5
 N          .    1050   1050   1050   1050   1050   1050   1050
;
run;
proc simnormal data=_cov_ out=err_sim numreal=1050 seed=10000;
var Col1-Col7;
run;
proc corr data=err_sim COV ;
Var Col1-Col7;
Run;
```

FIGURE 8.25
Generating error terms based on multivariate normal distribution.

Covariance Matrix, DF = 1049

	COL1	COL2	COL3	COL4	COL5	COL6	COL7
COL1	0.2621163981	0.1983212325	0.1293671737	0.0713632050	0.0917198972	0.0197314773	0.0220872529
COL2	0.1983212325	0.5063660784	0.2024320144	0.1143919796	0.1598004682	0.0356944450	0.0468382950
COL3	0.1293671737	0.2024320144	0.3572896853	0.1086274740	0.1806351228	0.0479072334	0.0441452229
COL4	0.0713632050	0.1143919796	0.1086274740	0.1554775620	0.1465265953	0.0427715360	0.0517942022
COL5	0.0917198972	0.1598004682	0.1806351228	0.1465265953	0.6703197431	0.1195104693	0.1525247103
COL6	0.0197314773	0.0356944450	0.0479072334	0.0427715360	0.1195104693	0.0893136562	0.0762924128
COL7	0.0220872529	0.0468382950	0.0441452229	0.0517942022	0.1525247103	0.0762924128	0.2637088143

Pearson Correlation Coefficients, N = 1050

	COL1	COL2	COL3	COL4	COL5	COL6	COL7
COL1	1.00000	0.54436	0.42273	0.35350	0.21881	0.12896	0.08401
COL2	0.54436	1.00000	0.47592	0.40769	0.27429	0.16785	0.12818
COL3	0.42273	0.47592	1.00000	0.46089	0.36911	0.26818	0.14382
COL4	0.35350	0.40769	0.46089	1.00000	0.45388	0.36296	0.25579
COL5	0.21881	0.27429	0.36911	0.45388	1.00000	0.48843	0.36277
COL6	0.12896	0.16785	0.26818	0.36296	0.48843	1.00000	0.49712
COL7	0.08401	0.12818	0.14382	0.25579	0.36277	0.49712	1.00000

FIGURE 8.26
Variance–covariance and correlation matrix for simulated dataset (CORR procedure output).

observation have a very small correlation of 0.05. In addition, the mean of every error term is defined to be zero and a different variance for the error term is assigned every week. The SIMNORMAL procedure in Figure 8.25 is used to simulate seven error terms per subject. The CORR procedure (the last procedure in Figure 8.25) outputs the variance–covariance and correlation matrix for the simulated dataset (see Figure 8.26). As expected, the correlations based on the simulated dataset (Figure 8.26) are similar to the values initially assigned (see the data step in Figure 8.25).

The SAS code in Figure 8.27 transforms the outcome of the SIMNORMAL procedure to be suitable for merging with the earlier generated dataset in Figure 8.24. Figure 8.28 shows the final structure of the dataset for analysis.

Figure 8.29 shows implementation of the repeated measures analysis using the MIXED procedure. Note that the variables Visit, Treatment, and Center were used as categorical covariates (as they are part of the CLASS statement), but the variable Baseline was used as a continuous covariate. All other statements were explained earlier in Section 8.2.2. The statement LSMEANS (LSMeans Treatment Visit*Treatment/cl diff;) provides overall estimates for the outcome by treatment and also for every treatment and week separately.

Option R in the REPEATED statement of Figure 8.29 requests output of the variance–covariance matrix by default for subject 1, but, as was described in Section 8.2, the variance–covariance matrix is set to be the same for all subjects. Comparing the estimated matrix from Figure 8.30 based on the model with the results from Figure 8.26 based on the simulations, we can

```
Proc Transpose data=err_sim out=err_sim_tr;
Var Col1-Col7;
By Rnum;
Run;

Data _errors_;
Set err_sim_tr;
ID= Rnum;
E1=Col1;
Keep ID E1;
Run;

Data mixed_ds1;
Merge mixed_ds _errors_;
Y=Y1+E1;
By ID;
Keep Y Baseline ID Visit Treatment Center;
Run;
```

FIGURE 8.27
Adding error terms to the outcome variable.

Patient-Reported Outcomes

ID	Visit	Treatment	Center	Baseline	Y
1	1	1	1	3.5707351	2.2774557
1	2	1	1	3.5707351	2.833129
1	3	1	1	3.5707351	1.9372473
1	4	1	1	3.5707351	1.4951632
1	5	1	1	3.5707351	1.5136012
1	6	1	1	3.5707351	1.0013326
1	7	1	1	3.5707351	1.1298376
2	1	1	1	2.9747287	2.6545671
2	2	1	1	2.9747287	1.7090414
2	3	1	1	2.9747287	1.8442144
2	4	1	1	2.9747287	0.838238
2	5	1	1	2.9747287	0.977405
2	6	1	1	2.9747287	0.9930507
2	7	1	1	2.9747287	0.5128065

FIGURE 8.28
Structure of the dataset for the repeated measures analysis (first two subjects are shown).

```
Proc Mixed data=mixed_ds1;

    class Visit Treatment ID Center;
    model Y = Baseline Visit Treatment Visit*Treatment Center/
solution ddfm=kr;
    Repeated Visit / Subject=ID Type=UN R;
    LSMeans Treatment Visit*Treatment / CL diff;

Run;
```

FIGURE 8.29
Implementation of the repeated measures model.

```
                    Estimated R Matrix for ID 1

Row   Col1      Col2      Col3      Col4      Col5      Col6      Col7

 1   0.2623    0.1987    0.1296    0.07137   0.09161   0.01978   0.02213
 2   0.1987    0.5063    0.2028    0.1138    0.1586    0.03588   0.04694
 3   0.1296    0.2028    0.3577    0.1087    0.1809    0.04820   0.04429
 4   0.07137   0.1138    0.1087    0.1551    0.1456    0.04286   0.05181
 5   0.09161   0.1586    0.1809    0.1456    0.6694    0.1195    0.1526
 6   0.01978   0.03588   0.04820   0.04286   0.1195    0.08975   0.07667
 7   0.02213   0.04694   0.04429   0.05181   0.1526    0.07667   0.2644
```

FIGURE 8.30
Estimated variance–covariance matrix from model.

see that the MIXED procedure provides close estimates (as expected) for the variance–covariance structure of error terms.

Figure 8.31 shows the estimated means at every week and for every treatment. It is seen that for treatment 1 at week 1, the estimated urge to smoke was 1.8580. The *exact* mean score for treatment 1 at week 1 can be calculated from Equation 8.10 (excluding the error term, e_{ijkz}, whose mean value is zero), which for this particular case can be rewritten as

$$Y = a + d \times (mean\ of\ x_i) + b_1 + r_1 + g_{11} + (mean\ of\ c_z).$$

Because x_i (the baseline score) is a continuous variable that was modeled in Figure 8.24 as

```
x = 3 + sqrt(0.1)*e;
```

the *(mean of x_i)* will be equal to 3. It is worthwhile to note that with real data the mean for this variable should be estimated based on all data from all subjects. On the other hand, center was used as a categorical predictor with 5 levels, and, because of this, *(mean of c_z)* will be simply the mean of those 5 effects. Note that with real data this would imply as if there was the same number of subjects in every center. Recall from Figure 8.24 that the center effect was defined by the statement

```
Array c{1:5} (0.01 0.02 -0.025 -0.01 0.02);
```

Then *(mean of c_z)* = (0.01 + 0.02 − 0.025 − 0.01 + 0.02)/5 = 0.003. Also note (again from Figure 8.24) that

```
a = 3       (a = 3;        /* the overall mean   */)
d = 0.07    (d = 0.07;     /* baseline slope */)
b₁ = −0.25  (Array b{1:7} (-0.25 -0.50 ...)
r₁ = −1.00  (Array r{1:3} (-1.00 -0.5 -0.25)
g₁₁ = −0.10 (Array g{1:3,1:7} (-0.10 -0.20....)
```

$a = 3$, $d = 0.07$, $b_1 = -0.25$, $r_1 = -1.00$, $g_{11} = -0.10$

And, finally, the actual mean score of Y at week 1 and treatment 1 can then be calculated as

$$Y = 3 + 0.07 \times 3 + (-0.25) + (-1.00) + (-0.10) + 0.003 = 1.863.$$

The value of 1.863 matches well with the estimated value of 1.8580.

8.4.2 Random Coefficient Model

The current example illustrates a random coefficient model. Seven hundred and fifty patients with metastatic renal cell carcinoma were randomized to sunitinib (Sutent; 6-week cycles: 50 mg orally once daily for 4 weeks, followed by 2 weeks off treatment) or IFN-alfa (interferon-alfa; 9 MU subcutaneous

Least Squares Means

Effect	Visit	Treatment	Estimate	Standard Error	Pr > |t|	Lower	Upper
Treatment		1	1.1444	0.01937	<.0001	1.1064	1.1824
Treatment		2	1.8930	0.01937	<.0001	1.8550	1.9310
Treatment		3	2.1548	0.01936	<.0001	2.1168	2.1928
Visit*Treatment	1	1	1.8580	0.02738	<.0001	1.8042	1.9117
Visit*Treatment	1	2	2.4372	0.02738	<.0001	2.3835	2.4909
Visit*Treatment	1	3	2.6965	0.02738	<.0001	2.6428	2.7503
Visit*Treatment	2	1	1.4384	0.03804	<.0001	1.3638	1.5131
Visit*Treatment	2	2	2.1843	0.03803	<.0001	2.1097	2.2589
Visit*Treatment	2	3	2.4353	0.03803	<.0001	2.3607	2.5099
Visit*Treatment	3	1	1.1641	0.03197	<.0001	1.1014	1.2269
Visit*Treatment	3	2	1.9405	0.03197	<.0001	1.8777	2.0032
Visit*Treatment	3	3	2.1676	0.03197	<.0001	2.1049	2.2304
Visit*Treatment	4	1	0.8714	0.02105	<.0001	0.8301	0.9128
Visit*Treatment	4	2	1.6753	0.02105	<.0001	1.6340	1.7166
Visit*Treatment	4	3	1.9353	0.02105	<.0001	1.8940	1.9766
Visit*Treatment	5	1	0.8593	0.04374	<.0001	0.7735	0.9451
Visit*Treatment	5	2	1.6794	0.04373	<.0001	1.5936	1.7652
Visit*Treatment	5	3	1.9782	0.04373	<.0001	1.8924	2.0640
Visit*Treatment	6	1	0.9143	0.01602	<.0001	0.8829	0.9458
Visit*Treatment	6	2	1.6668	0.01602	<.0001	1.6354	1.6982
Visit*Treatment	6	3	1.9420	0.01601	<.0001	1.9106	1.9734
Visit*Treatment	7	1	0.9053	0.02749	<.0001	0.8513	0.9592
Visit*Treatment	7	2	1.6679	0.02749	<.0001	1.6140	1.7218
Visit*Treatment	7	3	1.9284	0.02748	<.0001	1.8745	1.9824

FIGURE 8.31
Least squares mean estimates.

injection, three times weekly) (Cella et al., 2008). PRO measures included the Functional Assessment of Cancer Therapy-General (FACT-G), the FACT-Kidney Symptom Index-15 item (FKSI-15), and the EuroQoL-5D (EQ-5D) utility index score and the EQ visual analog scale (EQ-VAS). In general, across these various PRO measures, higher scores indicated better outcomes (better quality of life or fewer symptoms).

A random coefficient model was fit for each PRO measure. Outcomes were PRO postbaseline scores (measured at the planned time (cycle) of assessment) and the predictors were the corresponding baseline PRO score, treatment, time (treated as a continuous variable), and treatment-by-time interaction. Intercept and time were considered as random effects particular to each subject. All available data for each patient were used in the analysis. All parameter estimates were obtained using restricted maximum likelihood. Estimated means scores were calculated for all PRO measures and compared between treatments over time, as no specific time point was considered primary. Estimates of these treatment effects were compared with minimally clinically important differences of 2 points for FKSI-DRS, 3 points for FKSI-15, 5 points for FACT-G, and 2 points for each of the four FACT-G subscales.

Patients receiving sunitinib reported higher (more favorable) FKSI-15 scores at each cycle than those receiving IFN-alfa with a significant difference of 3.27 ($p < 0.0001$) in the overall mean across time (Cella et al., 2008; Figure 8.32). Similarly, adjusted differences based on the model in estimated (predicted) means for FACT-G (and all its subscales), EQ-5D index,

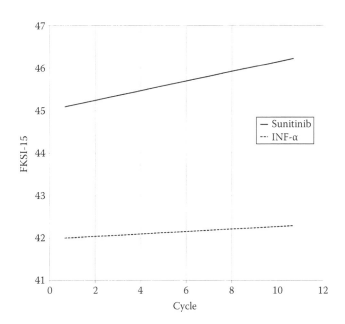

FIGURE 8.32
Estimated mean FKSI-15 score by treatment arm.

TABLE 8.2

Average Treatment Differences for PRO Instruments

Instruments	Overall Estimated Means		Difference[a] (95% Confidence Interval)
	Sunitinib	IFN-alfa	
FKSI-DRS	29.4	27.4	1.98 (1.46, 2.51)
FKSI-15	45.3	42.1	3.27 (2.36, 4.18)
FACT-G	82.3	76.8	5.58 (3.91, 7.24)
EQ-5D Index	0.76	0.73	0.04 (0.01, 0.06)
EQ-VAS	73.4	68.7	4.74 (2.60, 6.87)

[a] Difference between means may not equate exactly because of rounding error.

and EQ-VAS were all significantly favorable for sunitinib ($p < 0.01$; Table 8.2). Between-treatment differences in the estimated (predicted) mean scores were clinically meaningful, relative to pre-established thresholds, after cycle 4 for FKSI-DRS and at all assessments for FKSI-15, FACT-G, and the FACT-G functional well-being subscale.

The previous example can be simulated initially using the framework described in Section 8.3.2, which can serve as a starting point. As previously noted, the following predictors were in the model: subject's baseline PRO score, treatment, time, and treatment-by-time interaction, with intercept and time considered as random effects at the subject level. In the case of the two treatments, which pertain to this example, Equation 8.9 can be modified by adding subject's baseline PRO score, treatment, and treatment-by-time interaction as fixed effects:

$$Y_{ij} = a + b_1 \times x_i + b_2 \times r_i + b_3 \times t_{ij} + b_4 \times r_i \times t_{ij} + \alpha'_i + \beta'_i \times t_{ij} + e_{ij}, \tag{8.11}$$

where

Y_{ij} is the PRO score for subject i at the measurement occasion j ($i = 1, 2,...,750$; $j = 1, 2,...,n_i$; n_i represents the number of observations for subject i, n_i can range from just one observation to a maximum of 11 observations in this example)

a is the overall intercept

x_i is the baseline value of the PRO variable for subject i and b_1 is the slope for variable x_i

r_i is the treatment variable for subject i (with values of 1 for subjects on sunitinib and 0 for subjects on IFN-alfa) and b_2 is the slope for variable r_i

t_{ij} is the time of the assessment for subject i and b_3 is the slope for variable t_{ij}

b_4 is the slope for the treatment-by-time interaction effect

α'_i is the random intercept for subject i

β'_i is the random slope in time for subject i

e_{ij} is the error term for subject i at measurement occasion j

```
data _cov_ (type=corr);
input
_TYPE_ $   _NAME_ $    COL1      COL2       ;
datalines;
 CORR         COL1        1        0.4
 CORR         COL2        0.4      1
 MEAN         .           11       4
 STD          .           0.6      0.3
 N            .           750      750
;
run;

proc simnormal data=_cov_ out=err_sim numreal=750 seed=100;
var Col1-Col2;
run;

Data _tmp_1;
Set  err_sim;
sIntercept = Col1;
sSlope     = Col2;

ID=_N_;

Treatment=0;
If _N_>375 Then Treatment=1;

Keep sIntercept sSlope ID Treatment;
Run;
```

FIGURE 8.33
Simulating values of the individual intercepts and slopes.

Figures 8.33 through 8.36 represent the same technique used to generate the simulated dataset described in Section 8.3 with one exception. In Section 8.4.1, the SIMNORMAL procedure was introduced to generate random but correlated data. For this example, the SIMNORMAL procedure was used to generate 750 intercepts and slopes with predefined standard deviations (0.6 for intercept and 0.3 for slope), means (11 for intercept and 4 for slope), and a correlation of 0.4 between intercepts and slopes (see Figure 8.33). Subsequent to the SIMNORMAL procedure is the data step that adds subject ID and also assigns for the first half of the subjects treatment 0 and for the other half treatment 1.

For this example, 750 subjects are available and every subject can have up to 11 observations (NumberOfVisits=11; see Figure 8.36). The outcome variable Y is now based not only on values of Fixed_Intercept, Fixed_Slope, Random_Intercept, and Random_Slope, but also on other fixed effects introduced. Note that the SAS code line (Figure 8.36)

```
Y = Fixed_Intercept +
b1 * Baseline +
b2 * Treatment +
```

```
Data _tmp_1;
Set  _tmp_1;

Fixed_Intercept =    11;
Fixed_Slope     =     4;

Random_Intercept =   sIntercept    -    11;
Random_Slope =       sSlope        -     4;

Run;

Proc Corr data=_tmp_1 COV;
Var Random_Intercept Random_Slope;
Run;
```

FIGURE 8.34
Simulating values of the intercepts and slopes in terms of fixed and random effects.

```
Fixed_Slope * Cycle +
b4 * Cycle * Treatment +
Random_Intercept + Random_Slope* Cycle  + sqrt(0.3)*X5;
```

corresponds precisely to Equation 8.11. To be life-like, just five columns (Keep Y Baseline ID Cycle Treatment;) are kept as only they are needed to model these data. Figure 8.37 shows how the final simulated dataset will be displayed (data shown is for the first subject only).

Figure 8.38 represents the implementation of this random intercept–slope mixed effects model using the MIXED procedure. The implementation is very close to the implementation discussed in detail in Section 8.3.2.2. Note that the Treatment variable is not part of the Class statement. This is permissible only in the case of two treatments; for ease of interpretation, it is preferable to code Treatment with a value of 1 (for active treatment) and 0 (for the comparator or placebo). It was conducted for this example to provide ease of interpretation of the results. If a study has more than two treatments, treatment should be part of the Class statement.

Figure 8.39 shows results of the modeling for estimations of covariance parameters and fixed effects. Again, notice that the estimated parameters match very well the simulated values. For example, the modeled variance for the random intercepts is 0.3658, compared with the simulated value of 0.3778571853 (Figure 8.35). The residual parameter corresponds to e_{ij} in Equation 8.11 and to the last portion "+ sqrt(0.3)*X5" of the SAS code line to simulate outcome Y (Figure 8.36). This snippet of code informs that the variance for this residual term is defined as 0.3. The modeled variance of the residual term is essentially 0.3 (Residual 0.2965; Figure 8.39).

Solutions for fixed effects provide estimations for all other parameters of the model, which align as expected with their respective simulated values. The first parameter is the intercept with an estimated value of 11.1 (Intercept 11.0722...; see Figure 8.39)—which is defined in the simulation as a fixed intercept equal

```
Covariance Matrix, DF = 749
                         Random_
                         Intercept          Random_Slope

Random_Intercept    0.3778571853           0.0818019020
Random_Slope        0.0818019020           0.0920603024

                           Simple Statistics

Variable                N        Mean        StdDev           Sum       Minimum       Maximum

Random_Intercept      750    -0.00899       0.61470      -6.74209      -2.35449       1.94666
Random_Slope          750     0.00575       0.30341       4.31239      -0.97224       1.06087

        Pearson Correlation Coefficients, N = 750
              Prob> |r| under H0: Rho=0

                        Random_            Random_
                        Intercept           Slope

Random_Intercept        1.00000           0.43859
                                          <.0001

Random_Slope            0.43859           1.00000
                        <.0001
```

FIGURE 8.35

Means, variances, and covariance for random intercepts and slopes.

```
Data _tmp_2;
Set _tmp_1;

retain  seed3 5  seed4 6 seed6 1000;

   NumberOfVisits=11;

   b1=2;   /* Baseline effect slope */
   b2=2;   /* Treatment effect slope */
   b4=0.5; /* Cycle*Treatment interaction slope */

call rannor(seed6, X6);
Baseline = 10 + 30 * X6;

Call ranuni(seed3, X4);
Do Cycle=1 to (1+Int(NumberOfVisits * X4));

    call rannor(seed4, X5);

    Y = Fixed_Intercept +

    b1 * Baseline +

    b2 * Treatment +

    Fixed_Slope * Cycle +

    b4 * Cycle * Treatment +

    Random_Intercept + Random_Slope* Cycle + sqrt(0.3)*X5;

output;
End;

Keep Y Baseline ID Cycle Treatment;

Run;
```

FIGURE 8.36
Generating dataset for the analysis.

	ID	Treatment	Baseline	Cycle	Y
1	1	0	17.0322044	1	50.4572205
2	1	0	17.0322044	2	53.4570611
3	1	0	17.0322044	3	58.5910413
4	1	0	17.0322044	4	62.8645394
5	1	0	17.0322044	5	66.0364293
6	1	0	17.0322044	6	71.0559929
7	1	0	17.0322044	7	74.1786281
8	1	0	17.0322044	8	79.3806792
9	1	0	17.0322044	9	83.8165334
10	1	0	17.0322044	10	87.4831502
11	1	0	17.0322044	11	90.7673735

FIGURE 8.37
Structure of the dataset (first subject is shown).

```
Proc Mixed data=_tmp_2;

   Class ID;

   Model Y = Baseline Cycle Treatment Cycle*Treatment / Solution
ddfm=kr;

   Random INTERCEPT Cycle / Subject=ID Type=UN;

Run;
```

FIGURE 8.38
Implementation of the random intercept–slope mixed model.

```
Covariance Parameter Estimates

CovParm        Subject      Estimate
UN(1,1)        ID             0.3658
UN(2,1)        ID            0.08166
UN(2,2)        ID            0.09090
Residual                     0.2965

              Solution for Fixed Effects

                            Standard
Effect             Estimate    Error    DF   t Value   Pr> |t|

Intercept          11.0722   0.04139   692   267.51    <.0001
Baseline            1.9987  0.000951   719  2102.04    <.0001
Cycle               3.9995   0.01824   626   219.25    <.0001
Treatment           1.9062   0.05750   705    33.15    <.0001
Cycle*Treatment     0.5000   0.02581   631    19.37    <.0001
```

FIGURE 8.39
Covariance parameters and fixed effects estimates.

to 11 (`Fixed_Intercept = 11`; see Figures 8.33 and 8.34). The next parameter is the slope for the baseline covariate, with an estimated value of 2.0 (`Baseline 1.9987`)—which is defined in the simulation as a corresponding slope value equal to 2 (`b1 = 2;`/* Baseline effect slope*/; see Figure 8.36). The fixed effect for time was estimated as 4 (`Cycle 3.9995`; Figure 8.39)—which is defined in the simulation as a corresponding slope value of 4 (`Fixed_Slope = 4`; see Figures 8.33 and 8.34). The treatment effect (slope) was estimated as 1.9 (`Treatment 1.9062`; Figure 8.39)—which is defined in the simulation as a corresponding slope value equal to 2 (`b2 = 2;`/* `Treatment effect slope` */; see Figure 8.36). The last parameter is the slope for the time-by-treatment (or cycle-by-treatment) interaction term that was estimated as 0.5 (`Cycle*Treatment 0.5000`; Figure 8.39)—which is defined in the simulation as a corresponding slope value equal to 0.5 (`b4 = 0.5;`/* `Cycle*Treatment interaction slope` */; see Figure 8.36).

8.5 Summary

This chapter focuses on longitudinal models for examining effects in the context of a single-group design or parallel multiple-group design. The conceptual and practical importance of PRO measures assessed longitudinally is highlighted by a detailed description on the implementation of the two approaches generally referred to as random coefficient models and repeated measures models. The repeated measures model is presented with time as a categorical covariate and, separately, as a continuous covariate. Covariance structures of the residual error terms over time are given consideration. The random coefficient model is presented through explanation of its characteristics. Simulated examples in SAS, motivated by real-world applications and by the content stressed in the chapter, illustrate and implement the methods discussed. The methodologies are also illustrated with published applications from clinical studies on renal cell carcinoma and smoking cessation.

References

Brown, H. and R. Prescott. 2006. *Applied Mixed Models in Medicine*, 2nd edition. Chichester, England: John Wiley & Sons.

Cella, D., Li, J.Z., Cappelleri, J.C., Bushmakin, A., Charbonneau, C., Kim, S.T., Chen, I., Michaelson, M.D., and R.J. Motzer. 2008. Quality of life in patients with metastatic renal cell carcinoma treated with sunitinib versus interferon-alfa: Results from a phase III randomized trial. *Journal of Clinical Oncology* 26:3763–3769.

Fairclough, D.L. 2004. Patient reported outcomes as endpoints in medical research. *Statistical Methods in Medical Research* 13:1135–1138.

Fairclough, D.L. 2005. Analysing longitudinal studies of QoL. In: Fayers, P. and Hays, R. (editors). *Assessing Quality of Life in Clinical Trials*, 2nd edition. New York, NY: Oxford University Press, Chapter 3.

Fairclough, D.L. 2010. *Design and Analysis of Quality of Life Studies in Clinical Trials*, 2nd edition. Boca Raton, FL: Chapman & Hall/CRC.

Fitzmaurice, G.M., Laird, N.M., and J.H. Ware. 2011. *Applied Longitudinal Analysis*, 2nd edition. Hoboken, NJ: John Wiley & Sons.

Gonzales, D., Rennard, S.I., Nides, M., Oncken, C., Azoulay, S., Billing, C.B., Watsky, E.J., Gong, J., Williams, K.E., and K.R. Reeves. 2006. Varenicline, an alpha4beta2 nicotinic acetylcholine receptor partial agonist, vs sustained-release bupropion and placebo for smoking cessation: A randomized controlled trial. *JAMA* 296:47–55.

Hedeker, D. and R.D. Gibbons. 2006. *Longitudinal Data Analysis*. Hoboken, NJ: John Wiley & Sons.

Kenward, M.G. and J.H. Roger. 1997. Small sample inference for fixed effects from restricted maximum likelihood. *Biometrics* 53:983–997.

Littell, R.C., Milliken, G.A., Stroup, W.W., Wolfinger, R.D., and O. Schabenberber. 2006. *SAS System for Mixed Models*, 2nd edition. Cary, NC: SAS Institute Inc.

Newsom, J.T., Jones, R.N., and S.M. Hofer (co-editors). 2012. *Longitudinal Data Analysis: A Practical Guide for Researchers in Aging, Health, and Social Sciences.* New York, NY: Taylor & Francis Group.

SAS Institute Inc. 2011. *SAS/STAT® 9.3 User's Guide*, 2nd edition. Cary, NC: SAS Institute Inc.

Singer, J.D. and J.B. Willett. 2003. *Applied Longitudinal Data Analysis: Modeling Change and Event Occurrence.* New York, NY: Oxford University Press.

Vonesh, E.F. 2012. *Generalized Linear and Nonlinear Models for Correlated Data: Theory and Applications Using SAS®*. Cary, NC: SAS Institute Inc.

Weiss, R.L. 2005. *Modeling Longitudinal Data*. New York, NY: Springer-Verlag.

9

Mediation Models

A mediation model is one that seeks to identify and explain the mechanism that underlies an observed relationship between a predictor or independent variable (e.g., treatment group) and an outcome or dependent variable (e.g., sleep disturbance) via the inclusion of a third explanatory variable (e.g., pain), known as a mediator variable. Any of these three variables may be a patient-reported outcome (PRO) measure (e.g., sleep disturbance and pain may be PRO measures; an independent variable may also be a PRO measure). Mediation modeling is gaining currency in the application of PRO measures (Fairclough, 2010), and at least two full-length monographs have been devoted to mediation analysis (Iacobucci, 2008; MacKinnon, 2008). In pharmaceutical studies, for example, mediation models can help to elucidate the mechanism of action of a drug.

Rather than hypothesizing a direct causal relationship between the predictor and the outcome, a mediation model postulates that the predictor variable not only affects the outcome variable directly, but also affects the mediator variable, which in turn also affects the outcome variable. The mediator variable, therefore, serves to clarify the nature of the relationship between predictor and outcome variables. The postulated underpinning for a mediation model is driven by the theoretical or conceptual framework and the research objective.

It should be emphasized that no technique, including mediation models and other forms of structural equation models, can prove causation. Rather, the purpose of mediation analysis (and path analysis in general) is to determine whether the hypothesized causal inferences by a researcher are harmonious with the data. If the mediation model does not fit the data, then revisions are needed because then one or more of the model assumptions are not correct or need to be refined. If the mediation model is consistent with the data, this does not prove causation. Instead, it shows that the assumptions made are not contradicted and *may be valid*. It *may only be valid* because other models and assumptions may also fit the data. Making causal inferences between variables is a tricky business and a serious subject. The extent that one variable may cause another depends on the research design, including in part the temporal sequence of the variables and the plausibility of relations as informed by knowledge of the subject matter.

The approaches discussed in this chapter assume that the mediator and outcome are continuous variables. The predictor may be a categorical (e.g., binary) variable, as well as continuous. Mediation models with categorical data are discussed elsewhere (Iacobucci, 2008; MacKinnon, 2008). In this chapter, the basic elements of single mediator models are described and then extended to cover multiple mediator models, latent variable mediation models, multiple-outcome mediation models, and longitudinal mediation models. Concepts are illustrated with real-life examples and with computer simulations.

9.1 Single Mediator Model

9.1.1 Basics

Research has often focused on the relation between two variables, say, X and Y. Such research includes situations where the explanatory (predictor) variable X can be considered a possible cause of the outcome variable Y, as when, for example, subjects are randomized to interventions of the treatment group variable X. A theoretical premise may posit that an intervening (mediator) variable is an indicative measure of the process through which a predictor is thought to affect an outcome. The objective is to assess the extent to which the effect of the predictor variable on the outcome variable is indirect via the mediator or, alternatively, is otherwise direct, which captures all other effects.

As diagrammed in Figure 9.1, mediation in its simplest form is represented by a third variable (M, the mediator), so that the predictor X influences the

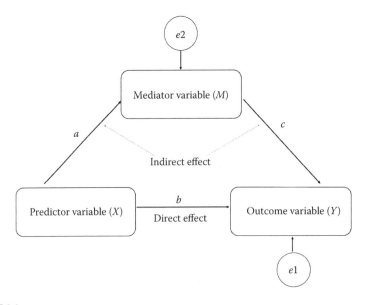

FIGURE 9.1
Basic mediation model: the predictor X influences the outcome variable Y directly and via the mediator (M).

mediator M, which, in turn, influences the outcome Y (X affects M and then M affects Y). Therefore, a natural question arises: What fraction of the total effect of X on Y is the direct effect and what fraction of the total effect of X on Y is the indirect effect mediated through the mediator M? The direct effect represents all other possible effects other than those attributed to the mediator.

The mediation model portrayed by Figure 9.1 for the subject j can be denoted by the following equations:

$$Y_j = i_1 + b \times X_j + c \times M_j + e_{1j}, \tag{9.1}$$

$$M_j = i_2 + a \times X_j + e_{2j}, \tag{9.2}$$

where

Y_j and M_j are the outcomes for subject j

i_1 and i_2 are the overall intercepts in Equations 9.1 and 9.2, respectively

a is the overall slope in Equation 9.2, representing the effect of the independent variable X on the mediator variable M

b is the overall slope in Equation 9.1, representing the direct effect of the independent variable X on the variable Y

c is the overall slope in Equation 9.1, representing the effect of the mediator variable M on the variable Y

e_{1j} and e_{2j} are the error terms, assumed independent, taken from a normal distribution with mean 0 and variance σ_1^2 and σ_2^2 (i.e., $e_{1j} \sim N(0, \sigma_1^2)$ and $e_{2j} \sim N(0, \sigma_2^2)$)

It should be emphasized that it is assumed that the mediation model is correctly specified to answer the research question of interest from a well-defined hypothesis. Under this hypothesis framework, the data provide empirical evidence regarding the postulated interrelationship among variables. If the hypothesis changes to include or exclude certain variables, with possible changes in the linkages between variables, then the model formulation would need to be modified accordingly. Hence, the model formulation should be fully aligned to its hypothesized framework.

Replacing M_j in Equation 9.1 by M_j from Equation 9.2 allows Y_j to be represented as

$$Y_j = i_1 + b \times X_j + c \times (i_2 + a \times X_j + e_{2j}) + e_{1j},$$

$$Y_j = (i_1 + c \times i_2) + (b + c \times a) \times X_j + (c \times e_{2j} + e_{1j}). \tag{9.3}$$

Equation 9.3 can be considered as the representation of the total effect of the variable X on variable Y, after accounting for the presence of the mediator M. The first part ($i_1 + c \times i_2$) is constant and represents the intercept, the second part $(b + c \times a)$ represents the slope, and the third part $(c \times e_{2j} + e_{1j})$ represents the error term. If variable X_j represents treatment with values of 0 for placebo and value of 1 for the active treatment, then $(b + c \times a)$ represents the total effect of active treatment on the outcome Y after accounting for placebo. Coefficient b represents the direct effect of X_j on variable Y_j. It is worthwhile to note that the term *direct effect* is somewhat misleading—this effect actually represents all other possible paths (excluding the path through the mediator M) from the independent variable X to the outcome Y. The expression $c \times a$ represents the indirect effect of X on Y through the mediator M. Note that the sum of the indirect effect $(c \times a)$ of X on Y via M and the direct effect (b) of X on Y equals the total effect of X on Y. The mediation modeling can be viewed as an attempt to decompose the total effect of X on Y to better understand the mechanism of action of X.

Now we are ready to answer the main question: What fraction of the total effect of X on Y is the direct effect and what fraction of the total effect of X on Y is the indirect effect mediated through the mediator M? The percentage of the total effect that is the direct effect (*the direct effect of X on Y*) can be expressed as follows:

$$direct\ effect = 100\left(\frac{b}{b + c \times a}\right). \tag{9.4}$$

In Equation 9.4, the fraction was multiplied by 100 to represent the effect as a percentage of the total effect.

The percentage of the total effect that is an indirect effect of X on Y (*the indirect effect of X on Y*) via the mediator M can be expressed as follows:

$$indirect\ effect = 100\left(\frac{c \times a}{b + c \times a}\right). \tag{9.5}$$

Complete mediation is the case in which the variable X no longer directly affects Y, so the path coefficient b is zero. On the other hand, no mediation occurs when the total effect of X on Y exists entirely through the direct effect, so that the coefficient b is nonzero and $c \times a$ is zero. Partial mediation is the case in which the direct path b and indirect path $c \times a$ are both nonzero.

9.1.2 Implementation of the Mediation Model Using the SAS MODEL Procedure

9.1.2.1 Simulated Dataset

A simulated dataset is used to illustrate the implementation of a mediation model. Consider a hypothetical clinical study with 200 subjects and two treatment arms. Each subject is randomized to an active drug or placebo.

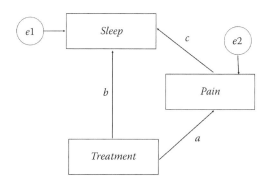

FIGURE 9.2
Mediation model: *Treatment* affects *Sleep* directly and indirectly via *Pain*.

The continuous outcome variables are PRO measures of Pain and Sleep, which could be, either cross-sectional or averaged over certain periods of time, depending on the question asked. In our synthetic study, the active agent is known to be efficacious in reducing pain. But it was observed as well that subjects on active drug also had improvements in sleep quality. A plausible hypothesis in such a study is that subjects sleep better while on active drug simply because they have less pain. The alternative hypothesis could be that drug affects sleep quality not only via reduction in pain, but also directly from other sources.

This hypothesis can be investigated with a mediation model (see Figure 9.2). Treatment variable is assigned a value of 1 for the active treatment arm and a value of 0 for the placebo arm. The treatment variable *Treatment* affects the sleep variable *Sleep* directly and also via variable *Pain*, which plays the role of the mediator in this model. Equations 9.1 and 9.2 for a subject *j* can then be written as

$$Sleep_j = i_1 + b \times Treatment_j + c \times Pain_j + e_{1j}, \tag{9.6}$$

$$Pain_j = i_2 + a \times Treatment_j + e_{2j}, \tag{9.7}$$

where

$Sleep_j$ and $Pain_j$ are the PRO measures for subject *j* representing, respectively, sleep and pain

i_1 and i_2 are the overall intercepts in Equations 9.6 and 9.7, respectively

a is the overall slope in Equation 9.7, representing the effect of active treatment (vs placebo) on pain

b is the overall slope in Equation 9.6, representing the direct effect of active treatment on sleep

c is the overall slope in Equation 9.6, representing the effect of pain on sleep

e_{1j} and e_{2j} are the error terms, assumed independent, taken from a normal distribution with mean 0 and variance σ_1^2 and σ_2^2 (i.e., $e_{1j} \sim N(0, \sigma_1^2)$ and $e_{2j} \sim N(0, \sigma_2^2)$)

The SAS code in Figure 9.3 generates the dataset with 200 observations (100 subjects per treatment arm). The SAS code lines

```
i1=2; i2=1;   /* Intercepts */
a=1.5;        /* effect of treatment on pain */
b=.5;         /* Direct effect of treatment on sleep*/
c=1 ;         /* effect of pain on sleep */
```

```
/*
Data with two continuous outcomes (Pain and Sleep) and one
categorical variable (Treatment) for mediation model.
-----------------------------------------------------------------
For this example we have 100 subjects (NumberOfRows) for every
treatment arm.
There are 2 treatment arms (NumberOfTreatments = 2;)
-----------------------------------------------------------------
*/

options nofmterr nocenter pagesize=2000 linesize=256;

%Let NumberOfRows      = 100;
%Let NumberOfTreatments = 2;

Data _mediation_1;

Retain seed1 100 seed2 200 ;

   i1=2; i2=1;   /* intercepts */

   a=1.5;        /* effect of treatment on pain */
   b=.5;         /* direct effect of treatment on sleep */
   c=1 ;         /* effect of pain on sleep */

      ID=0;
      Do Treatment=0 to (&NumberOfTreatments-1);
      Do i=1 To &NumberOfRows;

             ID=ID+1;

             Call rannor(seed2,X2);
             Pain = i2 + a*Treatment    + sqrt(0.5)*X2;

             Call rannor(seed1,X1);
             Sleep = i1 + b*Treatment + c*Pain + sqrt(0.2)*X1;

             output;

      End;
      End;
Keep ID Pain Sleep Treatment;

Run;
```

FIGURE 9.3
Generating dataset for the analysis.

ID	Treatment	Pain	Sleep
1	1	0	1.08614634	3.61472428
2	2	0	1.13765088	3.21591488
3	3	0	1.65626682	4.42535122
4	4	0	0.62077119	2.95922508
5	5	0	0.92054667	2.87004898
6	6	0	1.05774993	2.93029495
7	7	0	0.42588925	2.29645
8	8	0	0.11844797	2.04660944
9	9	0	1.80270644	4.53480665
10	10	0	0.67550108	2.44460741

FIGURE 9.4
Simulated dataset (data for the first 10 subjects are shown).

define the overall means and slopes, which correspond to the parameters i_1, i_2, a, b, and c in Equations 9.6 and 9.7. The SAS code lines

```
Call rannor(seed2,X2);
Pain = i2 + a*Treatment              + sqrt(0.5)*X2;
Call rannor(seed1,X1);
Sleep = i1 + b*Treatment + c*Pain + sqrt(0.2)*X1;
```

represent Equations 9.6 and 9.7. In this example, we model the different error terms in Equations 9.6 and 9.7. For example, in Equation 9.6 the variance is 0.2 (`Call rannor(seed1,X1); ... + sqrt(0.2)*X1;`) and in Equation 9.7 the variance is 0.5 (`Call rannor(seed2,X2); ... + sqrt(0.5)*X2;`).

Here, four columns (see Figure 9.3; "Keep ID Pain Sleep Treatment;") were kept in the final dataset. Although only Pain, Sleep, and Treatment are needed for the analysis, it is customary to keep subject ID as a part of a dataset. If some outliers are found in the dataset, for example, with values outside of the possible range for the variables under investigation, it could help to go back to the original data source and examine data for those subjects. Figure 9.4 shows, for the first 10 subjects, a portion of the final simulated dataset.

9.1.2.2 Implementation

Figure 9.5 represents implementation of the mediation model using the MODEL procedure (SAS, 2011). The SAS code line

```
Exogenous Treatment;
```

defines that treatment is an independent variable in this model (after all, the meaning of the word *exogenous* is originating from the outside). The next SAS code line

```
Parms i1 i2 a b c;
```

```
Proc Model Data=_mediation_1 CONVERGE=1e-7 MAXITER=100 SINGULAR=1E-10;

    Exogenous  Treatment;
    Parms i1 i2 a b c;

    Sleep  = i1 + b*Treatment + c*Pain;
    Pain   = i2 + a*Treatment          ;

    h.Pain = E2;
    h.Sleep = E1;

    Fit Sleep Pain / fiml;

    Estimate "Indirect Path" 100*c*a/(b+c*a);
    Estimate "Direct Path"   100*b/(b+c*a);
Run;
Quit;
```

FIGURE 9.5
Implementation of the mediation model using SAS MODEL procedure.

defines the parameter to be estimated in this model. Note that in this model two additional parameters, which are error terms, are also defined. The SAS code lines

$$h.Pain \ = E2;$$
$$h.Sleep = E1;$$

instruct SAS to estimate error terms. Note that the dataset should not have any columns with names i1, i2, a, b, c, E1, and E2. The SAS code lines

$$Sleep = i1 + b * Treatment + c * Pain; \qquad (9.8)$$

$$Pain = i2 + a * Treatment; \qquad (9.9)$$

correspond exactly to Equations 9.6 and 9.7. The SAS code line

$$Fit \ Sleep \ Pain \ / \ FIML;$$

instructs that Equations 9.8 and 9.9 should be fitted simultaneously using full information maximum likelihood (FIML), an approach to the estimation of simultaneous equations (SAS, 2011). FIML also assumes that the errors are normally distributed. The SAS code lines

$$Estimate \ "Indirect \ Path" \ 100*c*a/(b+c*a);$$

$$Estimate \ "Direct \ Path" \ 100*b/(b+c*a);$$

correspond to Equations 9.4 and 9.5 and provide key results in our example.

Figure 9.6 shows the results of modeling for estimation of the mediation model parameters. With this exercise, we can find how close the estimated modeled parameters are to the values we assigned for those parameters when data were simulated. From the Figure 9.6, for instance, the estimated modeled intercepts are close to 2.0 and 1 (i1 = 1.950863; i2 = 0.967249) and the

```
                Nonlinear FIML Parameter Estimates

                                Approx                  Approx
      Parameter      Estimate   Std Err    t Value      Pr> |t|

      i1             1.950863   0.0619      31.51       <.0001
      i2             0.967249   0.0741      13.05       <.0001
      a              1.528891   0.1048      14.59       <.0001
      b               0.48147   0.0924       5.21       <.0001
      c              1.041096   0.0434      23.99       <.0001
      E2             0.549241   0.0549      10.00       <.0001
      E1             0.206949   0.0207      10.00       <.0001
```

FIGURE 9.6
Partial output of the SAS MODEL procedure: Mediation model parameters.

true simulated values are 2 and 1 (i1 = **2**; i2 = **1**; /* Intercepts */; Figure 9.3), the estimated modeled variances σ_1^2 and σ_2^2 of the error terms are 0.21 and 0.55 (E1 0.206949; E2 0.549241) and the true simulated values are 0.2 and 0.5 (…+ sqrt(**0.5**)*X2; …+ sqrt(**0.2**)*X1; see Figure 9.3). Modeled values for *a*, *b*, and *c* are also close to the values defined in the simulations.

Figure 9.7 represents the key results for the mediation modeling—that is, the estimated percentages of the total effect that are direct and indirect. These estimated direct and indirect effects are 23.2% and 76.8%, respectively. The results here indicate that in this hypothetical study active treatment improves sleep mostly indirectly via improvements in pain. The direct effect of the active treatment (over and above placebo) on sleep accounts only for 23.2% of the total effect that the active treatment has on sleep. Again, because the values for *a*, *b*, and *c* are known from the simulations (a = **1.5**; b = **.5**; c = **1**; see Figure 9.3), and with knowledge of Equations 9.4 and 9.5, the true direct and indirect effects can be calculated as

$$direct\ effect = 100\frac{0.5}{0.5 + 1 \times 1.5} = 25\%$$

```
                  Nonlinear FIML Estimates

                          Approx           Approx
      Term        Estimate Std Err t Value Pr> |t|   Label

      Indirect Path  76.77638   4.1729   18.40   <.0001   100*c*a/(b+c*a)

                  Nonlinear FIML Estimates

                          Approx           Approx
      Term        Estimate Std Err t Value Pr> |t|   Label

      Direct Path    23.22362   4.1729    5.57   <.0001   100*b/(b+c*a)
```

FIGURE 9.7
Partial output of the SAS MODEL procedure: Estimates of direct and indirect effects.

and

$$indirect\ effect = 100\frac{1\times 1.5}{0.5+1\times 1.5} = 75\%,$$

showing that the modeled values of 23.2% and 76.8% are close to the true values of 25% and 75% for this mediation model.

9.1.3 Example with Multiple Independent Variables

In clinical studies, it is common to have more than just two treatment arms. As an illustration, interrelationships among several treatments (predictors), pain (mediator), and sleep outcomes were examined using mediation models for patients with fibromyalgia (Russell et al., 2009). The questions analogous to questions in Section 9.1.2 are investigated here. Do patients have reduced sleep disturbance only because they have reduced pain from the study medication? If so, the effect of study medication on reduced sleep disturbance would be wholly mediated and accounted for by reduced pain; if not, the study medication has an independent effect, above and beyond pain reduction, which contributes to reduced sleep disturbance.

While several mediation analyses were implemented and reported (Russell et al., 2009), the focus here involves one study in which 745 patients were randomized to placebo or three different doses of study medication. Specifically, we consider the direct and indirect effects of treatment with pregabalin 300 mg, 450 mg, and 600 mg (each vs placebo) on patient-reported sleep disturbance (range: 0–100, where higher scores reflect more sleep disturbance) from the Medical Outcomes Study Sleep Scale. This outcome, which had a 1-week recall period in this study, was assessed at the last week of treatment (week 14).

The mediator was a patient-reported daily diary pain score, based on a 11-point numeric rating scale (0 = no pain to 10 = worst possible pain) and averaged over the last 7 days of treatment. A set of simultaneous linear multiple regression equations was postulated to quantify treatment-related improvements in sleep disturbance that appeared to be due to reductions in pain (indirect treatment effect) and treatment-related improvements in sleep outcomes that were not explained, or mediated, by reductions in pain (direct treatment effect).

Relative to placebo, pregabalin 300 mg, 450 mg, and 600 mg reduced (improved) average sleep disturbance scores respectively by approximately 9.9, 12.7 and 17.8 points, which were the total effects of pregabalin (relative to placebo) on sleep disturbance scores at end of treatment. The mediation model showed that, for these total effects, approximately 80%, 73%, and 75.6% (all significantly different from zero, two-sided $p < 0.0001$) of the reduction in sleep disturbance were direct effects of the treatments themselves, while the remaining 20% (not significant) for 300 mg, 27% ($p = 0.0153$) for 450 mg, and 24.4% ($p < 0.0027$) for 600 mg were mediated via pain (Figure 9.8). The direct effect of study mediation on sleep disturbance reflects the effect of study medication independent of changes

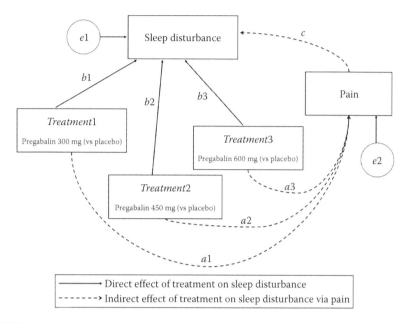

FIGURE 9.8

Direct and indirect effects of pregabalin on sleep disturbance with pain as the mediator.

in pain, while the indirect effect of the medicine on sleep disturbance represents the part mediated via pain (prompted by the analgesic effects of the medicine).

9.1.3.1 Simulated Dataset

A simulated dataset is used to illustrate the implementation of a mediation model with several independent variables. As described previously in Section 9.1.3, consider a clinical study with four treatment arms. Suppose that each subject is randomized to pregabalin 300 mg, 450 mg, 600 mg, or placebo (186 subject per treatment arm, for a total of 744 subjects). The outcome variables are PRO measures of Pain and Sleep. The mediation model is depicted by Figure 9.8. Three binary treatment variables (*Treatment1*, *Treatment2*, and *Treatment3*) are now needed to describe the four treatment arms. For example, for a subject on placebo all three treatment variables will be assigned a value of 0, for a subject on pregabalin 300 mg variable *Treatment1* will be assigned a value of 1 and the other two treatment variables will be assigned a value of 0 (*Treatment1=1, Treatment2=0, and Treatment3=0*).

Equations 9.1 and 9.2 for a subject j in this simulation can be written as

$$Sleep_j = i_1 + b1 \times Treatment1_j + b2 \times Treatment2_j$$

$$+ b3 \times Treatment3_j + c \times Pain_j + e_{1j}, \tag{9.10}$$

$$Pain_j = i_2 + a1 \times Treatment1_j + a2 \times Treatment2_j$$

$$+ a3 \times Treatment3_j + e_{2j}, \tag{9.11}$$

where

Sleep$_j$ and Pain$_j$ are PRO measures for subject j, representing sleep disturbance and pain, respectively

i_1 and i_2 are the overall intercepts in Equations 9.10 and 9.11, respectively

$a1$, $a2$, and $a3$ are the overall slopes in Equation 9.11, representing effects of
pregabalin 300 mg, 450 mg, 600 mg (each vs placebo) on pain

$b1$, $b2$, and $b3$ are the overall slopes in Equation 9.10, representing direct
effects of pregabalin 300 mg, 450 mg, 600 mg (each vs placebo) on sleep
disturbance

c is the overall slope in Equation 9.10 representing the effect of pain on
sleep disturbance

e_{1j} and e_{2j} are the error terms, assumed independent, taken from a normal
distribution with mean 0 and variance σ_1^2 and σ_2^2 (i.e., $e_{1j} \sim N(0, \sigma_1^2)$ and
$e_{2j} \sim N(0, \sigma_2^2)$)

The SAS code in Figure 9.9 is similar to that in Figure 9.3 (which has only
two treatments and therefore only one binary treatment variable), with one
important difference: based on the arm of the study (represented by the variable
TreatmentArm), the exogenous variables *Treatment1, Treatment2, and Treatment3*
are assigned a value of 0 or 1. The following SAS code lines illustrate this:

```
If TreatmentArm=1 Then Do; Treatment1=0; Treatment2=0;
Treatment3=0; End;
If TreatmentArm=2 Then Do; Treatment1=1; Treatment2=0;
Treatment3=0; End;
If TreatmentArm=3 Then Do; Treatment1=0; Treatment2=1;
Treatment3=0; End;
If TreatmentArm=4 Then Do; Treatment1=0; Treatment2=0;
Treatment3=1; End;
```

Figure 9.10 illustrates the structure of the dataset for the analysis and highlights the layout and values of variables for subjects from different treatment
arms. The subjects with ID = 1, 2, and 3 are from the placebo arm, subjects
with ID = 187 and 188 are from the first active treatment arm (simulating
pregabalin 300 mg), and so forth.

9.1.3.2 Implementation

The fraction representing the direct effect in the case of several treatment arms
is unique for every active treatment arm and can be expressed as:

$$direct\ effect\ for\ active\ treatment\ arm\ k = 100 \frac{b_k}{b_k + c \times a_k}, \tag{9.12}$$

```
/*
----------------------------------------------------------------
For this example we have 744 subjects
with 186 (NumberOfRows) for every treatment arm.
There are 4 treatment arms.
----------------------------------------------------------------
*/

options nofmterr nocenter pagesize=2000 linesize=256;

%Let NumberOfRows      = 186;

Data _mediation_1;

Retain seed1 100 seed2 200;

  i1=2; i2=1;        /* Intercepts */

  a1=0.4;            /* effect of 300 mg on pain */
  b1=0.8;            /* direct effect of 300 mg on sleep*/

  a2=0.45;           /* effect of 450 mg on pain */
  b2=0.7;            /* direct effect of 450 mg on sleep*/

  a3=0.5;            /* effect of 600 mg on pain */
  b3=0.75;           /* direct effect of 600 mg on sleep*/

  c=0.5 ;            /* effect of pain on sleep */

    ID=0;
    Do TreatmentArm=1 to 4;
    Do i=1 To &NumberOfRows;

    ID=ID+1;

  If TreatmentArm=1 Then Do; Treatment1=0; Treatment2=0;
Treatment3=0; End;
  If TreatmentArm=2 Then Do; Treatment1=1; Treatment2=0;
Treatment3=0; End;
  If TreatmentArm=3 Then Do; Treatment1=0; Treatment2=1;
Treatment3=0; End;
  If TreatmentArm=4 Then Do; Treatment1=0; Treatment2=0;
Treatment3=1; End;

            Call rannor(seed2,X2);
            Pain = i2 + a1*Treatment1 + a2*Treatment2 +
a3*Treatment3 + sqrt(0.05)*X2;

            Call rannor(seed1,X1);
            Sleep = i1 + b1*Treatment1 + b2*Treatment2 +
b3*Treatment3 + c*Pain + sqrt(0.1)*X1;

                output;

        End;
        End;
Keep ID Pain Sleep Treatment1 Treatment2 Treatment3;

Run;
```

FIGURE 9.9
Generating dataset for the analysis with four independent variables.

	ID	Treatment1	Treatment2	Treatment3	Pain	Sleep
1	1	0	0	0	1.0272419	2.887382
2	2	0	0	0	1.043529	2.5771055
3	3	0	0	0	1.2075298	3.1475897
				•••		
187	187	1	0	0	1.4642922	3.1733836
188	188	1	0	0	1.30744	3.2678548
				•••		
379	379	0	1	0	1.6409317	3.057832
380	380	0	1	0	1.5610803	3.3589318
				•••		
742	742	0	0	1	1.242234	3.5547042
743	743	0	0	1	1.5581368	3.6214557
744	744	0	0	1	1.4672426	3.14924

FIGURE 9.10
Simulated dataset for the mediation modeling in a study with four treatment arms.

$$indirect\ effect\ for\ active\ treatment\ arm\ k = 100\frac{c \times a_k}{b_k + c \times a_k}, \qquad (9.13)$$

where
  k represents a particular active treatment arm vs placebo (where $k = 1$ for
    pregabalin 300 mg, $k = 2$ for pregabalin 450 mg and $k = 3$ for 600 mg,
    with each of them vs placebo)
  a_k, b_k, and, c correspond to parameters $a1$, $a2$, $a3$, $b1$, $b2$, $b3$, and c in Equations
    9.10 and 9.11

Essentially this means that, although there is one integrated and unified
mediation model (with parameters emanating from it), the direct and indirect effects for every treatment should be calculated separately, as if only one
particular arm were present.

Figure 9.11 represents the implementation of the mediation model using the
MODEL procedure in SAS (SAS, 2011). The implementation is similar to that in
Figure 9.5 for two treatments (represented by one binary treatment variable).
It is worth mentioning that for the current implementation six `Estimate`
statements are needed to assess the direct and indirect effects, which repre-
sent Equations 9.12 and 9.13 for each of the three active treatment arms.

Figure 9.12 shows the corresponding partial output of the modeling. All estimated parameters ($i1$, $i2$, $a1$, $a2$, $a3$, $b1$, $b2$,...) are close to the values used in the
simulations. As was the case for the direct effects based on one treatment comparison, the hypothetical true direct effects are known (from Figure 9.9): 80%
[$= 100*0.8/(0.8+0.5\times0.4)$], 75.7% [$=100*0.7/(0.7+0.5\times0.45)$] and 75% [$=100* 0.75/$
$(0.75+0.5\times0.5)$] for pregabalin 300 mg, 450 mg, and 600 mg, respectively. From
Figure 9.12, the corresponding estimated values from the model are 77.58971%,
74.8279%, and 73.8851%, which closely match their corresponding true values.

```
Proc Model Data=_mediation_1 CONVERGE=1e-7 MAXITER=100 SINGULAR=1E-10;

    Exogenous Treatment1 Treatment2 Treatment3;
    Parms i1 i2 a1 a2 a3 b1 b2 b3 c;

    Sleep = i1 + b1*Treatment1 + b2*Treatment2 + b3*Treatment3 + c*Pain;
    Pain = i2 + a1*Treatment1 + a2*Treatment2 + a3*Treatment3   ;

    h.Pain = E2;
    h.Sleep = E1;

    Fit Sleep Pain / fiml ;

    Estimate "Indirect Path (300mg)" 100*c*a1/(b1+c*a1);
    Estimate "Direct Path (300mg)" 100*b1/(b1+c*a1);

    Estimate "Indirect Path (450mg)" 100*c*a2/(b2+c*a2);
    Estimate "Direct Path (450mg)" 100*b2/(b2+c*a2);

    Estimate "Indirect Path (600mg)" 100*c*a3/(b3+c*a3);
    Estimate "Direct Path (600mg)" 100*b3/(b3+c*a3);
Run;
Quit;
```

FIGURE 9.11
Implementation of the mediation modeling in a study with four treatment arms.

9.2 Model Invariance

Section 9.1 focused on the application of mediation models to the entire dataset, considering it as a single sample. Even in the case of multiple active treatments, we considered the entire sample as a whole. In this section, we will apply and examine mediation models across distinct groups and across time to address two key objectives. One key objective is to understand and examine whether the direct and indirect effects, expressed as a percentage of a total effect, are different among particular groups—in short, whether the mediation model is group invariant. The second key objective addresses whether the mediation model is time invariant.

The term *model invariance* should not be confused with *interaction* terms such as a treatment-by-group interaction effect typically considered in statistical analysis. For instance, the total effect between groups may be the same (i.e., no treatment-by-group interaction) but the proportion of total effect attributed to the direct effect (or indirect effect) may differ between groups (not model invariant). Alternatively, the total effect between groups may be different (i.e., treatment-by-group interaction) but the proportion of total effect attributed to the direct effect (or indirect effect) may not differ between groups (model invariant).

It is important to note that to answer the first objective, about group invariance, data for at least two distinct groups of subjects are needed. For example, a researcher could be interested whether a mediation model is gender invariant.

Parameter	Estimate	Std Err	t Value	Pr> |t|
i1	1.986162	0.0556	35.71	<.0001
i2	0.994318	0.0165	60.30	<.0001
a1	0.419551	0.0233	17.99	<.0001
a2	0.436764	0.0233	18.73	<.0001
a3	0.507617	0.0233	21.77	<.0001
b1	0.764016	0.0388	19.67	<.0001
b2	0.682891	0.0393	17.37	<.0001
b3	0.755381	0.0415	18.21	<.0001
c	0.52597	0.0510	10.32	<.0001
E2	0.050577	0.00262	19.29	<.0001
E1	0.097736	0.00507	19.29	<.0001

Nonlinear FIML Estimates

Term	Estimate	Approx Std Err	t Value	Approx Pr> |t|	Label
Indirect Path (300mg)	22.41029	2.4885	9.01	<.0001	100*c*a1/(b1+c*a1)

Nonlinear FIML Estimates

Term	Estimate	Approx Std Err	t Value	Approx Pr> |t|	Label
Direct Path (300mg)	77.58971	2.4885	31.18	<.0001	100*b1/(b1+c*a1)

Nonlinear FIML Estimates

Term	Estimate	Approx Std Err	t Value	Approx Pr> |t|	Label
Indirect Path (450mg)	25.1721	2.7854	9.04	<.0001	100*c*a2/(b2+c*a2)

Nonlinear FIML Estimates

Term	Estimate	Approx Std Err	t Value	Approx Pr> |t|	Label
Direct Path (450mg)	74.8279	2.7854	26.86	<.0001	100*b2/(b2+c*a2)

Nonlinear FIML Estimates

Term	Estimate	Approx Std Err	t Value	Approx Pr> |t|	Label
Indirect Path (600mg)	26.1149	2.8059	9.31	<.0001	100*c*a3/(b3+c*a3)

Nonlinear FIML Estimates

Term	Estimate	Approx Std Err	t Value	Approx Pr> |t|	Label
Direct Path (600mg)	73.8851	2.8059	26.33	<.0001	100*b3/(b3+c*a3)

FIGURE 9.12
Partial output: The mediation modeling in a study with four treatment arms.

That is, do males and female differ with respect to their direct (and indirect) effects, expressed as a percentage of the total effect for males and, separately, the total effect for females? While the study of time invariance is performed on the same subjects, data are needed for at least two time points. A natural question then becomes, do direct (and indirect) effects differ between time 1 and time 2?

9.2.1 Group Invariance

As an illustration of group invariance, the example described in detail in Section 9.1 is used as a starting point. Suppose that a researcher is interested whether the mediation model is invariant relative to gender (male—Group 1; female—Group 2). Then Equations 9.6 and 9.7 can be written as

$$Sleep_n = i_{11} + b1 \times Treatment_n + c1 \times Pain_i + e_{11n}, \tag{9.14}$$

$$Pain_n = i_{21} + a1 \times Treatment_n + e_{21n}, \tag{9.15}$$

$$Sleep_m = i_{12} + b2 \times Treatment_m + c2 \times Pain_m + e_{12m}, \tag{9.16}$$

$$Pain_m = i_{22} + a2 \times Treatment_m + e_{22m}. \tag{9.17}$$

Equations 9.14 and 9.15 represent a subject n from Group 1; Equations 9.16 and 9.17 represent a subject m from Group 2. Figure 9.13 depicts the mediation model.

The objective is to test whether the difference between direct effects (and indirect effects) from those two groups, expressed as a percentage of the group's respective total effect (males have their own total effect and females

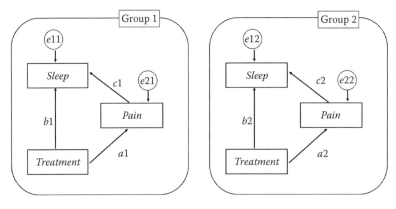

FIGURE 9.13
Mediation model to test group invariance.

have their own total effect), is statistically different from zero. These differences can be expressed as follows:

difference of direct effects (Group 1 vs Group 2)

$$= 100 \left(\frac{b1}{b1 + c1 \times a1} - \frac{b2}{b2 + c2 \times a2} \right) \tag{9.18}$$

difference of indirect effects (Group 1 vs Group 2)

$$= 100 \left(\frac{c1 \times a1}{b1 + c1 \times a1} - \frac{c2 \times a2}{b2 + c2 \times a2} \right) \tag{9.19}$$

A simulation of a dataset for this example can be based on the dataset created in Section 9.1.2 (specifically in Figure 9.3). Figure 9.14 adds the variable Group to the dataset with value of 1 (Group 1) and value of 2 (Group 2) randomly assigned to subjects with equal (50/50) probability.

The datasets representing Group 1 and Group 2 are independent. Thus, Equations 9.14 and 9.15 can be fit separately from Equations 9.16 and 9.17 in two subsequent applications of the SAS MODEL procedure. However, in this situation, a statistical significance of a difference represented by Equations 9.18 and 9.19 cannot be readily obtained. Fortunately, the MODEL procedure in SAS has a built-in capacity to handle several different models simultaneously. Figure 9.15 showcases the implementation of the two simultaneous mediation models using the "If ... Then ..." statement.

Figure 9.16 gives the partial output. Recall that the true indirect and direct effects, based on the parameters in the simulation, were 75% and 25% respectively (Section 9.1.2.2; Figure 9.3; Equations 9.4 and 9.5). Results for both groups are close to those values. The difference between direct effects of those two groups is 2.48363% (= 78.33674% − 75.85311%), with a nonsignificant p-value of 0.7684. This same p-value is obtained (as it should be) for the difference between indirect effects (2.48363% = 24.14689% − 21.66326%). These results support the conclusion that mediation models for Group 1 and Group 2 are gender invariant in this sample.

```
Data   _mediation_1;
Set    _mediation_1;
Group=1;
If ranuni(1000)>0.5 Then Group=2;
Run;
```

FIGURE 9.14
Adding group variable.

```
Proc Model Data=_mediation_1 CONVERGE=1e-7 MAXITER=100
SINGULAR=1E-10;

        Exogenous      Treatment;
        Parms i11 i21 i12 i22
              a1 b1 c1
              a2 b2 c2;

    If Group=1 Then
    Do;
        Sleep = i11 + b1*Treatment + c1*Pain;
        Pain = i21 + a1*Treatment;

        h.Pain = E21;
        h.Sleep = E11;
    End;

    If Group=2 Then
    Do;
        Sleep = i12 + b2*Treatment + c2*Pain;
        Pain = i22 + a2*Treatment;

        h.Pain = E22;
        h.Sleep = E12;
    End;

        Fit Sleep Pain / fiml;

        Estimate "Indirect (Group 1)" 100*c1*a1/(b1+c1*a1);
        Estimate "Direct (Group 1)" 100*b1/(b1+c1*a1);

        Estimate "Indirect (Group 2)" 100*c2*a2/(b2+c2*a2);
        Estimate "Direct (Group 2)" 100*b2/(b2+c2*a2);

        Estimate "Diff (Indirect)" 100*(c1*a1/(b1+c1*a1)-c2*a2/
        (b2+c2*a2));
        Estimate "Diff (Direct)" 100*(b1/(b1+c1*a1)-b2/(b2+c2*a2));

    Run;
    Quit;
```

FIGURE 9.15
Mediation model implementation for testing group invariance.

9.2.2 Longitudinal Mediation Models and Time Invariance

In Section 9.1.2, the example of the cross-sectional mediation model was discussed. An extension to the case of a longitudinal mediation model requires that outcomes be collected for subjects at more than one occasion during a study. Equations 9.20 through 9.23 define the longitudinal mediation model for a study when sleep disturbance and pain were collected at two time points:

$$Sleep_{j1} = i_{11} + b1 \times Treatment_j + c1 \times Pain_{j1} + e_{11j}, \tag{9.20}$$

```
                              Nonlinear FIML Estimates

                               Approx              Approx
Term               Estimate    Std Err   t Value   Pr > |t|   Label
Indirect (Group 1) 75.85311    5.6938    13.32     <.0001     100*c1*a1/(b1+c1*a1)

                              Nonlinear FIML Estimates

                               Approx              Approx
Term               Estimate    Std Err   t Value   Pr > |t|   Label
Direct (Group 1)   24.14689    5.6938    4.24      <.0001     100*b1/(b1+c1*a1)

                              Nonlinear FIML Estimates

                               Approx              Approx
Term               Estimate    Std Err   t Value   Pr > |t|   Label
Indirect (Group 2) 78.33674    6.2084    12.62     <.0001     100*c2*a2/(b2+c2*a2)

                              Nonlinear FIML Estimates

                               Approx              Approx
Term               Estimate    Std Err   t Value   Pr > |t|   Label
Direct (Group 2)   21.66326    6.2084    3.49      0.0006     100*b2/(b2+c2*a2)
```

FIGURE 9.16
Mediation model implementation for testing group invariance: Partial output.

(*continued*)

```
                          Nonlinear FIML Estimates

                            Approx            Approx
Term              Estimate  Std Err  t Value  Pr> |t|   Label

Diff (Indirect)   -2.48363  8.4240   -0.29    0.7684    100*(c1*a1/(b1+c1* a1)-c2*a2/(b2+c2*a2))

                          Nonlinear FIML Estimates

                            Approx            Approx
Term              Estimate  Std Err  t Value  Pr > |t|  Label

Diff (Direct)     2.483632  8.4240    0.29    0.7684    100*(b1/(b1+c1*a1) - b2/(b2+c2*a2))
```

FIGURE 9.16 (continued)
Mediation model implementation for testing group invariance: Partial output.

$$Pain_{j1} = i_{21} + a1 \times Treatment_i + e_{21j}, \qquad (9.21)$$

$$Sleep_{j2} = i_{12} + b2 \times Treatment_j + c2 \times Pain_{j2} + e_{12j}, \qquad (9.22)$$

$$Pain_{j2} = i_{22} + a2 \times Treatment_j + e_{22j}, \qquad (9.23)$$

where

$Sleep_{j1}$ and $Pain_{j1}$ are the PRO measures for subject j representing a sleep disturbance measure and a pain measure at time point 1, and $Sleep_{j2}$ and $Pain_{j2}$ are the same PRO measures for the same subject j at time point 2

i_{11} and i_{21} are the overall intercepts at time point 1 for Sleep and Pain, respectively, and i_{12} and i_{22} are the corresponding overall intercepts at time point 2

$a1$ is the overall slope for subject j in Equation 9.21, representing the effect of the treatment (vs placebo) on Pain at time point 1, and $a2$ is the overall slope for the same subject j in Equation 9.23, representing the effect of the treatment (vs placebo) on Pain at time point 2

$b1$ is the overall slope for subject j in Equation 9.20, representing the direct effect of the treatment on Sleep at time point 1, and $b2$ is the overall slope for the same subject j in Equation 9.22, representing the direct effect of the treatment on Sleep at time point 2

$c1$ is the overall slope for subject j in Equation 9.20, representing the effect of Pain on Sleep at time point 1, and $c2$ is the overall slope for subject j in Equation 9.22, representing the effect of Pain on Sleep at time point 2

e_{11j}, e_{21j}, e_{12j}, and e_{22j} are the error terms assumed to be from a normal distribution with mean 0 and corresponding variances σ_{11}^2, σ_{21}^2, σ_{12}^2, and σ_{22}^2 (i.e., $e_{nm} \sim N(0, \sigma_{nm}^2)$)

In the previous section on group invariance, the error terms were considered independent, because they were the part of the equations describing mediation models for two independent groups. In the case of a longitudinal mediation model, however, the assumption of independence of error terms is not valid. To account for this, it is assumed that error terms e_{11j} and e_{12j} covary over time within a subject, that is, $cov(e_{11j}, e_{12j}) = \sigma_1$ for any subject j (Equations 9.20 and 9.22). The same is true for the error terms e_{21j} and e_{22j}, with $cov(e_{21j}, e_{22j}) = \sigma_2$ for any subject j (Equations 9.21 and 9.23).

Note that the error terms e_{11j} and e_{21j} associated with two different measures (Sleep and Pain) at the same time (time 1) are assumed to be independent (Equations 9.20 and 9.21), as are the error terms e_{12j} and e_{22j} at time 2 (Equations 9.22 and 9.23). Hence, $cov(e_{11j}, e_{21j}) = 0$ and $cov(e_{12j}, e_{22j}) = 0$. The overall relationship between error terms for this example can therefore be expressed by the following variance–covariance matrix (with column

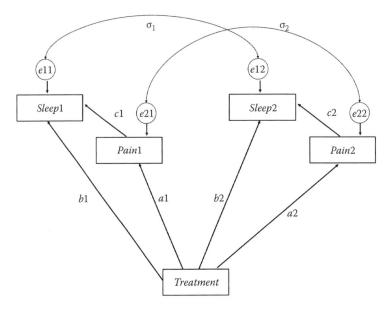

FIGURE 9.17
Illustrative longitudinal mediation model.

variables and row variables each represented by e_{11j}, e_{21j}, e_{12j}, and e_{22j}, in that order):

$$\begin{bmatrix} \sigma_{11}^2 & 0 & \sigma_1 & 0 \\ 0 & \sigma_{21}^2 & 0 & \sigma_2 \\ \sigma_1 & 0 & \sigma_{12}^2 & 0 \\ 0 & \sigma_2 & 0 & \sigma_{22}^2 \end{bmatrix}. \tag{9.24}$$

Matrix 9.24 also indicates that corresponding error terms for the two measures (Sleep and Pain) between time points are also assumed to be independent, with $\text{cov}(e_{21j}, e_{12j}) = 0$ (Equations 9.21 and 9.22) and $\text{cov}(e_{11j}, e_{22j}) = 0$ (Equations 9.20 and 9.23). Figure 9.17 depicts a visual diagram of Equations 9.20 through 9.23 and Matrix 9.24 for this longitudinal mediation model with two observations for a subject.

9.2.2.1 Simulated Dataset

A simulated dataset is used to illustrate the implementation of a longitudinal mediation model. The simulated study was described in Section 9.1.2. The additional aspect for the current example is that we will simulate two observations for every subject.

In Chapter 8 (specifically in Section 8.4), the simulation was described on how the SIMNORMAL procedure in SAS can be used to generate error

```
options nocenter;

data _cov_ (type=corr);
input
_TYPE_ $    _NAME_ $    COL1       COL2       COL3       COL4;
datalines;
  CORR        COL1        1          0          0.5        0
  CORR        COL2        0          1          0          0.6
  CORR        COL3        0.5        0          1          0
  CORR        COL4        0          0.6        0          1
  MEAN        .           0          0          0          0
  STD         .           0.2        0.5        0.1        0.4
  N           .           200        200        200        200
;
run;

proc simnormal data=_cov_ out=err_sim numreal=200 seed=10000;
var Col1-Col4;
run;

proc corr data=err_sim COV ;
Var Col1-Col4;
Run;
```

FIGURE 9.18
Generation of error terms.

from a multivariate normal distribution. Figure 9.18 generates four error terms for each of 200 subjects. The first step is to create a dataset with Type=CORR, which defines the correlations between error terms. Note that the structure of the dataset corresponds to the structure of the variance–covariance Matrix 9.24.

We also define that the mean of every error term should be zero, and also different variances for every error term should be assigned. The CORR procedure (Figure 9.18) outputs the variance–covariance and correlation matrix for the simulated dataset (Figure 9.19). As expected, the correlations based on the simulated dataset of 200 subjects (Figure 9.19) are close to the values initially assigned to them (see the data step in Figure 9.18).

The subsequent SAS code (Figure 9.20) generates the simulated data for subsequent analysis, and Figure 9.21 shows the structure of this dataset. Note that the following SAS code lines (from Figure 9.20)

```
Pain1   = i21 + a1*Treatment                 + COL2;
Sleep1 = i11 + b1*Treatment + c1*Pain1 + COL1;

Pain2   = i22 + a2*Treatment                 + COL4;
Sleep2 = i12 + b2*Treatment + c2*Pain2 + COL3;
```

correspond to Equations 9.20 through 9.23 with variables COL1, COL2, COL3, and COL4 representing error terms e_{11j}, e_{21j}, e_{12j}, and e_{22j}, respectively.

```
          Covariance Matrix, DF = 199

              COL1          COL2          COL3          COL4

COL1    0.0402797214   -.0011792336   0.0099440625   -.0010528310
COL2    -.0011792336   0.2842887133   0.0002735075   0.1340826629
COL3    0.0099440625   0.0002735075   0.0097006592   -.0028097042
COL4    -.0010528310   0.1340826629   -.0028097042   0.1672712039

          Pearson Correlation Coefficients, N = 200

              COL1          COL2          COL3          COL4

COL1       1.00000       -0.01102       0.50306       -0.01283
COL2      -0.01102        1.00000       0.00521        0.61487
COL3       0.50306        0.00521       1.00000       -0.06975
COL4      -0.01283        0.61487      -0.06975        1.00000
```

FIGURE 9.19
Variance–covariance and correlation matrix for simulated dataset (CORR procedure output).

```
Data _mediation_1;
Set  err_sim;

    i11=2;   i21=1;      /* Intercepts at time point 1*/
    i12=2.1; i22=.9;     /* Intercepts at time point 2*/

    a1=1.5;   /*  effect of treatment on pain at time point 1*/
    b1=.5;    /*  direct effect of treatment on sleep at time point 1*/
    c1=1 ;    /*  effect of pain on sleep at time point 1 */

    a2=1.6;   /*  effect of treatment on pain at time point 2*/
    b2=.4;    /*  direct effect of treatment on sleep at time point 2*/
    c2=1.1 ;  /*  effect of pain on sleep at time point 2*/

    ID=_N_;

    Treatment=0;
    If ranuni(100)>0.5 Then  Treatment=1;

    Pain1   = i21 + a1*Treatment              + COL2;
    Sleep1  = i11 + b1*Treatment + c1*Pain1 + COL1;

    Pain2   = i22 + a2*Treatment              + COL4;
    Sleep2  = i12 + b2*Treatment + c2*Pain2 + COL3;

Keep ID Pain1 Sleep1 Pain2 Sleep2 Treatment;

Run;
```

FIGURE 9.20
Generating simulated dataset for longitudinal mediation modeling.

ID	Treatment	Pain1	Sleep1	Pain2	Sleep2
1	0	1.8379204	3.9849221	1.491982	3.8123896
2	0	0.745216	2.7096785	1.2809588	3.5169493
3	1	2.914288	5.2956426	2.6852534	5.3450042
4	1	1.9902719	4.5552898	2.5628266	5.3723076
5	0	1.0678038	3.1900836	1.3246762	3.5583033
6	1	2.295673	5.1081378	2.6984872	5.5829397
7	0	0.2394783	2.5954151	0.3676703	2.4352158
8	0	0.5086551	2.490292	1.1380157	3.3161842
9	1	3.2005387	5.8700602	2.1371162	4.8804735
10	1	2.3962369	4.582331	2.843539	5.4966192
11	1	2.633023	5.1386184	2.6191967	5.2733402
12	0	0.936019	2.4715519	1.1893864	3.2469247

FIGURE 9.21
Structure of the simulated dataset for longitudinal mediation modeling.

9.2.2.2 Implementation

To account for covariation of error terms, the SAS CALIS procedure (introduced in Chapter 5) is used in this example (Figure 9.22). The equations under the LINEQS key word correspond to Equations 9.20–9.23. The statements under the STD key word define that variances for error terms, and the exogenous variable will be estimated. The statements under the COV key word define that covariances between e11 and e12, as well as between e21 and e22, should also be estimated.

Figure 9.23 represents partial output from the model. The part labeled "Manifest Variable Equations with Estimates" gives results for the estimated slopes $a1$, $b1$, $c1$, $a2$, $b2$, and $c2$ in Equations 9.20–9.23, which can be compared with the values used to generate the simulated dataset. For example, the modeled estimate of $a1$ is equal to 1.5594 based on 200 subjects (Figure 9.23) and in the simulation its true value is 1.5 (Figure 9.20). The estimated modeled covariance between the error terms e_{11} and e_{12} is 0.00985 (under "Covariances Among Exogenous Variables"; Figure 9.23). From the simulation setup its value is 0.0099440625 when based on 200 subjects (Figure 9.19) corresponding to correlation of 0.50306 (true value of correlation is 0.5; Figure 9.18).

Estimated differences of direct and indirect effects between time point 1 and time point 2 can be implemented by the following equations analogous to Equations 9.18 and 9.19 by replacing *Group 1* by *Time Point 1* and *Group 2* by *Time Point 2*. But the output of the CALIS procedure also provides already estimated total and indirect effects (Figure 9.24). From Figure 9.24, the indirect effect of treatment on sleep (expressed as a percentage of the total effect) at time point 1 can simply be calculated as 100*1.536478199/2.090265072 = 73.5% and at time point 2 as 100*1.700301068/2.142781549 = 79.4%.

The noticeable omission in our results is the absence of statistical inference for estimates of direct effects and indirect effects, along with their

```
Proc Calis cov data=_mediation_1 G4=1000 GCONV=1E-10 All
TECHNIQUE=LEVMAR;

/*----------------*/
LINEQS

Sleep1 = b1 Treatment + c1 Pain1 + e11,
Pain1 = a1 Treatment + e21,

Sleep2 = b2 Treatment + c2 Pain2 + e12,
Pain2 = a2 Treatment + e22
;
/*----------------*/
STD
Treatment = vartrt,

e11 = var11,
e21 = var21,
e12 = var12,
e22 = var22
;
/*----------------*/
COV
e11 e12 = COV1,
e21 e22 = COV2
;

Run;
```

FIGURE 9.22
Longitudinal mediation model implementation using SAS CALIS procedure.

respective differences between the two time points. The CALIS procedure does not provide a simple and direct way to calculate p-values or 95% confidence intervals for expressions based on combinations of the estimated model parameters. One way to estimate confidence intervals is via the bootstrap methodology. In Section 9.4, SAS code is provided and discussed demonstrating the implementation of the bootstrap simulations to estimate 95% confidence intervals for direct effects and indirect effects, along with their respective differences between two time points.

9.3 Advanced Example

9.3.1 Background

An advanced real-data example is now illustrated. The relationship between the physiological aspects of treatment for erectile dysfunction (ED) (i.e., erection hardness and erection maintenance) in a randomized, double-blinded, placebo-controlled trial of sildenafil was documented in previous research

```
Manifest Variable Equations with Estimates

Pain1     =    1.5594*Treatment +  1.0000 e21
               a1
t Value        20.6756
Sleep1    =    0.9853*Pain1      +  0.5538*Treatment +  1.0000 e11
               c1                   b1
t Value        40.6454              11.7193
Pain2     =    1.5713*Treatment +  1.0000 e22
               a2
t Value        27.1340
Sleep2    =    1.0821*Pain2      +  0.4425*Treatment +  1.0000 e12
               c2                   b2
t Value        69.9875              15.8127

Variances of Exogenous Variables
                                          Standard
Variable   Parameter      Estimate          Error    t Value

Treatment  vartrt          0.25035        0.02510      9.97
e11        var11           0.04005        0.00402      9.97
e21        var21           0.28341        0.02841      9.97
e12        var12           0.00961      0.0009630      9.97
e22        var22           0.16706        0.01675      9.97

Covariances Among Exogenous Variables

Var1      Var2     Parameter     Estimate    Standard Error    t Value

e11       e12      COV1          0.00985           0.00156       6.33
e21       e22      COV2          0.13451           0.01813       7.42
```

FIGURE 9.23
Longitudinal mediation model (partial output).

```
                           Total Effects

                Treatment              Pain1               Pain2

Pain1       1.559412343         0.0000000000        0.000000000
Sleep1      2.090265072         0.9852930856        0.000000000
Pain2       1.571281557         0.0000000000        0.000000000
Sleep2      2.142781549         0.0000000000        1.082111007

                         Indirect Effects

                Treatment              Pain1               Pain2

Pain1       0.000000000                    0                   0
Sleep1      1.536478199                    0                   0
Pain2       0.000000000                    0                   0
Sleep2      1.700301068                    0                   0
```

FIGURE 9.24
Estimated total and indirect effects.

(Claes et al., 2010). It was found that sildenafil treatment (relative to placebo) significantly improved erection maintenance, a physiologic requirement for satisfactory sexual performance. Approximately half of the effect of sildenafil on erection maintenance was estimated to be driven through the direct effects of treatment. The remaining effect of sildenafil on erection maintenance was substantially driven by erection hardness (the mediator).

The same study is now used to address a more involved and advanced objective: to test a psychosocial paradigm of ED by using mediation modeling to define the relationship of both the physiological aspects (erection hardness and erection maintenance) and the associated psychosocial aspects (confidence, sexual relationship satisfaction) of ED (Althof et al., 2010).

For pedagogical and illustrative purposes, only a selected portion of the entire published analysis is presented here (Althof et al., 2010). The dataset was derived from a multinational (Republic of Korea, Russian Federation, Spain, and Sweden), parallel-group, randomized (1:1:1), double-blind, placebo-controlled trial of fixed-dose sildenafil (100 or 50 mg, 8 weeks). In the mediation analysis, the two doses of sildenafil were combined into one treatment group. Medication was taken as needed for sexual activity but not more than once daily.

To assess erection hardness, at each occasion of sexual activity, the patient completed the Erection Hardness Score (EHS), a single-item PRO for assessing erection hardness ("How would you rate the quality [hardness] of your erection?") on an ordinal scale of 0 (no erection at all) to 4 (completely hard). As a proxy to assess erection maintenance, Item 4 of the International Index of Erectile Function (IIEF) was used ("During sexual intercourse, how often were you able to maintain your erection after you had penetrated [entered] your partner?" which is scored on an ordinal scale from 1 (almost never/never) to 5 (almost always/always); a score of 0 was assigned if intercourse was not attempted).

As a proxy to assess male confidence and sexual relationship satisfaction, the 14-item Self-Esteem And Relationship (SEAR) questionnaire, which has a 4-week recall (like the IIEF), was completed by patients. Items are scored on a 5-point scale from 1 (almost never/never) to 5 (almost always/always) for positive statements and in reverse order for negative statements. Item scores were separately summed for its two domains: the eight-item Sexual Relationship Satisfaction domain and the six-item Confidence domain (and its two constituent subscales, the four-item Self-Esteem subscale and the two-item Overall Relationship Satisfaction).

Then each domain and subscale score was transformed onto a 0-to-100 scale, with higher scores being more favorable. Like data from the EHS and the maintenance item (Item 4 from the IIEF), data from the SEAR questionnaire covered the last 4 weeks of the double-blind study for the purpose of the mediation modeling. In separate bivariate analyses, sildenafil treatment (vs placebo treatment) was substantially related to higher (more favorable) scores on EHS, on each SEAR domain and subscale, and on erectile maintenance (IIEF Item 4).

9.3.2 Mediation Model and Analysis

A mediation model is a type of path analysis or structural equation model. Figure 9.25 exemplifies this and diagrams the particular mediation model that became the final model (Althof et al., 2010). The mediation model includes one predictor (treatment: sildenafil vs placebo), two mediators (EHS and maintenance, with EHS in turn affecting maintenance), one manifest variable (performance anxiety, from 0 ("no anxiety") to 4 ("extremely anxious") and four latent outcomes (sexual relationship satisfaction, confidence, self-esteem, and overall relationship satisfaction) of which two (sexual relationship satisfaction, confidence) are of primary interest. Figure 9.25 exemplifies and depicts the final mediation model

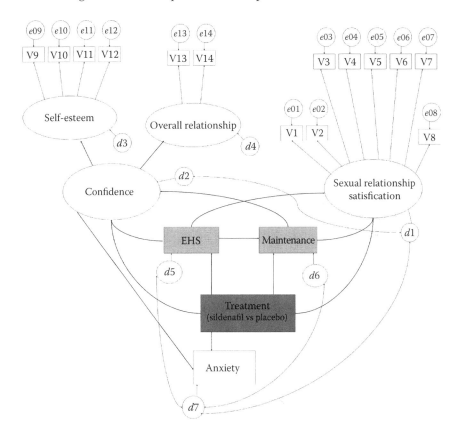

FIGURE 9.25

Mediation model depicting the inter-relationships among physiological and psychosocial variables in erectile dysfunction. (*Note*: Abbreviated item description—V1 = Relaxed about initiating sex, V2 = Confident erection would last long enough, V3 = Satisfied with sexual performance, V4 = Felt sex could be spontaneous, V5 = Was likely to initiate sex, V6 = Confident performing sexually, V7 = Satisfied with sex life, V8 = Partner unhappy with sexual relations (reverse-scored), V9 = Had good self-esteem, V10 = Felt like a whole man, V11 = Inclined to feel a failure (reverse-scored), V12 = Felt confident, V13 = Partner satisfied with relationship, and V14 = Subject satisfied with relationship.)

emanating from the investigation (Althof et al., 2010). In effect, sexual relationship satisfaction with its eight indicators (items) is represented by a first-order measurement model. Confidence is represented by a second-order measurement model, with self-esteem (embodied by four indicators) and overall relationship satisfaction (embodied by two indicators) factors represented by a first-order measurement model.

Model 9.25 depicts the sole independent or predictor variable (treatment, shaded dark gray), the two mediator variables (EHS and erection maintenance, shaded light gray), and the four dependent or outcome variables (sexual relationship satisfaction, confidence, and its lower order factors self-esteem and overall relationship satisfaction). In the figure, V1 through V14 represent the 14 items of the SEAR questionnaire, where ordinal categorical responses range from 1 = almost never/never to 5 = almost always/always; $e01$ through $e14$ represent their corresponding random error (residual) terms. Each of the two mediators and the six outcomes has its own disturbance or random error term (denoted $d1$ through $d6$ in Figure 9.25).

Note that, rather than having the two primary outcomes (confidence, sexual relationship satisfaction) be unrelated or having one affect the other (unidirectional arrow), the two primary outcomes were linked by allowing their disturbance terms to covary (as illustrated by the bidirectional arrow between $d1$ and $d2$ in Figure 9.25).

The results from the mediation modeling for the effects of treatment on confidence and on sexual relationship satisfaction are reported, respectively, in Figures 9.26 and 9.27. Results also include 95% confidence intervals for the effects, with these intervals obtained from bootstrap simulations. The model estimated that erection hardness mediated 43.7% (95% confidence interval [CI]: 29.3%, 62.4%) of the effect of treatment onto confidence and 45.9% (95% CI: 32.2%, 61.8%) of the effect of treatment onto sexual relationship satisfaction; erection maintenance mediated 23.0% (95% CI: 10.1%, 39.1%) of the effect of treatment onto confidence and 22.4% (95% CI: 10.1%, 36.5%) of the effect of treatment onto sexual relationship satisfaction. Therefore, collectively, erection hardness and erection maintenance mediated approximately two-thirds of the effect of treatment onto confidence and onto sexual relationship satisfaction.

9.4 Bootstrapping Methodology Implementation

The dataset "_mediation_1" created earlier (see Figures 9.18 and 9.20) is used to illustrate the bootstrap methodology for longitudinal mediation modeling in order to obtain 95% confidence intervals for the difference in direct effects between time points 1 and 2 and, separately, in indirect effects between the

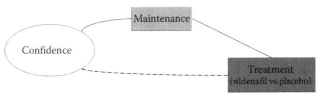

Via maintenance
 Indirect effect, % (95% confidence interval): 23.0 (10.1, 39.1)
 Direct effect, % (95% confidence interval): 33.0 (12.5, 49.3)

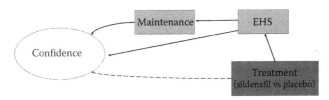

Via erection hardness
 Indirect effect, %: 43.7 (29.3, 62.4)
 Direct effect, %: 33.3 (12.5, 49.3)

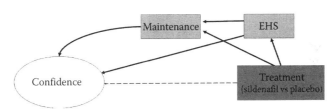

Via erection hardness and maintenance
 Indirect effect, %: 66.7 (50.7, 87.5)
 Direct effect, %: 33.3 (12.5, 49.3)

FIGURE 9.26
Effect (and 95% confidence interval) of sildenafil treatment on confidence (SEAR Confidence domain) indirectly (solid line) via the mediator variables (erection hardness [EHS] and erection maintenance [IIEF Item 4]) and directly (dashed line).

same time points. The structure of this dataset is shown in Figure 9.21. The SAS code (with comments) below shows step-by-step implementation of the bootstrap simulations (Figure 9.28).

After calculations are finished, a dataset with 10,000 observations should appear as shown in Figure 9.29. This dataset will be now used to produce a 95% confidence interval for the difference of the two direct effects between the two time points and, separately, for the difference of the two indirect

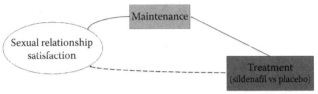

Via maintenance
   Indirect effect, % (95% confidence interval): 22.4% (10.1, 36.5)
   Direct effect, % (95% confidence interval): 31.7 (15.1, 46.5)

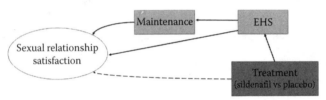

Via erection hardness
   Indirect effect, %: 45.9 (32.2, 61.8)
   Direct effect, %: 31.7 (15.1, 46.5)

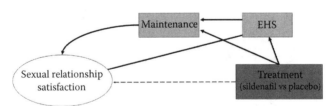

Via erection hardness and maintenance
   Indirect effect, %: 68.3% (53.5, 84.9)
   Direct effect, %: 31.7% (15.1, 46.5)

FIGURE 9.27
Effect (and 95% confidence interval) of sildenafil treatment on sexual relationship satisfaction
(SEAR Sexual Relationship Satisfaction domain) indirectly (solid line) via the mediator variables
(erection hardness [EHS] and erection maintenance [IIEF Item 4]) and directly (dashed line).

```
/*--------------------------------------------------------------
Could be useful to block log and output during the simulations.
*/

proc printto log="NUL:" print="NUL:";
Run;

%macro Bootstrap_Mediation(NumberOfSimulations) ;

%do i=1 %to &NumberOfSimulations;

/*--------------------------------------------------------------
---*/
/*
Proc SURVEYSELECT will produce the dataset of the same size as
the initial dataset based on the method of unrestricted random
sampling (METHOD=URS), which selects units with equal probability
and with replacement.

This new dataset will provide new data will be used by Proc CALIS.

Note that we need to have N=200 (i.e. number of observations) as a
part of the Proc SURVEYSELECT - the original dataset "_mediation_1"
has 200 observations
*/
            Proc SURVEYSELECT NOPRINT
            data=_mediation_1
            METHOD=URS
            SEED=-1
            OUTHITS
            N=200
            Out=_mediation_tmp;
            Run;
/*--------------------------------------------------------------
---*/
Proc Calis cov data=_mediation_tmp G4=1000 GCONV=1E-10 All
TECHNIQUE=LEVMAR
PRIVEC;

/*----------------*/
LINEQS

Sleep1 = b1 Treatment + c1 Pain1 + e11,
Pain1 = a1 Treatment + e21,

Sleep2 = b2 Treatment + c2 Pain2 + e12,
Pain2 = a2 Treatment + e22
;
/*----------------*/
STD
Treatment = vartrt,

e11 = var11,
e21 = var21,
```

FIGURE 9.28
SAS code to perform bootstrap simulations.

(continued)

```
e12 = var12,
e22 = var22
;
/*----------------*/
COV
e11 e12 = COV1,
e21 e22 = COV2
;

/*
Results of the CALIS procedure will be saved in the three
datasets: TotalEffects, IndirectEffects, and Estimates
*/
ods output
TotalEffects=TotalEffects
IndirectEffects=IndirectEffects
Estimates=Estimates;

Run;
/*----------------------------------------------------*/
/* Extract total effect of the treatment on sleep at time point
1*/
Data Total1;
Set  TotalEffects;
Total1=Treatment; Where RowName="Sleep1";
Keep Total1;
Run;

/* Extract total effect of the treatment on sleep at time point
2*/
Data Total2;
Set  TotalEffects;
Total2=Treatment; Where RowName="Sleep2";
Keep Total2;
Run;

/* Extract indirect effect of the treatment on sleep at time
point 1*/
Data Indirect1;
Set IndirectEffects;
Indirect1=Treatment; Where RowName="Sleep1";
Keep Indirect1;
Run;

/* Extract indirect effect of the treatment on sleep at time
point 2*/
Data Indirect2;
Set IndirectEffects;
Indirect2=Treatment; Where RowName="Sleep2";
Keep Indirect2;
Run;
```

FIGURE 9.28 (continued)
SAS code to perform bootstrap simulations.

```
/* Extract direct effect of the treatment on sleep at time
point 1*/
Data Direct1;
Set Estimates;
Direct1=Estimate; Where Parameter="b1";
Keep Direct1;
Run;

/* Extract direct effect of the treatment on sleep at time
point 2*/
Data Direct2;
Set Estimates;
Direct2=Estimate; Where Parameter="b2";
Keep Direct2;
Run;

/* Merge effects */
Data _effects_tmp;
Merge Total1 Total2 Indirect1 Indirect2 Direct1 Direct2;
Run;

/*-- Add results of a current simulation to the dataset
"_effects_" */
PROC APPEND BASE=_effects_ DATA=_effects_tmp;
Run;

%End;

%mend Bootstrap_Mediation;

/* Test code with just a few simulations first, and after
that only perform 10000 or more simulations*/
%Bootstrap_Mediation(10000) ;

/* turn on log and output */
proc printto;
Run;
```

FIGURE 9.28 (continued)
SAS code to perform bootstrap simulations.

effects between the two time points, with each effect expressed as a percentage of the total effect. For example, if interest centers on calculating the 95% confidence interval for the difference between the *indirect effect at time point 1* and the *indirect effect at time point 2*, the SAS code in Figure 9.30 can be executed. The outcome of those calculations is presented by Figure 9.31. In Section 9.2.2.2, the indirect effect of the treatment on the sleep outcome was estimated as 73.5% at time point 1 and 79.4% at time point 2. The 95% confidence interval for the difference between 73.5% and 79.4% is

	Total1	Total2	Indirect1	Indirect2	Direct1	Direct2
9990	2.1881	2.1599	1.6559	1.741	0.5322	0.4189
9991	2.0564	2.0622	1.5087	1.6259	0.5477	0.4363
9992	1.9913	2.0433	1.3977	1.5231	0.5935	0.5201
9993	2.0563	2.1279	1.5216	1.6922	0.5347	0.4357
9994	2.0608	2.1597	1.5074	1.7594	0.5534	0.4003
9995	2.1156	2.1961	1.6049	1.7872	0.5108	0.4089
9996	2.1186	2.2193	1.4405	1.7351	0.6781	0.4843
9997	2.0881	2.0902	1.5839	1.6742	0.5042	0.416
9998	2.0385	2.1731	1.4917	1.7235	0.5468	0.4496
9999	2.119	2.1749	1.5436	1.7229	0.5754	0.452
10000	2.315	2.2919	1.683	1.8311	0.6319	0.4608

FIGURE 9.29
Partial results of the bootstrap calculations (11 simulations out of 10,000).

```
Data _tmp_;
Set _effects_;

Diff = 100*(Indirect1/Total1 - Indirect2/Total2);

Keep Diff;
Run;

Proc Univariate data=_tmp_;
. Var Diff;
output out=pctscorepctlpts=2.597.5pctlpre=CI;
Run;

Data pctscore;
Set pctscore;
CI= "(" || compress(round(CI2_5,0.01)) || ";" ||
compress(round(CI97_5,0.01)) || ")";
Run;

Proc Print data=pctscore NOOBS;
Var CI;
Run;
```

FIGURE 9.30
Estimation of the 95% confidence intervals for the difference between the indirect effect at time point 1 and the indirect effect at time point 2.

```
           CI
      (-10.34;-1.34)
```

FIGURE 9.31
95% confidence interval estimation.

from −10.34% to −1.34% and does not include 0, indicating that the hypothesis that indirect effect at time point 1 and indirect effect at time point 2 are equal should be rejected.

9.5 Summary

In this chapter, fundamental elements of single mediator models are described and then expanded to cover the more advanced topics of multiple mediator models, latent variable mediation models, multiple-outcome mediation models, and longitudinal mediation models. In its simplest form, mediation analysis enables the total effect of a predictor variable on an outcome variable to be partitioned into an indirect effect via a mediator variable and a direct effect attributed to everything else. The formulation of and results from a mediation model depend on the postulated framework posed by the research objective. Concepts are explained and quantified through simulated examples in SAS having pedagogical steps and practical implications. As is also true for simulated examples presented in other chapters, assumptions made to certain values in the simulations of this chapter can be changed in order to deepen appreciation of the methodology and to cater to the specific applications of different readers. Concepts are also illustrated with a published real-life example with several treatments and also with an advanced real-life example with multiple latent outcomes and multiple mediators.

References

Althof, S.E., Berner, M.M., Goldstein, I., Claes, H.I.M., Cappelleri, J.C., Bushmakin, A.G., Symonds, T., and G. Schetzler. 2010. Interrelationship of sildenafil treatment effects on the physiological and psychosocial aspects of erectile dysfunction of mixed or organic etiology. *Journal of Sexual Medicine* 7:3170–3178.

Claes, H.I.M., Goldstein, I., Althof, S.E., Berner, M., Cappelleri, J.C., Bushmakin, A.G., Symonds, T., and G. Schnetzler. 2010. Understanding the effects of sildenafil treatment on erection maintenance and erection hardness. *Journal of Sexual Medicine* 7:2184–2191.

Fairclough, D.L. 2010. *Design and Analysis of Quality of Life Studies in Clinical Trials*, 2nd edition. Boca Raton, FL: Chapman & Hall/CRC.

Iacobucci, D. 2008. *Mediation Analysis*. Thousand Oaks, CA: Sage Publications.

MacKinnon, D.P. 2008. *Introduction to Statistical Mediation Analysis*. New York, NY: Taylor & Francis.

Russell, I.J., Crofford, L.J., Leon, T., Cappelleri, J.C., Bushmakin, A.G., Whalen, E., Barrett, J.A., and A. Sadosky. 2009. The effects of pregabalin on sleep disturbance symptoms among individuals with fibromyalgia syndrome. *Sleep Medicine* 10:604–610.

SAS Institute Inc. 2011. *SAS/ETS 9.3 User's Guide*. Cary, NC: SAS Institute Inc.

10

Missing Data

Missing assessment of patient-reported outcome (PRO) measures is the rule rather than the exception, especially in longitudinal studies. Missing data are inevitable for many reasons. Among them are when a patient dies, misses a specific appointment, drops out because this individual is no longer ill, or states being too ill to complete the questionnaire. Staff may also contribute to missing patient data by forgetting to administer the questionnaire or by not wanting to bother a patient perceived as too sick. A missing assessment is defined in this chapter to include a patient, who is not compliant based on a deviation from the planned data collection, as well as a patient dying or a patient being removed from the trial for reasons specified in the protocol.

Missing data can pose considerable challenges in the analysis of data from clinical trials and interpretation of results of these analyses for two main reasons: (1) potential loss of statistical power or sensitivity to detect clinically meaningful differences due to a reduced number of observations and, more seriously, (2) the potential bias in estimates of treatment effect (and other predictors) due to missing data. As indicated in the FDA (2009) guidance on PRO measures, "… missing data can introduce bias and interfere with the ability to compare effects in the test group with the control group because only a subset of the initial randomized population contributes, and these patient groups may no longer be comparable." This statement is apt whether or not the intention is to seek a label or promotional claim on a PRO measure.

Bias in treatment effect estimates is particularly suspect when respondents selectively dropout or skip items or instruments depending on their treatment. Further, if the missing data lead to a loss of a substantial number of subjects, the problem may be compounded by a loss of statistical power and precision of parameter estimates for treatment effect and other important predictors. Missing data can be a problem even if similar proportions of missing data are found between treatment groups and for the same reason.

No definitive rules exist for how much missing data is acceptable in a study. When the percentage of missing assessments is very small (say, <5%), the potential bias or impact on power may be minor or inconsequential. A percentage of missing assessments in the 5%–20% may or may not matter. Percentages of missing assessment above 20% may result in restricted conclusions and inferences (Fairclough, 2010). Any such recommendations need to be qualified because the seriousness of the problem depends on the reasons for the missing data, the objectives of the study, and intended use of the results. Results from trials influencing regulatory drug approval, for instance, require more stringent criteria than results used to design future studies. The best defense against missing data is to prevent it and, if not, to have solid evidence that the analyses are insensitive to missing data or to demarcate clear limits of missing data for the interpretation of results.

One approach to minimizing the occurrence of missing data is by taking appropriate steps during the design and conduct of the study. Nevertheless, missing data are still likely to occur due to patient death or dropout from the study and, therefore, plans should be in place on how to handle missing data during the analysis and reporting phases. These steps should be transparent and reportable, and prespecified especially in confirmatory clinical trials. In particular, the analysis plan should clearly state how the handling of missing data will be carried out when considering patient response.

For PRO measures, there are essentially two types of missing data: (1) item nonresponse when at least one item response is missing, but not all item responses are missing, from an otherwise complete questionnaire and (2) questionnaire nonresponse when all items from the questionnaire are missing. For a PRO label or promotional claim, rules should be specific for each PRO instrument, especially multi-item PRO instruments, and should be ideally determined during instrument development and validation phases. However, during these phases, a multi-item PRO instrument in use may not have imputation rules prepared when at least one but not all items are missing on the same scale; therefore, it becomes especially important to pay careful attention to the imputation strategy for such instruments to help ensure consistent reporting in the literature and systematic review of data.

Much has been published about missing data in general (Allison, 2002; Little and Rubin, 2002; Schafer and Graham, 2002; McKnight et al., 2007; Enders, 2010; Graham 2012; Carpenter and Kenward, 2013) and missing data in clinical trials (Molenberghs and Kenward, 2007; EMA, 2010; NRC, 2010; Mallinckrodt, 2013) including PRO measures (Fayers and Machin, 2007; Curran et al., 1998a,b; Fairclough et al., 1998a,b; Walters, 2009; Fairclough, 2010; Bell and Fairclough, in press; Izem et al., in press). Readers are encouraged to seek out these resources for an in-depth exposition of missing data.

In this chapter, intended as an overview, we highlight steps that need to be taken to minimize the occurrence of missing data in the design phase of a study, summarize alternative techniques that address various forms of missing data at the analysis stage, and present a simulated example on a particular analytic approach to address missing data.

10.1 Study Design to Minimize Missing Data

Although analytic strategies exist for missing data, their use is much less satisfactory than taking primary prevention and secondary prevention against missing data in the study design (Fairclough, 2010). While some missing data, such as that due to death, is not preventable, much can be done in terms of preventing missing data from reasons other than death. In terms of primary prevention, missing data can be minimized (or at least reduced) at the trial design stage and conduct stage of a clinical trial. For PRO measures, at least four steps have been recommended to minimize missing data at the design stage (Sloan et al., 2007; Fairclough, 2010).

First, PRO measures should be treated like any other endpoints in the trial, with the same accompanying due attention and oversight. They should not be perceived as an additional burden but, instead, as essential parts of the scientific goals that center on the patient.

Second, key personnel, such as a nurse or research coordinator, should be identified to oversee and coordinate the PRO aspects of the trial. Clearly specified procedures in the protocol for collecting PRO data are the first step in minimizing missing data. For instance, the protocol should include procedures on how to collect PRO data if the treatment schedule is disrupted and on how to complete a questionnaire when the patient requires assistance, as well as a system to prompt nurses or research coordinators that a PRO assessment is due. Education of all stakeholders (e.g., patients, research assistants, primary investigators) should be emphasized regarding the importance of collecting PRO assessments, noting that missing data can lead to a treatment effect distorted by selection bias.

Third, standard administration of the PRO instruments should be assured across sites, by training of personnel and review of data completeness (with remedial action taken when necessary). Adopting a common set of alternative methods to obtain follow-up data when patients do not complete questionnaires would be worthwhile and beneficial. The use of electronic data capture to collect responses from a PRO questionnaire, especially from diary data, may result in more complete and reliable data and also minimize missing data particularly at the item level (Stone et al., 2007; Byrom and Tiplady, 2010). Indeed, electronic data capture allows real-time monitoring of data, which can facilitate early intervention to prevent further missing data by a patient and to flag potential site issues.

Fourth, the presentation format and the conduct, timing, and duration of assessment burden should be considered from the patient's perspective in order to ensure that items are clear and that patients want to respond to them, thereby reducing patient burden. Items and their response choices need to be consistently understood, and, moreover, items need to be consistently administered. All respondents should have access to the information needed to answer the questions accurately.

While primary prevention of missing data is prudent, so is secondary prevention. Secondary prevention of missing data involves gathering information in the design and conduct stages—by prospectively documenting specific reasons for missing data—for subsequent use in the analysis and interpretation of the results. For example, adding reasons for missing data such as *Patient refusal due to poor health* and *Patient refusal unrelated to health* will be useful. Also useful is collecting auxiliary factors that may contribute to the missing assessments or predict (explain) them. Examples of such factors include concurrent data on toxicity and evaluations of patient health status by clinical staff or a caretaker. Collecting such information on PRO measures, whenever practical or to the largest extent possible, on participants who discontinue can be recorded and used subsequently in analyses.

This set of recommendations on reducing missing PRO data at the trial design and conduct stages is in agreement or consistent with a general set of recommendations given elsewhere (Burzykowski et al., 2009; Fairclough, 2010; NRC, 2010; Mallinckrodt, 2013). In addition, various design options and their tradeoffs can be considered (NRC, 2010; Mallinckrodt, 2013).

10.2 Missing Data Patterns and Mechanisms

Patterns of missing data can take essentially three forms. A terminal pattern of missing data occurs when no observations are made after a certain time. An intermittent pattern of missing data occurs when an observation is missing but at least one subsequent observation is observed. As a hybrid of those two patterns of missing data, a mixed pattern of missing data occurs when no observations are made after a certain time and an intermittent pattern exists prior to that time. For these three types of missing data patterns, the causes of missing data can be either related or unrelated to the patient's underlying health status. Three major mechanisms of missing data have been proposed for longitudinal data (Little and Rubin, 2002; Fairclough, 2010).

10.2.1 Missing Completely at Random

Data are *missing completely at random* (MCAR) if, conditional upon the covariates (e.g., baseline patient characteristics or treatment assignment), the probability of missingness on the outcome or dependent variable of interest (e.g., on a PRO measure) does not depend on either the observed responses or the unobserved response on the same outcome (e.g., the same PRO measure). In this scenario, it is assumed that randomization to treatments (in the case of a randomized controlled trial) is still preserved if the missing data are disregarded, a very strong assumption that is unrealistic in most practical applications. With MCAR, responses on the outcome of interest are not related to the probability of dropout. In the context of a PRO assessment, the basic assumption is that the reason for the missing PRO assessment is entirely unrelated to the particular health status measured by the PRO measure. Examples of MCAR include PRO data missing because the patient moved to a different geographic location, the staff forgot to administer the PRO questionnaire, and translations of the PRO questionnaire are not available in certain languages—events unrelated to the underlying PRO health status.

Identifying MCAR, or covariate-dependent missingness, involves exploring the missing data process to identify covariates that predict missing observations, for example, through correlational analysis and logistic regression analysis (with the outcome being missing or not missing). In general, because in MCAR missing responses are not related to observed or unobserved responses, the completed cases are assumed to be a random sample of the larger sample. In this case, estimation on parameters such as means and mean changes from baseline are preserved and are unbiased. Because of the reduction in sample size, though, the precision of those estimates will be lower (and the variability higher) than if all subjects had no missing data.

For MCAR data, it suffices to use analysis methods that use all available data, such as a univariate analysis of data from each time point that ignores data at other time points (e.g., a two-sample *t*-test or an analysis of covariance) and traditional multivariate analysis of variance. In this case, it would be appropriate to analyze the data on the completed cases or the available cases in the same way as if there were no missing data. Typically, however, the assumption of MCAR for PRO measures is rare and not tenable. Dropout related to side effects or lack of efficacy is likely to affect whether or not a PRO measure is missing and would not fit the MCAR assumption. As such, the resulting estimates that assume MCAR are likely to be biased.

10.2.2 Missing at Random

Data are *missing at random* (MAR) if, conditional upon the covariates and the observed responses of the dependent variable, the probability of missingness on the outcome (dependent) variable does not depend on the unobserved responses of the dependent variable itself. Thus, in the context of PRO data, the missingness on a PRO measure depends on its observed responses but not its missing responses (after conditioning on covariates). Missing or complete post-baseline PRO data at a given time may depend on the observed (and completed) PRO responses recorded at other times in the study (be they at baseline or postbaseline).

For instance, individuals who are experiencing better health and more favorable PRO responses may be generally more likely to be available for follow-up and therefore more likely to complete the subsequent self-evaluations. Suppose a patient had a meaningful improvement (reduction) in self-reported pain during the first 3 weeks of a 4-week study and then the patient had a marked worsening and dropped out. If the observation at the fourth week was obtained before the patient dropped out, then the missingness may be MAR (after adjusting or accounting for the previous set of responses on self-reported pain).

Differences between MCAR and MAR can be tested by examining the association of missing data with the observed PRO scores. Various approaches are available. They include graphical presentations, formal statistical tests, correlational analyses, and logistic regression. For instance, if subjects who dropped out earlier had poorer (lower) PRO scores at baseline, and scores were lower at the time of the assessment just prior to dropout (the last observation), then the data are not MCAR. A formal statistical test (Little, 1988) evaluates whether the means of the observed data are the same for each pattern of missing data—for example, those who complete only the first assessment, only up to the second assessment, only up to the third assessment, and so on.

A correlational analysis would involve the association (correlation) between a binary indicator of missingness (yes or no) and the observed data from the baseline PRO scores and subsequent PRO scores prior to the missingness. If these correlations are sizeable and meaningful, then the assumption of the MCAR is not warranted. Another analytic approach involves testing the baseline PRO score or prior PRO score (just before dropout) as predictors of missingness (dropout) in a logistic regression model (with the binary outcome of missing or not missing), after adjusting for the dependence on baseline covariates. If the adjusted odds ratios (adjusted for the set of baseline covariates) are sizeable and meaningful, evidence exists that the missingness is dependent on the observed PRO scores and, therefore, the assumption of MCAR is not valid.

In general, when missing data are MAR, the analytic methods that incorporate all available PRO assessments are needed. Unbiased estimates can be obtained from likelihood-based methods such as those found in the longitudinal models in Chapter 8, which consumes all available data simultaneously and over time. Relevant baseline covariates should also be considered as part of the model. If missingness is strongly dependent on a baseline covariate, and that covariate is ignored, the estimates of treatment effect may be biased.

10.2.3 Missing Not at Random

Data are *missing not at random* (MNAR) if the probability of missingness *does* depend on the unobserved responses of the dependent variable. In other words, the value of any unobserved response is a function of information that is not available and hence the prediction of a missing observation is open to appreciable bias. Suppose a patient had a meaningful improvement (reduction) in self-reported pain during the first 3 weeks of a 6-week study and then the patient had a marked worsening and dropped out. If the patient was lost to follow-up and there was no observation at the fourth week to reflect the worsened condition, the missingness is MNAR. When dropout rates differ by treatment group, it would be incorrect to automatically assume MNAR or that analyses assuming MCAR or MAR are invalid.

The missing data mechanism of MNAR has the least restrictive assumptions. Here the missing value is dependent on the unobserved value of the PRO measure at the time of the planned assessment. For instance, assessments are more likely to be missed when an individual is experiencing side effects of therapy, such as nausea or vomiting, then the missingness is MNAR. Alternatively, when assessments are more likely to be missed when an individual is experiencing the benefits of therapy and is less willing to return for follow-up, then the missingness is also MNAR.

Because the missing PRO scores are not observable, it is not possible to directly test a hypothesis between MNAR vs MAR, as the data needed to test the hypothesis are not available. Indirect approaches exist, however, to gather evidence suggestive of MNAR (Fairclough, 2010). One approach relies on fitting an underlying model in which a nonrandom missing data mechanism is assumed. Such a model may provide evidence that dropout is MNAR given a particular model. Neverthless, ruling out absence of evidence for MNAR (when the particular form of the nonrandom component is not evident) from one particular model does not rule out absence of evidence from other models in which a nonrandom mechanism is based under a different set of assumptions.

A second approach to examine MNAR is to gather measures of the disease or outcomes of treatment that are strongly associated with the PRO instrument (e.g., caregiver assessment, toxicity, and death). These auxiliary measures serve as surrogates to the PRO measure of interest and assume that the relationship between the observed PRO scores and the other (surrogate) measurements is similar to the relationship between the missing PRO scores and those other measurements. A more sophisticated way to proceed is to perform, at each planned PRO assessment, a logistic regression model with the binary assessment of progressive disease (yes or no) and death within 3 months prior to the planned assessment taken as the key predictors and with missingness (yes, no) taken as the outcome. The model can be adjusted for previous PRO score and also for baseline covariates such as age, performance status, and treatment assignment. If progressive disease or death remains strong predictors of missing assessments, then the evidence would suggest that the data are MCAR.

Again, however, the lack of such a relationship is not proof that the data are not MCAR. There could be, for instance, a selective bias such that, among those experiencing progressive disease, only those with little or no impact on the PRO attribute being measured actually complete the questionnaire (individuals with poor values on the PRO attribute do not complete the questionnaire).

A third approach to identify dependence on unobserved data comes from external sources. Clinicians and caregivers can provide anecdotal or ancillary information suggestive of nonrandom missing data.

The analysis of data suspected to be MNAR relies on strong untestable assumptions. Several models are available to address MNAR, such as pattern mixture models, selection models, and shared parameter models, and they are fully described elsewhere (Little, 1995; Hogan and Laird, 1997; Diggle et al., 2002; Little and Rubin, 2002; Molenberghs and Kenward, 2007; Fitzmaurice et al., 2008; Fairclough, 2010; Mallinckrodt, 2013). Analyses in the MNAR framework try in some manner to model or otherwise take into account the process or mechanism of the missing data. Fundamental issues surface in the analysis of MNAR data because the characteristics and statistical behavior of the missing data are unknown. Assumptions that need to be made cannot be verified and tested, because the data about which the assumptions are made are missing. In general, there is no reliable or guaranteed statistical technique for identifying the mechanism generating missing data. Plots of response over time for dropouts and completers may reveal a pattern. Nonetheless, MNAR is difficult to rule out in general, and sensitivity analyses should be implemented to examine the robustness of mean scores and other statistics on PRO measures even for minor MNAR scenarios.

10.3 Approaches for Missing Items within Domains or Measures

Data on PRO measures can occur as missing at the item level or for the entire questionnaire or for an entire domain within the questionnaire (when the questionnaire has multiple domains). A missing item involves the lack of a response for at least one specific item on the questionnaire; a missing domain or missing questionnaire involves patients who may fail to complete and return the whole domain or questionnaire. Instruments may include well-documented procedures by their developers on how to handle missing items, and such recommendations by developers are typically the preferred way to address missing items (Sloan et al., 2007; FDA, 2009).

For example, the European Organization for Research and Treatment of Cancer Quality of Life Questionnaire—Cancer-30 (EORTC QLQ-C30) consists of five functional scales (physical, role, cognitive, emotional, and social), three symptom scales (fatigue, pain, nausea and vomiting), a global health status scale, and 6 single-item scales (Fayers et al., 2001). The *EORTC QLQ-C30 Scoring Manual* has specified that under certain conditions missing values will be imputed for multi-item scales. Specifically, if at least half of the items from the scale have been answered, the missing items are assumed to have values equal to the average of those items that are present for the respondent. For example, the physical function subscale consists of five items and this scale can be estimated whenever at least three of its five constituent items are present.

Items or sets of items may be missing from a PRO instrument for various reasons, one of which may be by design (e.g., items may not be applicable as with those specific to employment among unemployed respondents). More problematic is when a respondent skips or forgets to respond to an item or items. Also, an individual might refuse to answer because of the sensitivity of the inquiry. These different reasons should be considered when planning for handling of missing data and for subsequent sensitivity analyses. Comparisons can be made to assess whether respondents with missing item nonresponse differ from those without missing item nonresponse across time points.

The simplest solution to dealing with missing items on a multi-item PRO measure is to treat the scale score as missing. This approach of course results in a loss of power and the threat of serious bias when the miss-ingness is informative regarding the patient's true PRO status. Single imputation methods, with varying degrees of complexity, exist for miss-ing item-level data (Fairclough, 2010). While reasonable, these methods make strong assumptions about the missing data mechanism, which may be unrealistic and may induce a systematic underestimate of the sampling variation in certain circumstances. The FDA (2009) guidance states that "the SAP can specify the proportion of items that can be missing before a domain is treated as missing." This approach requires rules that prespecify the number of items that can be missing to still consider the domain as adequately measured.

One typical approach is to prorate a scale score if at least half of the items from a PRO scale have been answered (Fairclough and Cella, 1996; Fairclough, 2010). If a subject completes at least half of the items being used to compute a multi-item scale or subscale (domain) of a PRO measure, this half-rule procedure of imputation takes the mean of a patient's observed responses and substitutes it for the missing values of the missing items on the same scale, as in the example given previously for the EORTC QLQ-30. The ensuing summated score (the simple sum of the observed and imputed values) is equivalent to taking the mean of the observed responses and mul-tiplying by the total number of items. A strength of the half-rule method is that it imputes a person-specific estimate for each missing item based on the average score across completed items on the same scale from the same person. Thus, unlike some other single imputation methods, the imputation of scores does not depend on data collected from other subjects, other trials, and even other domains or measures from the same subject. The half-rule method is well suited for multi-item scales where there is no clear ordering or hierarchy of item difficulty on the questions. Research has suggested that the approach, though simple, compares favorably (in terms of being most unbiased and precise) against regression-based and other single-imputation methods for item nonresponse (Fairclough and Cella, 1996).

The half-rule approach, however, should be used cautiously (or not used at all) when the questions have a strict hierarchy in terms of their diffi-culty as it occurs, for example, with the SF-36 physical functioning domain (Ware et al., 2000). In this case, if an individual responds *not limited at all* in performing rigorous activities (such as running, lifting heavy objects, participating in strenuous sports), this individual will also be *not limited at all* to walk one block and it would make sense to impute this response on performing rigorous activities to a missing response on whether or not an individual can walk one block. On the other hand, if an individual responds *not limited at all* to walking one block, this individual may or may not be lim-ited at all in performing rigorous activities and hence imputation of the for-mer to the latter (if the question on walking one block was completed and the question on rigorous activities was missing) would not be appropriate. In this case, special strategies may need to be adopted (Kosinski et al., 2000).

10.4 Approaches for Missing Entire Domains or Entire Questionnaires

A more complex situation than item-level missing on a domain or questionnaire is data missing from all items on a domain or questionnaire. Such missing questionnaires can happen for several reasons like dropout from the study or randomly failing to fill out an entire domain or questionnaire (e.g., by not realizing that there are more questions to complete on the next page of the form). In any of these situations, it is important to first analyze the rates (proportions) and reasons for missing data. Such information will help to gauge the severity of the nonresponse problem and the underlying mechanisms for missing data. There are at least four approaches to address data missing from forms pertaining to an entire domain or questionnaire (Fairclough, 2010), approaches that are highlighted in what follows.

10.4.1 Complete Case Analysis

One approach is to remove patients with missing or incomplete forms from the analysis and only analyze complete cases. This approach involves ignoring the missing data and performing analysis based on the complete cases. While the approach is not consistent with the intention-to-treat principle (where all subjects are analyzed according to their treatment assignment), an analysis based on only complete cases may, in some situations, have some value in a sensitivity analysis to examine the robustness of study findings.

While simple, a completers-only analysis is usually not recommended because it can break down initial randomization and reduce sample size and, in doing so, may produce biased results if the missing data are not MCAR. (As noted earlier in this chapter, missing completely at random (MCAR) on a PRO score occurs when the missingness is unrelated to what the PRO instrument is measuring, and hence its accompanying set of observed scores, as when, for example, a patient moves out of town or a staff member simply forgets to administer the questionnaire.)

Other methods that assume MCAR (though not based only on completers) are unweighted generalized estimating equations, summary statistics (a set of repeated measures on an individual is reduced to a single value such as the mean, slope, or area under the curve), and repeated univariate analyses (with repeated testing at each time point) (Fairclough, 2010; Bell and Fairclough, in press). Moreover, it should be noted that repeated univariate analyses do not take advantage of the longitudinal stream of data and involves using and comparing different groups of patients at each time point.

10.4.2 Imputation

A second approach to address missing entire domains or questionnaires is to impute the missing data, with a single value imputed for a particular missing data value. Different methods can be used for the imputation. The simplest way is to substitute the mean scores of patients with observed data for those with missing data (mean imputation). Unless the missing data are MCAR, which is typically not the case, this mean-imputation method may result in biased estimates and should be used cautiously. Another commonly used method is last observation carried forward, which replaces a patient's missing value with that patient's last completed observation. In the likelihood that data on a PRO instrument may not remain stable over time, last observation carried forward may also be suspect and result in a biased representation (Mallinckrodt et al., 2008; Bell and Fairclough, in press). This method is applicable when a constant mean response continues after time of dropout (i.e., on average, when patient response is assumed to remain the same after dropout as before dropout), which is improbable in many situations (like advanced progression in cancer).

Analogous to the last observation carried forward approach is the baseline observation carried forward approach, when all missing values for a subject are replaced by that subject's baseline observation. It is based on the assumption that initially randomized active medications have no effect after they are discontinued. Like last observation carried forward, baseline observation carried forward is prone to result in biased estimates of treatment effect for studies with informative missing data on outcome (e.g., if patients discontinue because of poor response to treatment that would have resulted in a poor PRO score if this score were not missing).

For either type of observation carried forward, the direction of bias can favor either the test-treated group or the control-treated group, depending on the circumstances (Mallinckrodt et al., 2008; Mallinckrodt, 2013). For example, if patients discontinue because of poor response to control treatment, last (or baseline) observation carried forward for an efficacy outcome will underestimate the superiority of a superior test treatment (with the bias therefore favoring the control treatment). If instead the patients discontinue because of poor response to test treatment, last (or baseline) observation carried forward for an efficacy outcome will underestimate the inferiority of an inferior test treatment (with the bias therefore favoring the test treatment). More sophisticated single-imputation techniques have been developed and they include regression imputation, hot deck imputation, and cold deck imputation (Little and Rubin, 2002).

A major limitation with single imputation methods is that variability estimates are generally too small, as the imputed values are treated as actual data when in fact they are not. However, this obstacle can be overcome by multiple imputations whereby several values are imputed instead of just one. Multiple imputation is intended to avoid the risk of underestimating variances. The multiple imputation method, which improves the accuracy of the estimated standard error belong to the treatment effect estimate, assumes that the missing data are MAR, where the missingness depends only on the observed data such as the most recently observed PRO value. The method involves, under MAR assumptions, combining estimates and standard errors obtained from multiple copies of the original data set in which missing values are replaced by randomly generated values based on a predictive model (Rubin, 1987; Little and Rubin, 2002; Carpenter and Kenward, 2013).

10.4.3 Maximum Likelihood Methods

A third approach to address the problem of missing data on an entire domain or questionnaire is through the application of a maximum likelihood-based approach using repeated-measures models or random coefficient models, which are detailed in Chapter 8 (Singer and Willett, 2003; Mallinckrodt et al., 2008; Fairclough, 2010; Fitzmaurice et al., 2011). In this approach, every subject would contribute the available (observed) measurements. Repeated measures models and random coefficient models employ a likelihood-based approach that is considered attractive because it can provide a valid estimate of treatment effects if missing data are MCAR or MAR, where the missing data are said to be ignorable (i.e., the data can be analyzed without explicitly modeling the missing data mechanism). Results from these two types of mixed-effect models may be quite robust when observed covariates (e.g., baseline scores on the PRO), as well as previous values of the outcome, are included and explain much of the missingness (Donaldson and Moinpour, 2005; Brown and Prescott, 2006).

Other methods that assume MAR (though not based strictly on maximum likelihood estimation) are extensions to generalized estimating equations (Bell and Fairclough, in press). An example is weighted generalized estimating equations where only observed data are used but are weighted to account for those who dropout, with the weights being the inverse of the predicted probability of being observed for each patient. These methods assume that the weighted model and the longitudinal outcome model are specified correctly.

10.4.4 MNAR Models

The fourth approach is especially relevant when missing data are *not missing at random* (MNAR) and hence depend on the (unknown) missing value. Three main types of MNAR models are pattern mixture models, selection bias, and shared random effects models (Fitzmaurice et al., 2008; Ibrahim and Molenberghs, 2009; Fairclough, 2010). In these three models, the joint distribution of the longitudinally measured outcome and either the dropout time or the missing data indicators are incorporated into the model. Each of these models seeks to convert the missing data problem to one in which the underlying assumption is that missing data are conditional MAR, given the model specified and assumptions imposed. When data are MNAR, the missing mechanism cannot be ignored and hence needs to be modeled explicitly.

Each of the three MNAR models that factorizes the full data (both observed data and missing data) in a different way. Of them, pattern mixture models are probably the best suited for practical applications of PRO data. When data are neither MCAR nor MAR, a MNAR model can be considered as a secondary model in sensitivity analyses. The benefit of MNAR methods is that they allow estimation without data under the assumption, of course, that the model is appropriate. The danger is that the appropriateness of the model and its assumptions cannot be verified from the data, because the relevant data are absent.

The idea behind pattern mixture models is to allow parameters to vary according to missing data patterns with respect to the outcome or dependent variable of interest (e.g., PRO measure), with the model being conditional upon membership in a particular dropout pattern (Hedeker and Gibbons, 1997). For example, three patterns can be identified: early dropouts, late dropouts, and completers. The estimates from each pattern or stratum are then combined using weights based on the proportion of individuals in each pattern. Various pattern mixture models can be fit, within the longitudinal modeling or repeated measures framework, depending on the number and characterization of the missing data patterns. Pattern mixture models have the advantage that a portion of the model specifying the missing data mechanism does not depend on the missing values. This advantage is offset by the need either to specify a set of restrictions to estimate all of the parameters or to create strata (patterns) where all parameters are estimable and missing values are assumed to be ignorable within each stratum. These models are well suited when the number of patterns is relatively small or can be combined as such. Section 10.6 goes into more detail about pattern mixture model with a simulated illustration.

As with MNAR models in general, selection models require a correct specification of the model for the full data (both observed and missing), the covariates, possibly auxiliary variables, and the dropout probability (Diggle and Kenward, 1994; Diggle et al., 2002; NRC, 2010). A selection model can be thought of as an integrated multivariate model where one central variable is the continuous efficacy outcome (e.g., PRO measure) from the primary analysis and another central variable is the binary outcome for dropout modeled via logistic regression that depends on covariates, previously observed values of the response or outcome variable (e.g., PRO measure), and the current measurement on the response variable (which is missing for all those who dropout and therefore relies on knowing the correct distribution of all values on outcome). The overall model links the measurement and missingness processes by having the outcome variable from the measurement model serve as a predictor in the dropout (missingness) model.

In shared parameter models, which are an overlap between selection models and pattern mixture models, time to dropout (or some other time to event, like survival time) and the longitudinal outcome (e.g., PRO measure) are modeled separately but they share common parameters, namely, random effects (Wu and Carroll, 1988; Wu and Bailey, 1989). A set of latent (unobserved) variables or classes are reflected in the random effects that are assumed to drive the measurement of outcome and the missing data as measured by time to dropout. Given the random effects, the measurement of outcome values (observed and unobserved) and time to dropout are assumed to be independent.

A shared parameter model can be thought of as an integrated multivariate model where one key variable is the continuous efficacy outcome (e.g., PRO measure) from the primary analysis and the second is time to dropout from (typically) the proportional hazards time-to-event analysis. The full data likelihood can be factored similar to a selection model (described in the previous paragraph) as the product of the marginal outcome distribution (of the observed or missing response given the random effect) and the conditional distribution of time to dropout (given the observed or missing response and the random effect). The dropout and measurement models are linked as the same random effects are in both outcome and dropout models. As with selection models, shared parameter models rest with untestable assumptions. In particular, shared parameter models assume that, conditional on the latent random effects, the outcome measurement and missingness are independent, which is not testable because the outcome is missing in every instance when time to dropout occurs prior to the end of the study.

10.5 Sensitivity Analyses

In general, the reliability of the available methods for handling missing data is dependent on the mechanism generating the missingness and the assumptions made. Defense of the assumptions should be made primarily on a clinical basis, not a statistical basis *per se*, with empirical or clinical evidence lending support whenever possible. Nonetheless, it can prove challenging to accurately determine why data are missing. It is good practice, therefore, to assess the robustness of a particular approach by repeating the analyses using alternative methods for different missingness scenarios. Sensitivity analyses are a series of analyses with different assumptions.

The aim of sensitivity analyses is to compare the results across the different analyses in order to better understand how much the inference about treatment effect relies on the assumptions regarding missing data. The degree to which inferential conclusions are stable or robust across such analyses provides an indication of the confidence that can be placed on the conclusions. The focus should compare the magnitude of treatment effect from the sensitivity analyses with that from the primary analysis; emphasis should be based on the magnitude of effect and not on p-values, which may be misleading. For PRO data, sensitivity analyses should be considered for a domain with missing item-level data as well as conducted for a PRO domain or questionnaire in which all items are missing.

The FDA (2009) guidance states that "sensitivity analyses in analyzing the PRO endpoints should be proposed in the protocol and the SAP to assess the robustness of statistical estimation for endpoints with the missing data imputed. We recommend that in the protocol the sponsor propose two or more sensitivity analyses with different methods for missing data imputation."

Indeed, a parsimonious set of logical and plausible set of sensitivity analyses should be prespecified. For example, for the analysis of longitudinal data, one recommendation is to consider a MAR-based analysis using a repeated measures model or random coefficient model as the main or primary model and a pattern mixture model as the secondary model in a sensitivity analysis. Pattern mixture models with varying but plausible identifying restrictions on parameters or patterns can be fit and compared.

While consensus does not currently exist on exactly how sensitivity analyses should be conducted and interpreted, the recent NRC guidance and other relevant sources on prevention and treatment of missing data have set forth principles and methods for consideration (Molenberghs and Kenward, 2007; Mallinckrodt et al., 2008; NRC, 2010; Mallinckrodt, 2013). As stated in the NRC report, "Sensitivity analyses should be part of the primary reporting findings from clinical trials. Examining sensitivity to the assumptions about the missing data mechanism should be a mandatory component of reporting."

10.6 Simulated Example Using SAS: Pattern Mixture Models

The main idea behind pattern mixture modeling is to account for the missing data by assigning subjects to several different strata or groups based on their pattern of missing data and with each stratum denoted by a distinct model. Different patterns can be uncovered and used in the analyses based on the research question, study design, drug effect, disease, and other considerations. One approach is to partition subjects into two groups: subjects who completed the trial (*completers*) vs subjects who did not (*dropouts*). This simple dichotomy makes two underlying assumptions: (1) any intermittent missing data between the first observation and the last observation for a subject are considered random and (2) for a subject to be a *completer* or *dropout* is informative and not a random event (meaning that we take stratum membership of *completer* or *dropout* as an informative and nonrandom effect). This pattern is applicable only if the number of dropouts is reasonably small. But in the case of many oncology studies, for instance, attrition typically plays a prominent role throughout the study, with attrition starting at the beginning of the study and continuing to the end of the study where only a relatively small percentage of subjects eventually complete the study and, hence, can be labeled *completers*.

In Section 8.4.2, we described an example based on a oncology study (Cella et al., 2008). Results from a random coefficient model were provided. A similar set of results was obtained using a pattern mixture model (Cella et al., 2008), suggesting that the results on treatment effect were not overly dependent upon the nature of missing data. In this model, each pattern (stratum) was defined by the time of last assessment. The first 2 cycles were combined as the first stratum and each subsequent stratum is based on a cycle whose subjects had data up until that cycle. As such, there was a separate stratum for each potential dropout time by cycle.

In the current section, we expand on that example using simulated data to illustrate pattern mixture modeling based on the empirical framework embodied in the example. Equation 8.11 from Chapter 8 can be extended to represent several patterns as follows:

$$Y_{ijp} = a + b_1 \times x_i + b_2 \times r_i + b_3 \times t_{ij} + b_4 \times r_i \times t_{ij} + a_p + b_{2p} \times r_i$$

$$+ b_{3p} \times t_{ij} + b_{4p} \times r_i \times t_{ij} + \alpha'_i + \beta'_i \times t_{ij} + e_{ij}, \qquad (10.1)$$

where

Y_{ijp} is the PRO score for subject i belonging to pattern p at measurement occasion j ($i = 1, 2,\ldots,750$; $j = 1, 2,\ldots,n_i$; n_i represents the number of repeated observations for subject i, where n_i can range from just one observation to a maximum of 11 observations in this example; $p = 1,2, \ldots, N_p$, N_p is the number of patterns or strata)

$a, b_1, x_i, b_2, b_3, b_4, \alpha'_i, \beta'_i, e_{ij}$ are the parameters described in detail in Section 8.4.2 (Equation 8.11)

a_p is the intercept parameter for pattern p

r_i is the treatment variable for subject i (with values of 1 for subjects on sunitinib and 0 for subjects on interferon-alfa) and b_{2p} is the slope for variable r_i for pattern p

t_{ij} is the jth time assessment for subject i and b_{3p} is the slope (over time) for variable t_{ij} for pattern p

b_{4p} is the slope for the treatment-by-time interaction effect for pattern p

Multiple ways exist to estimate the parameters of interest, all of which will result in the same set of results for any given hypothesis test. The model represented by Equation 10.1 is said to be *overparameterized*, meaning that there are more parameters to estimate relative to the degrees of freedom necessary for parameter estimation (i.e., relative to the number of values that are free to vary for parameter estimation). As a consequence, a unique solution would require that certain parameters should not be estimated but rather assigned fixed values *a priori*. In practice, a common approach for interpretation and presentation is to set the last pattern as the reference pattern by setting its parameters to zero; effects for all other patterns are defined relative to this last pattern.

Thus, in our illustration, the last pattern has a_{Np}, b_{2Np}, b_{3Np}, and b_{4Np} each fixed to equal zero (see Section 8.2.2.2 for additional details). This type of parameterization becomes relevant during the simulation of the data, because the estimation of the parameters for the subsequent modeling in this case will be simple to interpret, enabling them to be compared with the corresponding values defined in the simulation. Note that in SAS the MIXED procedure is implemented to use an overparameterized model. As a result, in the analysis of real data, referent parameterization is invoked automatically by the MIXED procedure during the modeling process.

Figure 10.1 uses the same approach to generate the simulated dataset described in Section 8.4.2 and incorporates several augmentations.

```
data _cov_ (type=corr);
input
_TYPE_ $    _NAME_ $    COL1       COL2        ;
datalines;
 CORR         COL1        1          0.4
 CORR         COL2        0.4        1
 MEAN         .           0          0
 STD          .           0.3        0.1
 N            .           750        750
;
run;

proc simnormal data=_cov_ out=err_sim numreal=750 seed=100;
var Col1-Col2;
run;

Data _tmp_1;
Set err_sim;
Random_Intercept = Col1;
Random_Slope     = Col2;

ID=_N_;

Treatment=0;
If _N_>375 Then Treatment=1;

r=ranuni(3000);
If r< 0.5            Then Pattern=1;
If r>=0.5 and r<0.9 Then Pattern=2;
If r>=0.9           Then Pattern=3;

Keep Random_Intercept Random_Slope ID Treatment Pattern;
Run;

Proc Means data=_tmp_1;
Var Random_Intercept Random_Slope;
Run;

Proc Corr data=_tmp_1 COV;
Var Random_Intercept Random_Slope;
Run;

Data _tmp_2;
Set  _tmp_1;

retain  seed3 5   seed4 6 seed6 1000;

   NumberOfVisits=11;
   b1=2;          /* Baseline effect slope*/
   Intercept=1 ;  /* intercept                       */
   Slope=2;       /* slope                           */
   b02=2;         /* Treatment effect slope          */
   b04=0.5;       /* Cycle*Treatment interaction slope */
```

FIGURE 10.1
Generating a dataset for the pattern mixture analysis.

(continued)

```
    Intercept1=10;   /*Pattern 1: intercept                     */
    Slope1=4;        /*Pattern 1: slope                         */
    b12=2;           /*Pattern 1: Treatment effect slope        */
    b14=0.5;         /*Pattern 1: Cycle*Treatment interaction slope*/

    Intercept2=5;    /*Pattern 2: intercept                     */
    Slope2=3;        /*Pattern 2: slope                         */
    b22=1.4;         /*Pattern 2: Treatment effect slope        */
    b24=0.3;         /*Pattern 2: Cycle*Treatment interaction slope*/

    Intercept3=0;    /*Pattern 3: intercept                     */
    Slope3=0;        /*Pattern 3: slope                         */
    b32=0;           /*Pattern 3: Treatment effect slope        */
    b34=0;           /*Pattern 3: Cycle*Treatment interaction slope*/

/*
call rannor(random number seed, variable name) returns a value
for the variable name specified that is generated from a normal
distribution with mean 0 and variance 1
*/
Call rannor(seed6, X6);

Baseline = 10 + 30 * X6;

/*
call ranuni (random number seed, variable name) returns a value
for the variable name specified that is generated from a uniform
distribution in the interval [0, 1]
*/
Call ranuni(seed3, X4);

If Pattern = 1 Then
Do;
LastCycle           = 1+Int(3 * X4) ;
Pattern_Intercept = Intercept1    ;
Pattern_Slope     = Slope1        ;
b2                = b12           ;
b4                = b14           ;

End;

If Pattern = 2 Then
Do;
LastCycle           = 4+Int(5 * X4) ;
Pattern_Intercept = Intercept2    ;
Pattern_Slope     = Slope2        ;
b2                = b22           ;
b4                = b24           ;
End;
```

FIGURE 10.1 (continued)
Generating dataset for the pattern mixture analysis.

```
If Pattern = 3 Then
Do;
LastCycle          = 9+Int (3 * X4)   ;
Pattern_Intercept = Intercept3        ;
Pattern_Slope      = Slope3           ;
b2                 = b32              ;
b4                 = b34              ;
End;

Do Cycle=1 to LastCycle;
    call rannor(seed4, X5);

    Y =   Intercept+ b1 * Baseline   +   b02 * Treatment + Slope *
Cycle   + b04 * Cycle * Treatment +      Pattern_Intercept +   b2 *
Treatment + Pattern_Slope * Cycle + b4 * Cycle * Treatment +
Random_Intercept + Random_Slope*
Cycle   + sqrt(0.05)*X5;

output;
End;

Keep Y  Baseline ID Cycle Treatment Pattern ;

Run;
```

FIGURE 10.1 (continued)
Generating dataset for the pattern mixture analysis.

In Section 8.4.2, data were modeled according to Equation 8.11, but now we introduce several patterns: 50% of the subjects are randomly assigned to pattern 1 (If r< 0.5 Then Pattern=1;), 40% of subjects are randomly assigned to pattern 2 (If r>=0.5 and r<0.9 Then Pattern=2;), and the remaining 10% of subjects are randomly assigned to pattern 3 (If r>=0.9 Then Pattern=3).

The next most important detail is the specification of the patterns. Subjects from the first pattern are the subjects who were in the trial at least during the first cycle but not more than 3 cycles (LastCycle = 1+Int(3 * X4);); in this pattern, subjects had at least one observation during the first 3 cycles but no observations thereafter. Subjects from the second pattern are those who had at least one observation between cycle 4 and cycle 8 (inclusive) but no observations after cycle 8 (LastCycle = 4+Int(5 * X4);). Note that subjects from the second pattern also could have any number of observations or none at all during the first 3 cycles. Subjects from the third pattern had at least one observation from cycle 9 to cycle 11 (inclusive). Note again that subjects from the third pattern could also have any number of observations (or none at all) during the first 8 cycles. For example, if a subject had only two observations with one observation at cycle 4 and another observation at cycle 10, this subject will belong to the third pattern. If a subject had only three observations at cycles 1, 2, and 8, this subject will belong to the second pattern. As a result, the additional variable Pattern is added to the dataset for the analysis (relative to the dataset from Section 8.4.2).

```
Proc Mixed data=_tmp_2;

   Class ID Pattern;

   Model Y = Baseline Cycle Treatment Cycle*Treatment Pattern
Cycle*Pattern Treatment*Pattern Cycle*Treatment*Pattern /
Solution ddfm=kr;

   Random INTERCEPT Cycle / Subject=ID Type=UN;

Run;
```

FIGURE 10.2
Implementation of the pattern mixture model.

Figure 10.2 represents the implementation of the pattern mixture model using a random intercept–slope mixed-effect model. Comparing this implementation (Figure 10.2) with the implementation presented by Figure 8.38, we see that additional elements were added to the Model statement, which correspond to Equation 10.1 (with the parameter *time* in Equation 10.1 represented by the variable *cycle* in Figure 10.2). Note that the intercept term in Equation 10.1 is automatically (a default) part of the Model statement and is therefore not specified there, but should be specified explicitly in the Random statement.

Figure 10.3 provides estimation of the fixed effects portion of the model, which are as expected close to their respective simulated values. For example, the fixed effect for time (cycle) associated with pattern 1 was estimated as 2.01 (Cycle 2.0113; see Figure 10.3) and defined in the simulation with a corresponding slope value of 2 (Slope=2; /*slope*/; see Figure 10.1). Pattern-specific estimates for pattern 1 and pattern 2 are relative to, or in comparison with, referent pattern 3. For example, the fixed effect for time associated with pattern 1 was estimated as 4.01 (Cycle*Pattern 1 4.0125; see Figure 10.3) and defined in the simulation with a corresponding slope value of 4 (Slope1=4; /*Pattern 1: slope */; Figure 10.1).

The fixed effect for treatment effect associated with pattern 1 was estimated as 1.94 (Treatment*Pattern 1 1.9405; Figure 10.3) and defined in the simulation with a corresponding slope value of 2 (b12=2; /*Pattern 1: Treatment effect slope */; Figure 10.1). The fixed effect for time-by-treatment interaction associated with pattern 1 was estimated as 0.45 (Cycle*Treatm*Pattern 1 0.4519; Figure 10.3), which is close to the corresponding slope value of 0.5 defined in the simulation (b14=0.5; /*Pattern 1: Cycle*Treatment interaction slope*/; Figure 10.1). Other estimates in Figure 10.3 share the same types of interpretation.

A natural question to ask is, "How can the model presented by Figure 10.2 be implemented with real data, where the values of variable *Pattern* are not known?" Creating patterns is the most critical part of pattern mixture models. In some cases, the simple dichotomy of *completers* and *dropouts* may suffice.

Solution for Fixed Effects

Effect	Pattern	Estimate	Standard Error	DF	t Value	Pr > |t|
Intercept		0.9873	0.05025	482	19.65	<.0001
Baseline		1.9995	0.000458	751	4367.51	<.0001
Cycle		2.0113	0.01607	312	125.15	<.0001
Treatment		2.0829	0.07262	476	28.68	<.0001
Cycle*Treatment		0.5094	0.02341	311	21.76	<.0001
Pattern	1	9.9833	0.06202	741	160.97	<.0001
Pattern	2	5.0903	0.05821	514	87.44	<.0001
Pattern	3	0	.	.	.	.
Cycle*Pattern	1	4.0125	0.02554	918	157.14	<.0001
Cycle*Pattern	2	2.9919	0.01884	340	158.78	<.0001
Cycle*Pattern	3	0	.	.	.	.
Treatment*Pattern	1	1.9405	0.08921	731	21.75	<.0001
Treatment*Pattern	2	1.1903	0.08458	513	14.07	<.0001
Treatment*Pattern	3	0	.	.	.	.
Cycle*Treatm*Pattern	1	0.4519	0.03684	924	12.27	<.0001
Cycle*Treatm*Pattern	2	0.2891	0.02741	341	10.55	<.0001
Cycle*Treatm*Pattern	3	0	.	.	.	.

FIGURE 10.3
Solution for fixed effects in the pattern mixture model.

If enough data are available, a much more ambitious strategy can be employed. In the example described in this section, every cycle can be defined as a separate pattern. For example, all subjects who have data up to the first cycle would be assigned to pattern 1, all subjects who have data up to the second cycle would be assigned to pattern 2, and so on. It is important to emphasize that such detailed strata will lead to many parameters requiring estimation in the model. In the case of the three patterns, 17 fixed parameters surfaced (17 = (number of effects across patterns or nonspecific pattern effects) + (number of pattern-specific effects)*(number of parameters per pattern) = 5 + 4*3; Figure 10.3). And if 11 patterns are created, the number of fixed parameters in the model will swell to 49 (= 5 + 4*11), which could easily lead to the inability of the model to converge to a set of solutions.

A more balanced approach can be based on the patterns based on the attrition of subjects. Drawing from the data generated in Figure 10.1, Figure 10.4 provides SAS code to calculate the number of subjects who have only data up

```
Proc Means NOPRINT data=_tmp_2;
Class ID;
Var Cycle;
OUTPUT OUT=Patterns MAX=Last_Cycle;
Run;

Proc Freq data=Patterns;
Tables Last_Cycle;
Where ID ne .;
Run;
```

FIGURE 10.4
SAS code to assess attrition of subjects.

```
Last_Cycle      Frequency
-----------------------------
        1           130
        2           126
        3           130
        4            54
        5            57
        6            54
        7            56
        8            58
        9            32
       10            27
       11            26
```

FIGURE 10.5
Number of subjects having data up and only to a certain cycle (attrition of subjects).

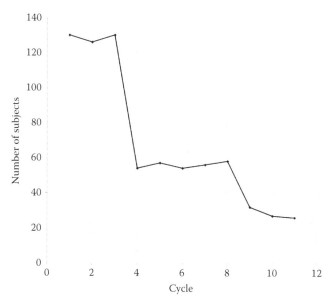

FIGURE 10.6
Attrition of subjects.

to a certain cycle. Figure 10.5 represents the results and Figure 10.6 depicts this information graphically for 750 subjects. Based on Figure 10.6, we can see a drop in the attrition graph after cycle 3 and after cycle 8. Based on this pattern of attrition, the evidence of three patterns can be proposed: subjects who have data (at least one observation) only up to cycle 3 can be classified into the first pattern; subjects who have at least one observation after cycle 3, but not beyond cycle 8, can be classified into the second pattern; and subjects who have at least one observation after cycle 8 can be classified into the third pattern.

10.7 Summary

Missing data are difficult to avoid in PRO research. A set of recommendations is highlighted on how to minimize (or at least reduce) missing data at the trial design stage and conduct stage of a clinical trial. The three major mechanisms of missing data for longitudinal data—MCAR, MAR, MNAR—are described in this chapter. Data on PRO scores can occur as missing at the item level or for the entire questionnaire or an entire domain within the questionnaire. A user of PRO instruments should consult with their developers for guidance on how to address item-level missing data. Simple imputation using the half-rule method can be useful when less than 50% of the items are missing in a domain or questionnaire. Four approaches are highlighted to address data missing on the whole domain or questionnaire: complete case analysis, imputation, maximum likelihood estimation, and specialized models when data are MNAR. Their merits and shortcomings are noted. Because it can prove quite challenging to accurately determine why data are missing, it is good practice to assess the robustness of a particular approach by repeating the analyses using alternative methods for different missingness scenarios. Finally, a simulated example using a pattern mixture model, a type of MNAR model, is illustrated.

References

Allison, P.D. 2002. *Missing Data*. Thousand Oaks, CA: Sage Publications.

Bell, M.L. and D.L. Fairclough. In press. Practical and statistical issues in missing data for longitudinal patient reported outcomes. *Statistical Methods in Medical Research*. Published online 19 February 2013. E-pub ahead of print. DOI: 10.1177/0962280213476378.

Brown, H. and R. Prescott. 2006. *Applied Mixed Models in Models*, 2nd edition. Chichester, England: John Wiley & Sons Ltd.

Burzykowski, T., Carpenter, J., Coens, C., Evans, D., France, L., Kenward, M., Lane, P. et al. of the PSI Missing Data Expert Group. 2010. Missing data: Discussion points from the PSI missing data expert group. *Pharmaceutical Statistics* 9:288–297.

Byrom, B. and B. Tiplady (editors). 2010. *ePro: Electronic Solutions for Patient Reported Data*. Surrey, England: Gower.

Carpenter, J.R. and M.G. Kenward. 2013. *Multiple Imputation and Its Application*. Chichester, England: John Wiley & Sons Ltd.

Cella, D., Li, J.Z., Cappelleri, J.C., Bushmakin, A., Charbonneau, C., Kim, S.T., Chen, I., Michaelson, M.D., and R.J. Motzer. 2008. Quality of life in patients with metastatic renal cell carcinoma treated with sunitinib versus interferon-alfa: Results from a phase III randomized trial. *Journal of Clinical Oncology* 26:3763–3769.

Curran, D., Bacchi, M., Schmitz Hsu, S.F., Molenberghs, G., and R.J. Sylvvester. 1998a. Identifying the types of missingness in quality of life data from clinical trials. *Statistics in Medicine* 17:739–756.

Curran, D., Molenberghs, G., Fayers, P.M., and D. Machin. 1998b. Incomplete quality of life data in randomized trials: Missing forms. *Statistics in Medicine* 17:697–709.

Diggle, P.J., Heagerty, P., Liang, K.Y., and S.L. Seger. 2002. *The Analysis of Longitudinal Data*, 2nd edition. Oxford, England: Oxford University Press.

Diggle, P.J. and M.G. Kenward. 1994. Informative dropout in longitudinal data (with discussion). *Applied Statistics* 43:49–93.

Donaldson, G.W. and C.M. Moinpour. 2005. Learning to live with missing quality-of-life data in advanced-stage disease trials. *Journal of Clinical Oncology* 23:7380–7384.

Enders, C.K. 2010. *Applied Missing Data Analysis*. New York, NY: Guilford Press.

European Medicines Agency (EMA), Committee for Medicinal Products for Human Use (CHMP). 2010. *Guideline on Missing Data in Confirmatory Clinical Trials*. http://www.ema.europa.eu/ema/ (Accessed on August 31, 2013).

Fairclough, D.L. 2010. *Design and Analysis of Quality of Life Studies in Clinical Trials*, 2nd edition. Boca Raton, FL: Chapman & Hall/CRC.

Fairclough, D.L. and D.F. Cella. 1996. Functional Assessment of Cancer Therapy (FACT-G): Non-response to individual questions. *Quality of Life Research* 5:321–329.

Fairclough, D.L., Peterson, H.F., Cella, D., and P. Bonomi 1998a. Comparison of several model-based methods for analyzing incomplete quality of life data in cancer clinical trials. *Statistics in Medicine* 17:781–796.

Fairclough, D.L., Peterson, H.F., and V. Chang. 1998b. Why are missing quality of life data a problem in clinical trials of cancer therapy? *Statistics in Medicine* 17:667–677.

Fayers, P.M., Aaronson, N.K., Bjordal, K., and M. Groenvold on behalf of the EORTC Quality of Life Study Group. 2001. *EORTC QLQ-C30 Scoring Manual*, 3rd edition. Brussels, Belgium: European Organisation for Research and Treatment of Cancer.

Fayers, P.M. and D. Machin. 2007. *Quality of Life: The Assessment, Analysis and Interpretation of Patient-Reported Outcomes*, 2nd edition. Chichester, England: John Wiley & Sons Ltd.

Fitzmaurice, G., Davidian, M., Verbeke, G., and G. Molenberghs (editors). 2008. *Longitudinal Data Analysis*. Boca Raton, FL: Chapman & Hall/CRC.

Fitzmaurice, G.M., Laird, N.M., and J.H. Ware. 2011. *Applied Longitudinal Analysis*, 2nd edition. Hoboken, NJ: John Wiley & Sons Ltd.

Food and Drug Administration (FDA). 2009. Guidance for industry on patient-reported outcome measures: Use in medical product development to support labeling claims. *Federal Register* 74(235):65132–65133. http://www.fda.gov/Drugs/DevelopmentApprovalProcess/DrugDevelopmentToolsQualificationProgram/ucm284399.htm. (Accessed on August 31, 2013).

Graham, J.W. 2012. *Missing Data: Analysis and Design*. New York, NY: Springer.

Hedeker, D. and R.D. Gibbons. 1997. Application of random-effects pattern-mixture models for missing data in longitudinal studies. *Psychological Methods* 2:64–78.

Hogan, J.W. and N.M. Laird. 1997. Mixture models for the joint distribution of repeated measures and event times. *Statistics in Medicine* 16:239–258.

Ibrahim, J.G. and G. Molenberghs. 2009. Missing data methods in longitudinal studies: A review. *Test* 18:1–43.

Izem, R., Kammerman, L.A., and S. Komo. In press. Statistical challenges in drug approval trials that use patient-reported outcomes. *Statistical Methods in Medical Research*. Published online 21 February 2013. E-pub ahead of print. DOI: 10.1177/0962280213476376.

Kosinski, M., Bayliss, M., Bjorner, J.B., and J.E. Ware. 2000. Improving estimates of SF-36 Health Survey scores for respondents with missing data. *Medical Outcomes Trust Monitor* 5:8–10.

Little, R.J.A. 1988. A test of missing completely at random for multivariate data with missing values. *Journal of the American Statistical Association* 83:1198–1202.

Little, R.J.A. 1995. Modeling the drop-out mechanism in repeated measures studies. *Journal of the American Statistical Association* 90:1112–1121.

Little, R.J.A. and D.B. Rubin. 2002. *Statistical Analysis with Missing Data*, 2nd edition. Hoboken, NJ: John Wiley & Sons Ltd.

Mallinckrodt, C.H. 2013. *Preventing and Treating Missing Data in Longitudinal Clinical Trials: A Practical Guide*. New York, NY: Cambridge University Press.

Mallinckrodt, C.H., Lane, P.W., Schnell, D., Peng, Y., and J.P. Mancuso. 2008. Recommendations for the primary analysis of continuous endpoints in longitudinal clinical trials. *Drug Information Journal* 42:303–319.

McKnight, P.E., McKnight, K.M., Sidani, S., and A.J. Figueredo. 2007. *Missing Data: A Gentle Introduction*. New York, NY: Guilford Press.

Molenberghs, G. and M.G. Kenward. 2007. *Missing Data in Clinical Studies*. Chichester, England: John Wiley & Sons Ltd.

National Research Council (NRC). 2010. *The Prevention and Treatment of Missing Data in Clinical Trials*. Panel on handling missing data in clinical trials. Committee on National Statistics, Division of Behavioral and Social Sciences and Education. Washington, DC: The National Academies Press.

Rubin, D.B. 1987. *Multiple Imputation for Nonresponse in Surveys*. New York, NY: John Wiley & Sons Ltd.

Schafer, J.L. and J.W. Graham. 2002. Missing data: Our view of the state of the art. *Psychological Methods* 7:147–177.

Singer, J.D. and J.B. Willett. 2003. *Applied Longitudinal Data Analysis: Modeling Change and Event Occurrence*. New York, NY: Oxford University Press.

Sloan, J.A., Dueck, A.C., Erickson, P.A., Guess, H., Revicki, D.A., Santanello, N.C., and the Mayo/FDA Patient-Reported Outcomes Consensus Meeting Group. 2007. Analysis and interpretation of results based on patient-reported outcomes. *Value in Health* 10 (Suppl. 2):S106–S115.

Stone, A., Shiffman, S., Atienza, A., and L. Nebeling. 2007. *The Science of Real-Time Data Capture*. New York, NY: Oxford University Press.

Walters, S.J. 2009. *Quality of Life Outcomes in Clinical Trials and Health-Care Evaluation: A Practical Guide to Analysis and Interpretation*. Chichester, England: John Wiley & Sons Ltd.

Ware, J.E., Snow, K.K., and M. Kosinski. 2000. *SF-36 Health Survey: Manual and Interpretation Guide*. Lincoln, RI: QualityMetric Incorporated.

Wu, M.C. and K.R. Bailey. 1989. Estimation and comparison of changes in the presence of informative right censoring: Conditional linear model. *Biometrics* 45:939–955.

Wu, M.C. and R.J. Carroll. 1988. Estimation and comparison of changes in the presence of informative right censoring by modeling the censoring process. *Biometrics* 44:175–188.

11

Enriching Interpretation

As discussed previously, to be useful to patients and other decision-makers (e.g., physicians, regulatory agencies, and reimbursement authorities), a patient-reported outcome (PRO) measure must undergo a validation process to confirm that it is measuring what it is supposed to be measuring and also undergo reliability testing to ensure it is accurately measuring what it is intended to measure (Fairclough, 2004). But more is needed: PRO results must also be interpreted by attaching meaning to them and applying methods to enrich their interpretation (Marquis et al., 2004; Schünemann et al., 2006; Revicki et al., 2007; McLeod et al., 2011; Cappelleri and Bushmakin, in press).

Unlike well-established clinical measurements such as survival and blood pressure, which are generally understood and can be measured directly, the latent (unobserved) concepts captured by PROs (and health measurement scales in general) may be unfamiliar to many healthcare professionals and patients. Patient-reported outcomes have been used to define and operationalize (through their constituent observed items) latent concepts (also known as factors, domains, or dimensions) like emotional well-being. Unlike survival and blood pressure, there may be insufficient data available or lack of experience or clinical understanding to draw from to properly interpret what, for example, a 5-point change means on a 0–30 PRO scale.

The problem has been compounded because, for every latent concept measured, there may be several PRO instruments that slightly differ or have different scoring systems. These subtleties can make it difficult to compare or build a body of evidence as to what a meaningful change means as has been done with, for instance, blood pressure where it is now known, after many years of use, what constitutes high or low blood pressure.

Given the prevalence and influence of PRO instruments in medical care, especially in chronic diseases, interpretation of scores and changes in scores from PRO measures is crucial for understanding the meaning and relevance of these scores for effective decision-making across different types of study designs. Useful interpretation of score values (e.g., score values above a certain threshold are considered a successful response) or score changes (e.g., change from baseline to end of study above a certain threshold is considered meaningful improvement) can be valuable in designing studies, evaluating interventions, educating consumers, and informing health policymakers in regulatory, reimbursement, and advisory agencies (e.g., the National Institute for Health and Clinical Excellence in the United Kingdom).

Thus an inherent and fundamental issue for a PRO measure centers on its meaning. In this chapter, the logic and rationale of the methods intended to enhance the interpretation of PRO scores are expressed generally. In addition, published examples are provided to show real-life implications of the methodologies, and simulated examples using SAS are also provided to accentuate understanding.

11.1 Anchor-Based Approaches

An anchor is a measure or criterion related to the targeted PRO under examination (Lydick and Epstein, 1993). As defined in this article, an anchor can be a measure different from or part of the PRO measure under consideration. The chosen anchor should be clearly understood in context and be easier to interpret than the PRO measure of interest, and the anchor should be appreciably or moderately correlated with the targeted PRO. An anchor-based approach links the targeted concept of the PRO instrument to the meaningful concept or criterion emanating from the anchor.

Anchor-based approaches are the preferred way to enhance the clinical interpretation to the targeted PRO measure. Considerations for anchor-based methods include the nature of the relationship (e.g., linear) between the anchor and the targeted PRO, the type of anchor, and the study population of interest. What follows are four ways that employ variations of the anchor-based approaches.

11.1.1 Percentages Based on Thresholds

One of the simplest forms of presentation and interpretation is to show the percentage of patients above and below some specified value, which is an anchored value with a meaningful criterion (Fayers and Machin, 2007). The method of percentages based on thresholds can be useful when the threshold on a PRO measure is chosen judiciously so that its value has relevance, rather than being some arbitrary cut point. For example, a score above 25 on the erectile function domain of the International Index of Erectile Function is regarded as having normal erectile function (Cappelleri et al., 1999). In comparative studies, the proportion of patients in each treatment group who fall into this normal category can be noted and compared.

Establishing a threshold or multiple thresholds on a PRO measure corresponding to disease severity levels is another example of the use of an anchor-based approach. Such was the case when disease severity levels were obtained on the Fibromyalgia Impact Questionnaire (FIQ), a disease-specific measure developed to capture the spectrum of problems related to fibromyalgia and responses to therapeutic intervention (Bennett et al., 2009).

The FIQ has a recall period of past week (7 days) and its total score ranges from 0 to 100, with higher scores indicating a greater impact of fibromyalgia. In this same investigation, using a pain diary, patients were asked to rate their pain in the past 24 h on an 11-point numerical scale, with the pain diary completed each morning upon awakening. The average of the last 7 daily entries was used to determine the baseline, weekly and endpoint pain score for each patient. As strong Pearson correlations across different assessments (average of 0.67) were found between the FIQ total scores and the average pain scores, it was reasonable to determine FIQ severity category cutoff scores using pain severity as an anchor. Based on previous research (Bennett et al., 2009), optimal cut points on pain severity were predetermined as 0–3 = mild, 4–6 = moderate, and 7–10 = severe based on an 11-point (0–10) numerical rating scale. A FIQ severity categorization was created corresponding to values of 3.5 and 6.5 on the pain scale taken as boundaries between pain severity categories (averaging pain over time transforms the original integer values from 0 to 10 to a continuous variable from 0 to 10): 0 to <3.5, mild pain; ≥3.5 to <6.5, moderate pain; and ≥6.5 to 10, severe pain. A repeated measures model was used to estimate the relationship between the FIQ total scores (as outcome) and the average pain scores (as predictor) assessed at pretreatment visit and posttreatment visits (with the two measures aligned with respect to their corresponding time assessments and recall periods). A FIQ total score from 0 to <39 was found to represent a mild impact, ≥39 to <59 a moderate impact, and ≥59 to 100 a severe impact (Figure 11.1). The severity bands can

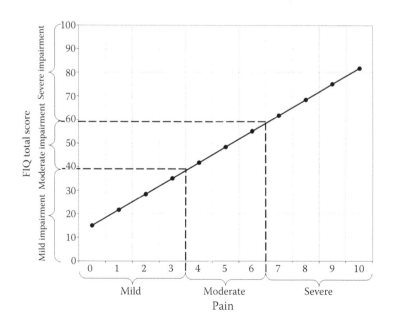

FIGURE 11.1
Severity categorization of FIQ total score using pain severity as an anchor.

```
%Let NumberOfRows        = 100;
%Let NumberOfVisits      = 7;

%Let s_error1 = 20;
%Let s_error2 = .2;

%Let seed1 = 1;
%Let seed2 = 2;
%Let seed3 = 3;

Data _mixed_1;

   b0=80;  /* Intercept for Score*/
   b1=-10; /* Visit effect for Score */

   a0=10;   /* Intercept for Pain*/
   a1=-1;   /* Visit effect for Pain*/

      ID=0;
      Do i=1 To &NumberOfRows;

         ID=ID+1;

         Do Visit=1 to (1+Int(&NumberOfVisits * ranuni(&seed1)));
           Score = b0 + b1*Visit + rannor(&seed2)*sqrt(&s_error1);
           Pain  = a0 + a1*Visit + rannor(&seed3)*sqrt(&s_error2);
           output;
         End;

      End;
Keep Score Pain ID Visit;

Run;

/*
As a result of modeling, the variable Pain might not be in the
range from 0 to 10 (usual range for Pain scale).
We use Proc Stdize to normalize Pain to be in the range from 0 to 1.
The same applies for the variable Score.
*/
Proc Stdize data=_mixed_1 out=_mixed_2 method=RANGE;
var Score Pain;
Run;

/*
This step will change the range of the variable Pain to be from
0 to 10 and the range of the variable Score to be from 0 to 100.
*/
Data _mixed_2;
Set  _mixed_2;
Pain  = Pain  * 10;
Score = Score * 100;
Run;
```

FIGURE 11.2
Simulating a dataset to examine the relationship between Score (outcome) and Pain (predictor).

be useful as a criterion for study inclusion, as an anchor itself to define clinically important scores for other PRO measures, and as a way to assess treatment differences (e.g., by calculating the percentage of patients who improve by at least one category on severity within each treatment group and then comparing these percentages between treatment groups).

11.1.2 Simulated Example: Severity Categorization

The simulated example illustrates how the type of severity categorization described in Figure 11.1 can be performed more generally by using a simulated dataset. A multivariate simulated dataset is created with a continuous outcome (here the variable Score will play the role of the FIQ total score in Figure 11.1), two covariates (Visit and Pain), and the variable ID for identification of subjects, as given in Figure 11.2. This example contains 100 subjects (defined by the variable NumberOfRows). For every subject, there are from 1 to 7 visits (NumberOfVisits = 7). The SAS code in Figure 11.2 generates the simulated dataset. The data layout in Figure 11.3 depicts the structure of the final simulated dataset. Note that Figure 11.3 represents the standard way a dataset could be structured for a repeated measures model and, in this case, one that focuses on the relationship between the outcome variable Score and the predictor variable Pain (more details on repeated measures models are given in Chapter 8).

Figure 11.4 shows implementation of the Mixed procedure (SAS, 2011) that is used to develop the severity categorization for the variable Score based on the variable Pain. Figure 11.5 provides the partial output. The first 11 lines of that output (beginning with Pain = 0) can be used to create a graph that resembles Figure 11.1; the last two lines give cutoff scores for severity categorization on the outcome variable Score. This simulation provides cutoff scores of 38.2 (38.1651) and 65.3 (65.2619), which are close to the results reported using real data earlier in this chapter.

ID	Visit	Score	Pain
1	1	86.477679987	9.4652601914
1	2	73.332337615	7.9678018435
2	1	84.024696292	8.9303289077
3	1	86.354397654	9.1243845085
3	2	70.958155512	6.6441290133
3	3	52.8051996	5.8536769545
3	4	43.765302507	4.6849460105
3	5	42.117163151	3.326784542
3	6	16.134948499	1.9310167857
3	7	15.65229953	0.8598846265

FIGURE 11.3
Final simulated dataset (data for the first three subjects are shown).

```
Proc Mixed data=_mixed_2;
     Class ID Visit ;
     Model Score = Pain / ddfm=kr s;

     Repeated Visit / Type=UN Subject=ID;

     Estimate " Pain =0 " Intercept 1 Pain 0 /cl;
     Estimate " Pain =1 " Intercept 1 Pain 1 /cl;
     Estimate " Pain =2 " Intercept 1 Pain 2 /cl;
     Estimate " Pain =3 " Intercept 1 Pain 3 /cl;
     Estimate " Pain =4 " Intercept 1 Pain 4 /cl;
     Estimate " Pain =5 " Intercept 1 Pain 5 /cl;
     Estimate " Pain =6 " Intercept 1 Pain 6 /cl;
     Estimate " Pain =7 " Intercept 1 Pain 7 /cl;
     Estimate " Pain =8 " Intercept 1 Pain 8 /cl;
     Estimate " Pain =9 " Intercept 1 Pain 9 /cl;
     Estimate " Pain =10" Intercept 1 Pain 10 /cl;

     Estimate " Pain =3.5 " Intercept 1 Pain 3.5 /cl;
     Estimate " Pain =6.5 " Intercept 1 Pain 6.5 /cl;
Run;
```

FIGURE 11.4
Implementation of the repeated measures mixed-effects model to quantify the relationship between the outcome variable Score and the predictor variable Pain.

Label	Estimate	Standard Error	Pr > |t|	Alpha	Lower	Upper
Pain =0	6.5523	1.8715	0.0024	0.05	2.6299	10.4746
Pain =1	15.5845	1.5984	<.0001	0.05	12.2173	18.9517
Pain =2	24.6168	1.3292	<.0001	0.05	21.7971	27.4364
Pain =3	33.6490	1.0668	<.0001	0.05	31.3650	35.9330
Pain =4	42.6812	0.8179	<.0001	0.05	40.9150	44.4475
Pain =5	51.7135	0.5995	<.0001	0.05	50.4335	52.9935
Pain =6	60.7457	0.4576	<.0001	0.05	59.8182	61.6733
Pain =7	69.7780	0.4679	<.0001	0.05	68.8473	70.7087
Pain =8	78.8102	0.6229	<.0001	0.05	77.5709	80.0495
Pain =9	87.8425	0.8465	<.0001	0.05	86.1555	89.5294
Pain =10	96.8747	1.0976	<.0001	0.05	94.6826	99.0669
Pain =3.5	38.1651	0.9400	<.0001	0.05	36.1427	40.1876
Pain =6.5	65.2619	0.4408	<.0001	0.05	64.3820	66.1417

FIGURE 11.5
Estimated means and 95% confidence intervals from the repeated measures mixed-effects model in Figure 11.4.

11.1.3 Criterion-Group Interpretation

A criterion-group interpretation, which is related to interpretation based on threshold percentages, involves the comparison of scores from the particular group of interest to a criterion group, a known group worthy of comparison that can serve as a yardstick for interpretation. One way to achieve this is by the use of a criterion contrast—or a yardstick approach—derived from groups in a representative clinical or practical setting that represent a familiar difference on the outcome of interest (Sechrest et al., 1996; Lipsey and Wilson, 2001).

This method of interpretation requires that meaningfully different groups be defined in the setting of interest. As a result, practitioners and other informed observers will readily comprehend the practical or clinical significance of the treatment effect generated from its contrast with well-defined and distinct clinical groups. Thus, the method requires a consensus of how meaningfully different groups are defined and who they are.

For instance, suppose the criterion effect on a PRO measure between the most severe group and the least severe group is 6 points, and the treatment difference on the same measure between active treatment and control treatment is 3 points. We can then gauge the magnitude and benefit of the active treatment as being conceptually equivalent to having the most severe patients improve to the point that they moved half way (3/6) to the level of the least severe patients.

In another variation of criterion-group interpretation, a PRO measure may use population-based reference values, which provide expected or typical scores that are called norms, to benchmark or anchor interpretation on a PRO measure (Marquis et al., 2004; Fayers and Machin, 2007). These normative data or reference values can be taken from a survey of randomly selected subjects from the general population, which includes subjects with chronic or acute illness as well as subjects who are healthy. While the general population is the most frequently used norm, the healthy population can be used to provide an indication of the "ideal" target value. Normative data can be also obtained for different disease groups.

Baseline scores on the Medical Outcomes Study (MOS) Sleep Scale from two trials for the treatment of fibromyalgia were compared with scores obtained from a nationally representative sample in the United States (Cappelleri et al., 2009a). Higher scores on the MOS Sleep Scale indicate more of the attribute being assessed (e.g., more sleep disturbance and more sleep adequacy). A one-sample z-test for the mean was also conducted to test whether the mean of each sleep subscale from each of the two trials differed statistically from the corresponding normative mean, taken as a fixed targeted value. Scores for each subscale of the MOS Sleep Scale were statistically ($p < 0.001$) and substantially poorer than the general population normative values in the United States, suggesting that patients with fibromyalgia have greater sleep problems relative to the general population (Figure 11.6). For instance,

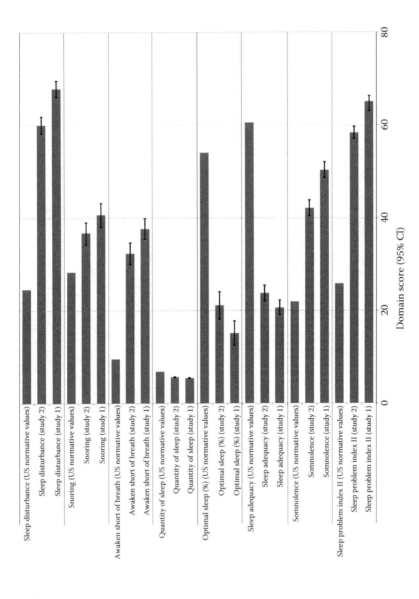

FIGURE 11.6
Baseline mean scores (95% confidence intervals) on the Medical Outcomes Study Sleep Scale for patients with fibromyalgia vs values from the US general population.

patients with fibromyalgia reported sleeping an average of 5.4 and 5.6 h per night in the two studies, whereas the general population reported an average of 6.8 h of sleep per night.

Consider a criterion-based method for interpretation that involves a comparison of PRO scores between a disease sample and a similar sample with respect to age, gender and other important factors but without the disease of interest. In addition to traditional statistical testing to compare these two independent samples before treatment (using a two-sample *t*-test) and, separately, after treatment (also using a two-sample *t*-test), equivalency testing can be applied to compare the disease group, before and after treatment, with the nondisease group to examine whether the disease group after treatment improved to "normal" ranges on the PRO measure of interest (Rogers et al., 1993; Kendall et al., 1999; Cappelleri et al., 2006).

Four classifications on statistical significance and clinical equivalence are possible (Table 11.1). The most compelling and desired transition is to show that the PRO scores from the disease sample before treatment are *both statistically different* and *not clinically equivalent* with the PRO scores from the nondisease sample (cell III in Table 11.1) and, subsequently, that the PRO scores from the disease sample after treatment are *both clinically equivalent* and *statistically not different* to PRO scores from the nondisease sample (cell II in Table 11.1). Such a change indicates that an intervention is associated with normalization of a health condition that the PRO instrument is measuring. It should be emphasized, however, that this ideal change is quite a high hurdle to achieve and an intervention can have a clinically meaningful change and be quite beneficial without moving to cell II (Table 11.1).

TABLE 11.1

Classification of Tests on Statistical Significance and Clinical Equivalence

		Statistical Significance Test	
		Statistically Significant from 0 (95% CI excludes 0)	*Not Statistically Significant from 0 (95% CI includes 0)*
Clinical Equivalence Test	*Clinically Equivalent (entire 90% CI within region of equivalence)*	**Cell I** Clinically equivalent and statistically significant	**Cell II** Clinically equivalent and not statistically significant
	Not Clinically Equivalent (entire 90% CI not within region of equivalence)	**Cell III** Not clinically equivalent and statistically significant	**Cell IV** Not clinically equivalent and not statistically significant

Note: CI, Confidence interval.

Statistical significance for a mean difference can be declared, for example, if the corresponding two-sided 95% confidence interval does not include zero. Clinical equivalence for a mean difference can be declared, for example, if the corresponding two-sided 90% confidence interval is contained completely within the range of equivalence. To maintain a 0.05 significance level for equivalence testing, a two-sided 90% confidence interval is generally used instead of a two-sided 95% CI (Westlake, 1981; Liu, 2003; Steiger, 2004). The rationale for this is that the estimated effect cannot be small in both directions, one for superiority and one for inferiority, so the confidence interval is relaxed to provide the same amount of power that would be obtained with a one-sided test. Two one-sided tests at the 0.05 level of significance, one side for superiority and the other side for inferiority, are the same as testing whether the entire 90% CI is within the equivalence interval. Other significance levels (other than 0.05) and confidence levels (other than 90% or 95%) may be considered, depending on the objectives of the study.

As an illustration, consider the Self-Esteem And Relationship (SEAR) questionnaire (range: 0–100, where higher scores are more favorable) between men with erectile dysfunction (ED) at baseline and a control group of age-similar men without ED, the latter group having been assessed on one occasion and not treated for ED (Cappelleri et al., 2006). "Control" group here represents the group without the condition of interest; it bears no relation to control treatment (this group was not given any treatment for ED by the study investigators). For each domain or subscale of the SEAR questionnaire, the equivalency interval was defined as within half a standard deviation (SD) of the score from the corresponding domain or subscale in the non-ED (control) sample.

For example, the mean self-esteem score in the control group without ED was statistically different from the mean self-esteem score in the pretreatment sample with ED (the difference in means was 31.9 points and the 95% CI for the difference in mean self-esteem scores ranged from 24.8 to 39.0, which excluded zero) and this pair of mean scores was also not clinically equivalent (the entire 90% CI (25.9–37.9) was outside the zone of equivalence) (Figure 11.7). In both settings, before and after treatment, the zone of equivalence on the self-esteem score is the same and taken as one half of its SD in the group without ED, that is, one half of 22.8, or 11.4.

In contrast, the mean self-esteem score in the control group without ED was not statistically different from the mean self-esteem score in the post-treatment sample with ED (the difference in means was 2.5 points and the 95% CI for the difference in mean self-esteem scores ranged from −4.0 to 9.0, which included zero) and this pair of mean scores was also clinically equivalent (the entire 90% CI (−2.9 to 7.9) was within the zone of equivalence) (Figure 11.7).

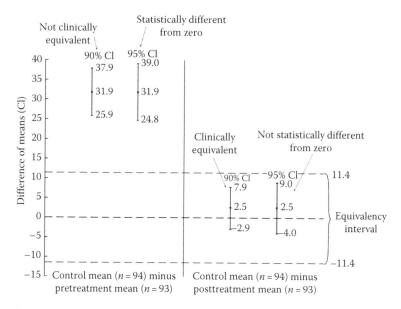

FIGURE 11.7

Difference of control mean vs pretreatment and posttreatment means on the self-esteem subscale of the Self-Esteem And Relationship questionnaire.

11.1.4 Content-Based Interpretation

A content-based interpretation of a multi-item PRO measure uses a representative item, along with its response categories, internal to this multi-item measure itself to understand the meaning of different scores on that measure (Ware et al., 1994, 2000; Cappelleri et al., 2007; Thompson et al., 2007). In addition to descriptive statistics, item response theory (Chapter 6; Hambleton et al., 1991; Chang and Reeve, 2005; de Ayala, 2009; Massof, in press), ordinal logistic regression (Lall et al., 2002; O'Connell, 2005; Arostegui et al., 2012), and binary logistic regression (Kleinbaum and Klein, 2010; Agresti, 2012; Hosmer et al., 2013) can be used for content-based interpretation. Here, a given multi-item domain score being a manifestation of an underlying construct (e.g., physical functioning) is linked to a probability of achieving the attribute embodied by an item (either an ordinal response variable or, if dichotomized, a binary response variable such as whether or not someone can walk around the block) internal to that multi-item domain.

For example, a content-based interpretation was applied using the Rasch model (Chapter 6), a type of item response theory model, on the six-item near-vision subscale of the German version of the 39-item National Eye Institute Visual Function Questionnaire in 200 patients with age-related macular degeneration (Thompson et al., 2007). Scores ranged from 0 (worst) to 100 (best).

For a given subscale score, an estimated probability of responding to each category of an ordinal item was obtained and the probabilities of responding to the two most favorable categories (no difficulty or little difficulty) were combined. For example, an individual with an estimated true score of 75 on the near-vision subscale was expected to have approximately a 27% likelihood of little or no difficulty with reading small print, a 94% likelihood of little or no difficulty with finding an object on a crowded shelf, and nearly a 100% likelihood of little or no difficulty with shaving/styling hair/applying makeup (Figure 11.8).

The Rasch model can also be used to assess item difficulties in relation to a patient's true state for a health condition assessed by the PRO measure, a relation that can also aid in interpretation (Hambleton et al., 1991; Chang and Reeve, 2005; Schünemann et al., 2006; Bond and Fox, 2007; Thompson et al., 2007; de Ayala, 2009; Luo et al., 2009; Massof, in press).

A content-based approach to interpretation requires that the model be appropriate and its assumptions met. If there is doubt about the suitability of the model when the response variable is an ordinal variable, it is advisable to also fit a binary logistic regression by collapsing the ordinal categories of the item-level response into two larger categories and to compare its results with the results from the ordinal model. A content-based approach is not advisable when there

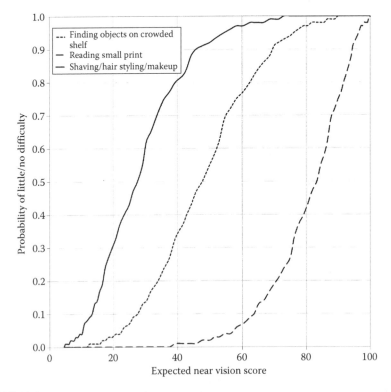

FIGURE 11.8
Probability of little or no difficulty on three illustrative items from near-vision subscale of the National Eye Institute Visual Function Questionnaire.

are only two or three items on the multi-item domain because interpretation then becomes circular and too redundant (Cappelleri et al., 2007).

11.1.5 Clinically Important Difference

Highly significant *p*-values indicate little about the magnitude of a difference; statistical significance does not imply clinical significance. While a small *p*-value makes it likely that a real difference exists, which may be driven solely by an adequate or a large sample size, the observed or real difference might in fact not be clinically relevant.

An anchor-based approach to quantify a clinically important difference (CID) on a PRO measure involves the use of an external measure—an anchor—which should be clearly interpretable and appreciably correlated with the targeted PRO measure (Testa and Simonson, 1996; Crosby et al., 2003; Guyatt et al., 2003; King, 2011). Responses on such an anchor can come from clinical measurements, clinician reports, or, preferably, patient reports. For example, patients can be asked to rate the extent of their change in their overall health status retrospectively since the beginning of the study on a 7-point scale (Patient Global Impression of Change [PGIC]): 1 = "very much improved," 2 = "much improved," 3 = "minimally improved," 4 = "no change," 5 = "minimally worse," 6 = "much worse," and 7 = "very much worse." Then the mean changes from baseline on the PRO instrument of interest can be obtained for each of the categories on the anchor, and the differences in mean changes on the PRO scores between adjacent categories on the anchor can be considered to represent a clinically important difference. Data used in the analysis would be pooled across all treatments.

An alternative (or in addition) to PGIC, which is asked only at follow-up, a question can be asked serially—for example, one at baseline and one at follow-up—about the severity of a patient's overall current condition (e.g., none, mild, moderate, and severe; or severity levels on the Clinical Global Impression—Severity [CGIS]), and the difference in the mean PRO scores between adjacent categories on the anchor can be examined for a clinically important difference on the PRO (data should also be pooled across treatments). Using such a serial anchor, which focuses on the current state (either at the time when asked or over a relatively short time frame until the present), may address potential recall issues that may arise from a retrospective assessment that require patients to compare their current state relative to the start of the study.

If the PRO score (or change in PRO score from baseline) is the outcome and the CGIS (or PGIC) is a continuous predictor in a regression model, an estimated clinically important difference as measured by the difference in mean PRO scores (or the difference in mean changes from baseline) between adjacent categories on the anchor measure will be a constant. If the anchor measure is taken instead as a categorical predictor in a regression model, and the functional relationships are similar to those when the anchor measure is taken as a continuous predictor, then the results from the anchor measure as continuous predictor would provide a more sensitive and parsimonious estimate of a clinically important difference.

Otherwise, a simple average of the mean PRO scores differences between every pair of adjacent categories on the anchor measure can be used as an estimate of a clinically important difference. If, however, a sparse number of patients are found for at least one level of a categorical anchor measure (most likely at either end or both ends), making estimation at that level unreliable, proportionally greater weights should be assigned to those categorical levels with a larger number of observations when arriving at an estimate of a clinically important difference.

As an example, reconsider the FIQ for patients with fibromyalgia (Bennett et al., 2009). A repeated measures model was used to estimate the mean change from baseline in FIQ total scores (range 0–100 points) corresponding to each category on the PGIC, the anchor taken as a continuous predictor (Figure 11.9). Differences in these mean changes between adjacent categories of PGIC corresponded to a clinically important difference of 8.1 (95% confidence interval (CI): 7.6–8.5; Figure 11.9).

An estimated clinically important difference may vary in different situations because of natural sampling variation, different study populations, type of anchor or external criterion, time of assessment, and other considerations. An instrument's clinically important difference should first be confirmed within a given population. However, findings may not necessarily be generalizable and, for the same reasons, a clinically important difference is not necessarily a minimally clinically important difference, which is a more challenging avenue to pursue (Copay et al., 2007; King, 2011).

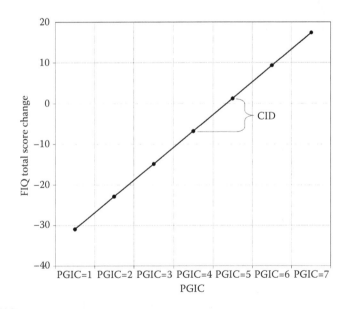

FIGURE 11.9
Estimate of clinically important difference on the FIQ total score using PGIC as an anchor. *Abbreviation*: FIQ, Fibromyalgia Impact Questionnaire; CID, clinically important difference; PGIC, Patient Global Impression of Change.

Moreover, a CID based on a one-category difference from a patient's global impression of change taken retrospectively or from severity levels taken serially, or from other anchors, could exceed a smaller but clinically relevant difference based on a less than a one-category difference (e.g., a one-half category difference). Less than one-category difference, however, is not measurable because a one-category difference is the smallest unit for which a patient can record a change.

It is possible that the level of the anchor suggesting no change can actually be associated with an improvement or deterioration on the targeted PRO of interest (see, e.g., Figure 11.9, which indicates improvement on the FIQ when the PGIC of 4 suggests no retrospective change). This noticeable incongruity can happen between the anchor measure and the targeted PRO because, though related, they are measuring different concepts; it can also happen because of measurement error. It is more important that improvements in the targeted PRO measure be associated with improvements across (as opposed to within) levels of the anchor and that a calibration occurs by taking differences in mean PRO scores between adjacent pairs of categories on the anchor.

A CID is often taken on an absolute scale (as a raw change) but can also be taken on a relative scale as a percent change, which we refer to as the Clinically Important Percent Change (CIPC) (see next section).

11.1.6 Simulated Example: Clinically Important Difference

The SAS code, presented in Figure 11.10 with annotated comments, creates a simulated dataset in order to obtain estimation of the clinically important difference. A few additional points should be addressed. There could be some issues in estimation of the CIPC if we have many subjects with an outcome score of zero at baseline. Additional checks (using *If* statements) should be added to avoid baseline zero values in the denominator of these calculations. Additional analyses should be applied to understand the number of excluded observations (by using frequency tables) and the possible impact on CIPC estimation (by using sensitivity modeling).

Figure 11.11 shows the structure of the simulated dataset (with data only for the first 5 subjects). This dataset has all the information needed for CID estimation. But this dataset also has, for example, variable "Treatment," *which will not be used in the CID estimations* as modeling for CID estimation is performed *across treatments*. (The variable "Treatment" will be reserved for use later in Section 11.2.4.)

The SAS implementation of the model to estimate the CID is presented in Figure 11.12. It is important to note that, while baseline observations (Visit = 0) are part of the simulated dataset (Figure 11.11), they should be excluded from the modeling calculations; only postbaseline observations should be used. The first data step in Figure 11.12 excludes those baseline observations from the dataset to be used by MIXED procedure. The variable "ChangeScore" is used as an outcome, and the variable PGIC is used as a predictor (anchor). We use

```
/*
Multivariate data with a continuous outcome (Y) and 2 covariates
(Visit, Treatment) for repeated measures modeling.
------------------------------------------------------------------
For this example we have 100 subjects (NumberOfRows) for every
treatment arm.
For every subject we have from 1 to 7 post-treatment visits
(NumberOfVisits = 7;) and one baseline visit.
There are 3 treatment arms (NumberOfTreatments = 3;)
------------------------------------------------------------------
Y represents the PRO variable of interest for which the estimated
clinically important difference (CID) is to be calculated.

PGIC represents an anchor - a one-category change on this anchor will
correspond to the estimated CID on the targeted PRO variable (Y).
------------------------------------------------------------------
*/

options nofmterr nocenter pagesize=2000 linesize=256;

%Let NumberOfRows       = 100;
%Let NumberOfVisits     = 7;
%Let NumberOfTreatments = 3;

%Let s_error = 1.5;
%Let s_error1 = 1;

%Let seed1 = 1;
%Let seed2 = 2;

Data _mixed_1;

    b0=10;     /* Intercept for Y*/
    b1=1.5;    /* Visit effect for Y */
    b2=2;      /* Treatment effect for Y */
    b3=.5;     /* Visit*Treatment interaction effect for Y */

    b00=0;     /* Intercept for PGIC*/
    b10=.5;    /* Visit effect for PGIC*/
    b20=1;     /* Treatment effect for PGIC*/
    b30=.7;    /* Visit*Treatment interaction effect for PGIC*/

      ID=0;
      Do Treatment=1 to &NumberOfTreatments;
      Do i=1 To &NumberOfRows;

         ID=ID+1;

         Do Visit=0 to (1+Int(&NumberOfVisits * ranuni(&seed1)));

            If Visit=0 Then
            Do;
            Baseline= b0 + rannor(&seed2)*sqrt(&s_error);
```

FIGURE 11.10
Creating a simulated dataset: Clinically important difference.

```
                Y=.;
                PGIC=.;
                output;
                End;
                Else
                Do;
                Y    =b0 + b1*Visit + b2*Treatment + b3*Visit*Treatment +
rannor(&seed2)*sqrt(&s_error);
                PGIC=b00 + b10*Visit + b20*Treatment + b30*Visit*Treatment +
rannor(&seed2)*sqrt(&s_error1);
                    output;
                    End;

              End;

        End;
        End;
Keep Y Baseline PGIC ID Visit Treatment;

Run;

/*
As a result of modeling, the predictor variable PGIC, which
serves as the anchor, will not be in the range from 1 to 7 (its
desired range).
We use Proc Stdize to normalize PGIC to be in the range from 0 to 1
*/
Proc Stdize data=_mixed_1 out=_mixed_2 method=RANGE;
var PGIC;
Run;

/*
This step will change the range of the variable PGIC to be from 1 to 7
with all values being integers (i.e., only values 1, 2, 3, 4, 5, 6, 7).

We also added two new variables (which will be used in CID
modeling). Variable "ChangeScore" will be used as outcome.
Variable ChangeScorePct also can be used as outcome if we would
like to estimate Clinically Important Percent Change (CIPC)
*/
Data _mixed_2;
Set  _mixed_2;
ChangeScore=Y-Baseline;
ChangeScorePct=100*(Y-Baseline)/Baseline; /*additional steps for
the PRO measures should be taken if scores at Baseline can be 0;
dividing by the value of 0 is not permissible*/
PGIC=Int(PGIC*6+1);

Run;
Proc Means Data=_mixed_2;
Run;
Proc Freq Data=_mixed_2;
Run;
```

FIGURE 11.10 (continued)
Creating a simulated dataset: clinically important difference.

ID	Treatment	Visit	Baseline	Y	PGIC	ChangeScore	ChangeScorePct
1	1	0	9.75601	.	.	.	.
1	1	1	9.75601	15.7728	1	6.016796888	61.6727353
1	1	2	9.75601	17.3098	2	7.553782138	77.4269789
2	1	0	10.6291	.	.	.	.
2	1	1	10.6291	13.8939	1	3.264826284	30.7159251
2	1	2	10.6291	16.0391	1	5.409958472	50.8976174
2	1	3	10.6291	17.6936	2	7.064543684	66.4641778
2	1	4	10.6291	19.0151	2	8.386011809	78.8967278
3	1	0	11.297	.	.	.	.
3	1	1	11.297	13.6029	1	2.305966046	20.4122409
3	1	2	11.297	15.3573	2	4.060369963	35.9420947
3	1	3	11.297	17.8058	2	6.508858139	57.615931
3	1	4	11.297	21.2385	2	9.941551256	88.0018766
3	1	5	11.297	22.7094	2	11.41240335	101.021751
3	1	6	11.297	21.6062	2	10.30918764	91.2561668
4	1	0	11.4949	.	.	.	.
4	1	1	11.4949	13.2274	1	1.732509369	15.0720212
4	1	2	11.4949	15.5836	1	4.088712435	35.5698858
4	1	3	11.4949	19.1823	1	7.687446885	66.8771924
4	1	4	11.4949	21.4507	2	9.955827217	86.6110403
4	1	5	11.4949	23.3353	2	11.84039842	103.005928
4	1	6	11.4949	22.335	2	10.84008614	94.3036794
5	1	0	9.84169	.	.	.	.
5	1	1	9.84169	13.5146	1	3.672902462	37.3198351
5	1	2	9.84169	16.7488	1	6.907063293	70.1816794
5	1	3	9.84169	17.0049	2	7.163168226	72.7839248
5	1	4	9.84169	20.6806	2	10.83886197	110.132122
5	1	5	9.84169	21.314	2	11.47227251	116.568115
5	1	6	9.84169	23.1386	2	13.29694792	135.108381
5	1	7	9.84169	25.3353	3	15.49361641	157.428414

FIGURE 11.11
Dataset structure to be used in mixed modeling to estimate the CID.

PGIC as a continuous predictor in this model, and hence we impose a linear relationship between the outcome and the anchor. Later we will use PGIC as a categorical predictor—with that model used in a sensitivity analysis. Note that no other covariates are needed (and actually should not be used).

By using the "Repeated" statement, we acknowledge that we can have more than one observation from the same subject. In this example, we use the First-Order Autoregressive Covariance Structure [AR(1)], which is applicable if time between visits can be considered the same. In the case of the uneven time periods between visits, Unstructured Covariance Structure [UN] or Spatial Covariance Structures [e.g., SP(POW)(c)] should be considered. If a CIPC is needed to be estimated, the variable ChangeScore in the Model statement should be replaced by the variable ChangeScorePct.

In Figure 11.12, the first estimate statement (Estimate "CID(One ...) will produce CID estimation. Other estimate statements will produce mean

```
Data _mixed_3;
 Set _mixed_2;
 Where Visit In (1 2 3 4 5 6 7);
 Run;

 Proc Mixed data=_mixed_3;
 Class ID Visit ;
 Model ChangeScore = PGIC / ddfm=kr s;
 Repeated Visit / Type=AR(1) /*UN*/ Subject=ID;

 Estimate "CID(One Category Change) = " PGIC 1 /cl;

 Estimate " PGIC=1 " Intercept 1 PGIC 1 /cl;
 Estimate " PGIC=2 " Intercept 1 PGIC 2 /cl;
 Estimate " PGIC=3 " Intercept 1 PGIC 3 /cl;
 Estimate " PGIC=4 " Intercept 1 PGIC 4 /cl;
 Estimate " PGIC=5 " Intercept 1 PGIC 5 /cl;
 Estimate " PGIC=6 " Intercept 1 PGIC 6 /cl;
 Estimate " PGIC=7 " Intercept 1 PGIC 7 /cl;

 Run;
```

FIGURE 11.12
Proc Mixed for longitudinal modeling: CID estimation.

values for the "ChangeScore" corresponding to different levels of the variable PGIC (to compare later with results of a sensitivity analysis using PGIC as a categorical anchor).

Figure 11.13 shows that the CID for the PRO measure Y is estimated as 4 points (3.9665; 95% CI: 3.8242 to 4.1088).

In the model depicted by Figure 11.12, we used PGIC as a continuous predictor to estimate the CID and, in doing so, we imposed a linear relationship between the outcome and the anchor. In the following sensitivity analysis (see Figure 11.14), we relax this linearity assumption and allow PGIC to be used as a categorical predictor and thereby do not impose any functional relationship between the outcome and the anchor. To achieve this, we added PGIC variable in the list of the class variables (Class ID Visit PGIC;).

Figure 11.15 shows mean values for the variable "ChangeScore" for every level of the PGIC. Figure 11.16 shows that the sensitivity analysis supports the linearity assumption as the results from both modeling calculations are close to each other. We note that, though, some difference at the PGIC value of 7 but this can be explained by knowing that we have only one (!) observation with the PGIC value of 7 in our simulated dataset (see Figure 11.17)—whose sparseness is quite typical for real data—as the PGIC distribution will most likely be skewed.

A different approach to estimate CID is based on a serially measured anchor such as CGIS. In this case, the outcome (PRO) variable will not be the change from the baseline but the value of the outcome at every visit (including at baseline as well as at follow-up visits). The variable Y from Figure 11.11 is an example of the PRO variable that should be used if the

Label	Estimate	Standard Error	Pr > |t|	Alpha	Lower	Upper
CID(One Category Change) =	3.9665	0.07249	<.0001	0.05	3.8242	4.1088
PGIC=1	4.9722	0.1417	<.0001	0.05	4.6939	5.2504
PGIC=2	8.9387	0.09874	<.0001	0.05	8.7445	9.1328
PGIC=3	12.9052	0.09970	<.0001	0.05	12.7090	13.1013
PGIC=4	16.8717	0.1437	<.0001	0.05	16.5893	17.1540
PGIC=5	20.8381	0.2046	<.0001	0.05	20.4363	21.2400
PGIC=6	24.8046	0.2712	<.0001	0.05	24.2719	25.3374
PGIC=7	28.7711	0.3403	<.0001	0.05	28.1028	29.4394

FIGURE 11.13
Estimated CID and means for the variable "ChangeScore" based on PGIC.

```
Proc Mixed data=_mixed_3;

  Class ID Visit PGIC ;

  Model ChangeScore = PGIC / ddfm=kr s;

  Repeated Visit / Type=AR(1) Subject=ID;

  Lsmeans    PGIC /cl;

  Run;
```

FIGURE 11.14
Proc Mixed for longitudinal modeling: Sensitivity analysis.

Least Squares Means

Effect	PGIC	Estimate	Standard Error	Pr > |t|	Alpha	Lower	Upper
PGIC	1	5.3561	0.1939	<.0001	0.05	4.9757	5.7365
PGIC	2	8.7256	0.1233	<.0001	0.05	8.4836	8.9677
PGIC	3	12.8642	0.1564	<.0001	0.05	12.5572	13.1713
PGIC	4	17.3115	0.2384	<.0001	0.05	16.8438	17.7792
PGIC	5	20.6988	0.3406	<.0001	0.05	20.0305	21.3672
PGIC	6	25.0653	0.5040	<.0001	0.05	24.0764	26.0542
PGIC	7	26.7490	2.3192	<.0001	0.05	22.1987	31.2993

FIGURE 11.15
Estimated means for the variable "ChangeScore" (PGIC as a categorical predictor).

anchor represents a serial measurement. The SAS implementation in this case is represented by Figure 11.18, assuming that the dataset "_mixed_" has variables ID, Visit, Y, and CGIS.

11.2 Distribution-Based Approaches

The method highlighted thus far to estimate the magnitude and meaning of an important difference on a patient-centered scale maps the responses on an anchor measure grounded with clinical manifestations from patients (e.g., PGIC, PGIS) or clinicians (e.g., CGIS) to the PRO responses.

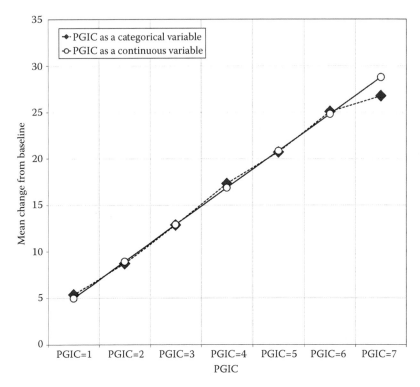

FIGURE 11.16
Mean changes in PRO measure as a function of PGIC.

PGIC	Frequency	Percent	Cumulative Frequency	Cumulative Percent
1	179	14.98	179	14.98
2	518	43.35	697	58.33
3	300	25.10	997	83.43
4	114	9.54	1111	92.97
5	57	4.77	1168	97.74
6	26	2.18	1194	99.92
7	1	0.08	1195	100.00

FIGURE 11.17
Frequencies on PGIC.

To complement such clinical input, approaches based on the empirical distribution of the data may prove useful. Such distribution-based methods can offer valuable insights about the magnitude of an effect. These methods also allow for a standardization of different scales with different ranges and ways of scoring. On the other hand, a limitation of distribution-based

```
Proc Mixed data=_mixed_;

Class ID Visit ;

Model Y = CGIS / ddfm=kr s;

Repeated Visit / Type=AR(1) Subject=ID;

Estimate "CID(One Category Difference) = " CGIS 1 /cl;

Estimate " CGIS =1 " Intercept 1 CGIS 1 /cl;
Estimate " CGIS =2 " Intercept 1 CGIS 2 /cl;
Estimate " CGIS =3 " Intercept 1 CGIS 3 /cl;
Estimate " CGIS =4 " Intercept 1 CGIS 4 /cl;
Estimate " CGIS =5 " Intercept 1 CGIS 5 /cl;
Estimate " CGIS =6 " Intercept 1 CGIS 6 /cl;
Estimate " CGIS =7 " Intercept 1 CGIS 7 /cl;

Run;
```

FIGURE 11.18
Proc Mixed for longitudinal modeling: Serial anchor.

methods should be noted: although their interpretation can be meaningful, they do not provide information about *clinical* meaningfulness (Hays et al., 2005). In this section, a few of the more useful distribution-based methods are described.

11.2.1 Effect Size

An effect size (ES) indicator can be an informative metric to gauge the magnitude of differences in a PRO measure within a group or between two groups. Effect sizes can take various forms and they are fundamental to sample size estimation (Fayers and Machin, 2007; Julious et al., 2009; Julious and Walters, in press). Here we define and restrict attention to a particular variant of ES expressed as a standard metric with difference in means between two groups (or, alternatively, mean changes within a single group) in its numerator and a measure of variability in its denominator. This form of ES is also known as the standardized mean difference, which is a kind of signal-to-noise ratio that quantifies the amount of effect relative to variability. Variations on this type of ES exist based on what is taken as a measure of variability in the denominator (Kazis et al., 1989; Crosby et al., 2003; Fayers and Machin, 2007; King, 2011).

When SDs differ in the denominator of the ES, results from different studies for the same PRO measure can give different ES values even though their differences in means (numerators) may be the same. The ES should therefore be accompanied by their constituent elements, namely, their means and SD in order to be aware of such a potential subtlety.

Values on ES from different scales on the same intervention render standardized changes whose magnitudes can be fairly compared on the same dimensionless scale, despite the scales having potentially different methods of scoring and different ranges of values. In addition, the ES provides a general set of thresholds or benchmarks through adjectival descriptors on the impact of an intervention, with values of 0.2 generally regarded as "small," 0.5 as "medium," and 0.8 as "large" (Cohen, 1988). In the case of two interventions, for instance, an ES of 0.5 indicates that the mean difference in scores between two interventions equals one-half of a standard deviation unit. In the case of a single intervention, an ES of 0.5 indicates that mean change in scores from baseline to follow-up is also one-half of a standard deviation unit. Thus ES can be useful for providing a benchmark for assessing the magnitude and, through this, the meaning of differences or changes in health status (Kazis et al.,1989).

For the impact of an intervention within a single group, values of ES have commonly appeared in at least two ways. One way is the mean of changes in the scores recorded by the same subjects at two different times, divided by the SD of these changes in scores. Note that the SD in this case will be affected by the effects of the intervention over time, which some researchers believe may cloud the interpretation of results. This approach, referred as the standardized response mean, corresponds closely to the method of calculating a paired *t*-test.

The second way is the same mean changes in scores but divided by the SD of the scores recorded at the first occasion. Here the focus is on changes in scores relative to background or natural variability of scores inherent to the PRO measure in the population sampled, variability that is free from an intervention's effect and extraneous events. For example, the responsiveness of the SEAR questionnaire for ED in a single intervention study of 93 men given sildenafil was based on an ES defined as the mean change in scores from baseline (to end of study) divided by the SD score at baseline (Althof et al., 2003). The magnitude of the change was quite high for most aspects of the SEAR questionnaire (Sexual Relationship Satisfaction, ES = 1.6; Confidence, ES = 1.0; Self-Esteem, ES = 1.1) and moderate for one (Overall Relationship Satisfaction, ES = 0.6), suggesting that the SEAR questionnaire is responsive for detecting psychosocial gains from a known beneficial intervention.

These two ways of computing an ES for a single group can be explained when comparing two interventions from two independent groups of participants. For two independent groups, the numerator can be the difference in mean changes from baseline to follow-up (or, alternatively, in means at follow-up) between two independent groups, and the denominator can be the corresponding pooled SD of changes in scores from the two groups. Alternatively, the denominator can be the baseline SD of scores pooled from the two groups, which some researchers may find preferable, where the magnitude of the mean difference between interventions is relative to the normal variability of measurement (before intervention).

For example, in a double-blind placebo-controlled study of sildenafil, which enrolled 256 subjects, sizeable treatment differences were observed and effect sizes on the SEAR questionnaire were calculated as the difference in the mean change scores between treatment groups divided by the pooled SD of scores at baseline (O'Leary et al., 2006). Large effect sizes of the differences in mean changes were obtained between active treatment and placebo treatment for the Self-Esteem subscale (ES = 0.84), the Sexual Relationship Satisfaction domain (ES = 1.02), and the Confidence subscale (ES = 0.86); a moderate-to-large ES was found for the Overall Relationship Satisfaction domain (ES = 0.63).

11.2.2 Probability of Relative Benefit

Differences between treatment groups at a specific follow-up time or change from baseline can be evaluated nonparametrically with the Wilcoxon rank-sum test using ridit analysis (Donaldson, 1998; Acion et al., 2006; Cappelleri et al., 2008). This type of analysis is well-suited for ordinal responses at the item level or subscale or total scale levels. The Mann–Whitney U statistic from the Wilcoxon rank-sum test gets converted, using ridit analysis, to a probability that represents the chance that a randomly selected patient from the treatment group has a more favorable response than a randomly selected patient from the control group. For instance, the method addresses the question, what is the likelihood that a randomly selected patient in the treatment group would have greater reduction in pain relative to a randomly selected patient in the control group?

As an illustration based on the literature, reconsider the SEAR questionnaire for men with ED. Data were combined from two 12-week, double-blind, placebo-controlled, flexible-dose sildenafil trials having identical protocols: one conducted in the United States and the other in Mexico, Brazil, Australia, and Japan (Cappelleri et al., 2008). Response categories of each SEAR item used a 4-week reference period and were based on a 5-point scale (1 = almost never/never, 2 = a few times, 3 = sometimes, 4 = most times, and 5 = almost always/always). The difference (sildenafil vs placebo) in the change from baseline to week 12 was evaluated with the Wilcoxon rank-sum test using ridit analysis (Donaldson, 1998; Acion et al., 2006; Cappelleri et al., 2008).

The probability of increased psychosocial benefit from baseline to week 12 was higher with sildenafil for each SEAR item (two-sided $p < 0.001$) and ranged from 0.60 ("My partner was unhappy with the quality of our sexual relations" [item reverse-scored]) to 0.72 ("I was satisfied with my sexual performance"). Across all items, the average probability was 0.67 (SD of 0.04) that a randomly selected patient in the sildenafil group would have a more favorable psychosocial change relative to a randomly selected patient in the placebo group (Cappelleri et al., 2008).

11.2.3 Responder Analysis and Cumulative Proportions

According to the FDA final guidance on PRO measures for a label claim, it is recommended to display individual responses using *a priori* responder definition: the threshold value on an individual's PRO change score that is to be interpreted as a treatment benefit (FDA, 2009; McLeod et al., 2011; Cappelleri et al., 2013). The proportion of subjects meeting the responder definition can then be reported for each treatment group and compared between groups. The responder definition is determined empirically and may vary by target population or other clinical trial design characteristics.

Responder analysis is a determined attempt to understand whether the effect of an intervention, shown to be statistically significant on a PRO measurement scale, has clinical significance. While it has defenders (Lewis, 2004), its limitations have been reported (Senn, 2003; Farrar et al., 2006; Snapinn and Jiang, 2007; Cappelleri et al., 2009b; Kunz, 2011). Limitations include the expected reduction in statistical power when moving from a continuous to binary outcome and, when not assessed empirically and justifiably, the potential for an arbitrary cutoff score to bifurcate or separate responders from nonresponders. Responder analysis is best positioned as a descriptive display and as an adjunct to—as a complement and supplement to—the main analysis based on the full original scale of measurement using established statistical methods (e.g., repeated measures or random coefficient models when the data are longitudinal).

By itself a responder analysis is strictly based on the distribution of the data. But when combined with an anchor-based method, which can give empirical justification for different responder levels, responder analysis can lend significant clinical import and context to PRO measures. Hence, anchor-based methods can provide empiric evidence for any responder definition. As described earlier, anchor-based methods explore the associations between the targeted concept of the PRO instrument and the concept measured by the anchor (or anchors). To be useful, the anchors chosen should be easier to interpret than the PRO measure itself and should correlate well with the PRO measure.

A cumulative distribution function (CDF) can display a continuous plot of the change from baseline on the horizontal axis and the cumulative percentage of patients experiencing up to that change on the vertical axis, which negates the need for a specific responder definition. Consider a situation where lower change or more negative scores are better or more favorable (Figure 11.19). Along the vertical axis in Figure 11.19, it can be seen that 70% of the subjects in the experimental group had scores of 10 or less (lower is better) compared with 55% of the subjects in the control group. The consistent horizontal separation between the distribution functions suggests that the experimental treatment was beneficial relative to control over the entire range of changes. Alternatively, a cumulative distribution plot can be portrayed as an inverse CDF (one minus the CDF) with a continuous plot

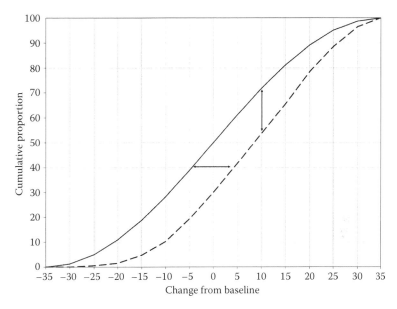

FIGURE 11.19
Illustrative cumulative distribution functions of two treatments groups where more negative
change scores are better (sold line, experimental group; dashed line, control group).

of a given change from baseline on the horizontal X-axis and the percent of
patients experiencing at least that change on the vertical Y-axis.

A key point here is that cumulative distribution plots, be they a CDF or one
minus it, be labeled and specified clearly to allow for easy and clear interpretation with respect to the directionality of score changes (e.g., do positive
changes indicate improvement or deterioration?) and their associated percentages of patients. Such cumulative distribution response curves, one for
each intervention (treatment) group, would allow for a variety of response
thresholds to be examined simultaneously and would encompass all data.

Cumulative distribution plots are most compelling and best suited for
interpretation when there is minimal overlap in the curves between treatments. When there is some or considerable overlap, the cumulative treatment
curves interact and interpretation gets clouded. In such a case, judgment is
needed on what cutoff scores are considered clinically most plausible. When
dropout is informative, a CDF with dropouts assigned the worst possible
score has merit, as does a nonparametric test (e.g., Wilcoxon's rank-sum test)
in which dropouts are assigned the worst ranks (Lachin, 1999).

Graphs on cumulative proportions based on improvement generally
define "improvement" based on changes on one side of zero in the favorable
direction, but some other number may be justified and chosen. In addition,
responder analysis and cumulative proportions need not be based necessarily on change scores; they can, in principle, be based on posttreatment scores.

Cumulative proportion of responder's analysis (CPRA) is a modification on a CDF analysis and considers only subjects who improved (Farrar et al., 2006). A CPRA graph presents the cumulative proportion of patients who achieved a specific response level as improvement from baseline, determined by levels of response from lowest to highest. The response level may be absolute change from baseline or percentage change from baseline; which one to use depends on the clinical and analytical context. Cut-off points for response levels can be shown on the X-axis (horizontal axis) and graphed against the percentage (or proportions) of responders that are equal to or more favorable than the particular level of response shown on the Y-axis (vertical axis).

As an adaptation of CPRA, the application of area under the curve (AUC) to a responder analysis has been proposed to encompass all relevant responder information and to enrich the interpretation of responder curves for different treatments (Cappelleri et al., 2009b). This AUC approach incorporates all available data on responders, not just a slice at a given cutoff or threshold score (e.g., proportion of patients with at least 50% pain improvement from baseline), and sweeps across all possible improvement scores and then integrates results. This approach invites CPRAs to be interpreted as if all responders in given intervention group have improved (on average) by a certain value (e.g., by a certain percentage if the responder metric is percentage change from baseline) in characterizing and profiling the average *responder*. In contrast, the typical or traditional responder analysis informs on the magnitude of the average *response* or, in other words, the average percentage of response among subjects who are taken to have responded (as defined to have improved by at least a certain response level).

A limitation of the CPRA approach and its AUC metric is that it considers only patients who were defined as responders and does not consider patients who did not respond on a PRO measure. For a balanced perspective, nonresponder profiles of subjects who did not respond (i.e., who worsened or otherwise fell short of meeting the responder criterion) within a given intervention group should also be depicted and summarized by considering only nonresponders (Bushmakin et al., 2011). An examination of both responder profiles and nonresponder profiles envelopes the entire span of the data in order to understand both treatment response and treatment nonresponse on a PRO measure.

11.2.4 Simulated Example: CDF Plots

In Section 11.1.6 (Figure 11.10) a simulated dataset was created to illustrate the SAS implementation of calculations for the CID. This dataset has all the information needed to create CDF plots. The first variable needed is ChangeScorePct, which represents percent change from baseline for the PRO measure of interest and which was originally intended in Section 11.1.6 to estimate the CIPC. Before creating these CDF plots, though, we need to select a particular time point. In the example in Figure 11.20, we selected the last visit (visit 7) from the previously simulated dataset in Figure 11.10. Note that the SAS code from Figure 11.20 should be run after the SAS code from Figure 11.10.

Figure 11.21 shows the resulting CDF plots for the three treatment groups, each of which resembles a step-function plot. These step-function plots were the result of a small number of available observations for the last visit in this simulated study. If the SAS code is changed by selecting data only from visit 3, for example, the CDF plots will be more smooth (see Figure 11.22) because more

```
Data _mixed_3_cdf;
Set  _mixed_2;
Where Visit=7;
Run;

    ods graphics on /HEIGHT=600PX WIDTH=1000PX IMAGEFMT=BMP;
    Proc Capability data=_mixed_3_cdf noprint;
       Class Treatment;
       cdf ChangeScorePct /overlay
              vref = 0 to 100 by 20
                                   ;

    Run;
    ods graphics off;
```

FIGURE 11.20
Creating CDF plots using SAS Proc Capability.

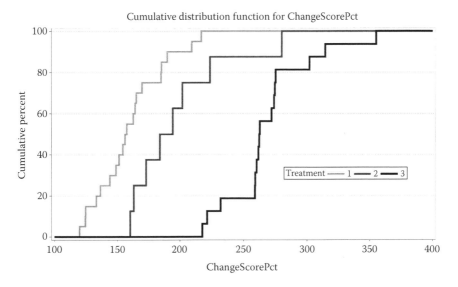

FIGURE 11.21
CDF plots at visit 7.

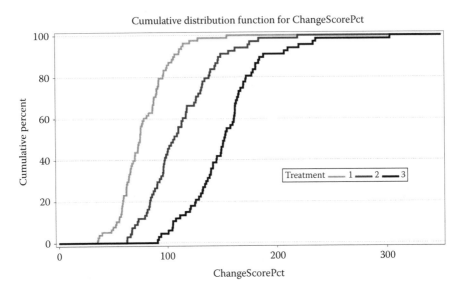

FIGURE 11.22
CDF plots at visit 3.

subjects are available for analysis. This depiction highlights the need to consider some kind of imputation technique for missing values if all subjects are to be included in the CDF analysis. Otherwise the CDF analysis will be based on only complete cases which would result in a biased representation if they (CDF plots) are not representative of all cases (those both missing and nonmissing).

11.3 Multiple Testing

It has been well-recognized, especially for regulatory purposes, that multiple comparisons of drug treatments can erroneously result in statistically significant findings. Because data on a particular PRO measure is usually measured over a number of time points, and because the same study may comprise multiple PRO instrument (or multiple subscales within the same PRO instrument) as well as non-PRO endpoints, it becomes important to describe in the statistical analysis plan how to deal with this multiplicity issue, especially if the evaluation in the clinical trial is intended for label claims based on PRO measures. Several methods can be applied to address the multiple testing (Dmitrienko et al., 2005, 2010; Fairclough, 2010).

One of the methods for inferential purposes is to use summary measures or summary statistics. For instance, a single measure can be constructed by aggregating data across different domains on the same questionnaire if such aggregation is justified clinically and statistically. Such a summary measure can be used as the primary endpoint for hypothesis testing and, consequently, prevents the concern of repeated statistical testing on multiple individual domains of the same instrument, which should be reported as well and considered supplemental.

Summary statistics can be constructed on a particular subscale or domain of an instrument to summarize its repeated observations over time on an individual and then across individuals in the same treatment group. Examples include, for each treatment group, the average of the within-subject posttreatment values, area under growth curve, and time to reach a peak or a prespecified value. The use of such summary statistics begins with the construction of a summary statistic for each individual, follows with the analysis of the summary statistic across individuals within the same group, and then continues with a corresponding between-group comparison. For instance, each individual has its own rate of change over time, these rates of change are then averaged (by taking their mean) across individuals within the same group, and finally these average rates of change are compared between treatment groups.

A potential problem with the use of summary score is that significant changes in some specific domains may be masked and what is really measured may become clouded or convoluted, resulting in low confidence about the effect of treatment as measured by the summary score.

Another way to minimize the problem of multiplicity is to restrict the number of key domains and time points, no more than a few. These key domains at specific time points should be prespecified in the statistical analysis plan as primary endpoints for statistical inference. Other domains at other time points may be regarded as secondary endpoints. While this recommendation provides a straightforward way to handle the multiplicity issue, a major challenge is how to select the most appropriate domains and time points. One way to address this challenge is to rely on substantive knowledge, well-grounded theory, and research objectives in tandem with the nature of the disease and the intended effects of the interventions.

Often several multiple endpoints, both PRO and non-PRO endpoints, would be of clinical interest for regulatory label claim. One suitable method is to test them using a gate-keeping strategy whereby secondary endpoints are analyzed and tested inferentially in a prespecified sequential order only after success on a primary endpoint (FDA, 2009). More generally, the key endpoints are ranked from most important to least important from the list of endpoints considered most relevant. This process can be done using a sequential method by testing additional endpoints in a defined sequence each at the usual alpha at the 0.05 level of statistical significance. The inferential analyses on a PRO measure for a regulatory claim cease when a failure (lack of significance) occurs. Analyses on any remaining endpoints, which are no longer part of the regulatory claim, should still be performed and reported for full disclosure and supplemental purposes. In the gate-keeping approach, then, it becomes important that the clinical trial protocol specify all relevant primary and secondary endpoints, and their order for inferential analysis and testing.

The issue of multiplicity can also be addressed in several other ways including through *p*-value adjustment (Dmitrienko et al., 2005, 2010; Fairclough, 2010). Three types of *p*-value adjustment are commonly considered: (1) the Bonferroni method, (2) the Bonferroni–Holm (step-down) method, and (3) the Hochberg (step-up) method. Of the three methods, the Bonferroni's procedure is the most conservative. In contrast, the Holm's procedure and Hochberg's method are generally more accurate and preferable.

11.4 Summary

Useful interpretation of score values or score changes on PRO measures can be valuable in designing studies, evaluating interventions, educating consumers, and informing health policymakers involved with regulatory, reimbursement, and advisory agencies. Unlike certain "objective" outcomes like blood pressure, subjective outcomes often lack the historical, empirical, and clinical thread to draw from for meaningful interpretation. This chapter focuses on enriching and enhancing the interpretation of PRO measures, a central topic commensurate with their impact. The logic and rationale of two broad methods—anchor-based and distribution-based—are elucidated. Several anchor-based approaches are highlighted: percentages based on thresholds, criterion-group interpretation, content-based interpretation, and clinically important difference. Distribution-based approaches include ES, probability of relative benefit, responder analysis, and cumulative proportions. Applications using published examples and simulated tutorials are provided to complement and supplement the exposition. Multiple testing of PRO measures can affect interpretation by rendering a false claim on a significantly significant result on a PRO measure between treatments. A general appreciation of multiple testing is highlighted.

Acknowledgment

This chapter draws directly in part from Cappelleri and Bushmakin, in press.

References

Acion, L., Peterson, J.L., Temple, S., and S. Arndt. 2006. Probabilistic index: An intuitive non-parametric approach to measuring the size of treatment effects. *Statistics in Medicine* 25:591–602.

Agresti, A. 2012. *Categorical Data Analysis*, 3rd edition. Hoboken, NJ: John Wiley & Sons.

Althof, S.E., Cappelleri, J.C., Shpilsky, A., Stecher, V., Diuguid, C., Sweeney, M., and S. Duttagupta. 2003. Treatment responsiveness of the Self-Esteem And Relationship (SEAR) questionnaire in erectile dysfunction. *Urology* 61:888–893.

Arostegui, I., Núñez-Antón, V., and J.M. Quintan. 2012. Statistical approaches to analyse patient-reported outcomes as response variables: An application to health-related quality of life. *Statistical Methods in Medical Research* 21:189–214.

Bennett, R.M., Bushmakin, A.G., Cappelleri, J.C., Zlateva, G., and A.B. Sadosky. 2009. Minimally clinically important difference in the Fibromyalgia Impact Questionnaire (FIQ). *Journal of Rheumatology* 36:1304–1311.

Bond, T.G. and C.M. Fox. 2007. *Apply the Rasch Model: Fundamental Measurement in the Human Sciences*, 2nd edition. Mahwah, NJ: Lawrence Erlbaum.

Bushmakin, A.G., Cappelleri, J.C., Zlateva, G., and A. Sadosky. 2011. Applying area-under-the-curve analysis to enhance interpretation of response profiles: An application to sleep quality scores in patients with fibromyalgia. *Quality of Life Research* 20:491–498.

Cappelleri, J.C. and A.G. Bushmakin. in press. Interpretation of patient-reported outcomes. *Statistical Methods in Medical Research*. Published online 19 February 2013. E-pub ahead of print. DOI: 10.1177/0962280213476377.

Cappelleri, J.C., Althof, S.E., O'Leary, M.P., and L.J. Tseng on behalf of the US and International SEAR Study Group. 2008. Analysis of single items on the Self-Esteem And Relationship questionnaire in men treated with sildenafil citrate for erectile dysfunction: Results of two double-blind placebo-controlled trials. *BJU International* 101:861–866.

Cappelleri, J.C., Bell, S.S., Althof, S.E., Siegel, R.L., and V.J. Stecher. 2006. Comparison between sildenafil-treated subjects with erectile dysfunction and control subjects on the Self-Esteem And Relationship questionnaire. *Journal of Sexual Medicine* 3:274–282.

Cappelleri, J.C., Bell, S.S., and R.L. Siegel. 2007. Interpretation of a self-esteem subscale for erectile dysfunction by cumulative logit model. *Drug Information Journal* 41:723–732.

Cappelleri, J.C., Bushmakin, A.G., McDermott, A., Dukes, E., Sadosky, A., Petrie, C.D., and S. Martin. 2009a. Measurement properties of the Medical Outcomes Study Sleep Scale in patients with fibromyalgia. *Sleep Medicine* 10:766–770.

Cappelleri, J.C., Bushmakin, A.G., Zlateva, G., and A. Sadosky. 2009b. Pain responder analysis: Use of area under the curve to enhance interpretation of clinical trial results. *Pain Practice* 9:348–353.

Cappelleri, J.C., Rosen, R.C., Smith, M.D., Quirk, F., Maytom, M.C., Mishra, A., and I.H. Osterloh. 1999. Some developments on the International Index of Erectile Function (IIEF). *Drug Information Journal* 33:179–190.

Cappelleri, J.C., Zou, K.H., Bushmakin, A.G., Carlsson, M.O., and T. Symonds. 2013. Cumulative response curves to enhance interpretation of treatment differences on the Self-Esteem And Relationship questionnaire for men with erectile dysfunction. *BJU International* 11:E115–E120.

Chang, C.H. and B.B. Reeve. 2005. Item response theory and its applications to patient-reported outcomes measurement. *Evaluation in the Health Professions* 28:264–282.

Cohen, J. 1998. *Statistical Power Analysis for the Behavioral Sciences*, 2nd edition. Hillsdale, NJ: Lawrence Erlbaum.

Copay, A.G., Subach, B.R., Glassman, S.D., Polly, D.W. Jr., and T.C. Schuler. 2007. Understanding the minimum clinically important difference: A review of concepts and methods. *The Spine Journal* 7:541–546.

Crosby, R.D., Kolotkin, R.L., and G.R. Williams. 2003. Defining clinically meaningful change in health-related quality of life. *Journal of Clinical Epidemiology* 56:395–340.

de Ayala, R.J. 2009. *The Theory and Practice of Item Response Theory*. New York, NY: Guilford Press.

Dmitrienko, A., Molenberghs, G., Chuang-Stein, C., and W. Offen. 2005. *Analysis of Clinical Trials Using SAS®: A Practical Guide*. Cary, NC: SAS Institute Inc.

Dmitrienko, A., Tamhane, A.C., and F. Bretz (editors). 2010. *Multiple Testing Problems in Pharmaceutical Statistics*. Boca Raton, FL: Chapman & Hall/CRC.

Donaldson, G.W. 1998. Ridit scores for analysis and interpretation of ordinal pain data. *European Journal of Pain* 2:221–227.

Fairclough, D.L. 2004. Patient-reported outcomes as endpoints in medical research. *Statistical Methods in Medical Research* 13:115–138.

Fairclough, D.L. 2010. *Design and Analysis of Quality of Life Studies in Clinical Trials*, 2nd edition. Boca Raton, FL: Chapman & Hall/CRC.

Farrar, J.T., Dworkin, R.H., and M.B. Max. 2006. Use of the cumulative proportion of responders analysis graph to present pain data over a range of cut-off points: Making clinical trial data more understandable. *Journal of Pain and Symptom Management* 31:369–377.

Fayers, F.M. and D. Machin. 2007. *Quality of Life: The Assessment, Analysis and Interpretation of Patient-Reported Outcomes*, 2nd edition. Chichester, England: John Wiley & Sons Ltd.

Food and Drug Administration (FDA). 2009. Guidance for industry on patient-reported outcome measures: Use in medical product development to support labeling claims. *Federal Register* 74(235):65132–65133. http://www.fda.gov/Drugs/DevelopmentApprovalProcess/DrugDevelopmentToolsQualificationProgram/ucm284399.htm. (Accessed on August 31, 2013)

Guyatt, G.H., Osoba, D., Wu, A., Wyrwich, K.W., Norman, G.R., and the Clinical Significance Consensus Meeting Group. 2003. Methods to explain the clinical significance of health status measures. *Mayo Clinic Proceedings* 77:371–383.

Hambleton, R.K., Swaminathan, H., and H.J. Rogers. 1991. *Fundamentals of Item Response Theory*. Newbury Park, CA: Sage Publications.

Hays, R.D., Farivar, S.S., and H. Liu. 2005. Approaches and recommendations for estimating minimally important difference for health-related quality of life measures. *Journal of Chronic Obstructive Pulmonary Disease* 2:63–67.

Hosmer, D.W., Jr., Lemeshow, S., and R.X. Sturdivant. 2013. *Applied Logistic Regression*, 3rd edition. Hoboken, NJ: John Wiley & Sons.

Julious, S.A. 2009. *Sample Size for Clinical Trials*. London, England: Chapman & Hall/CRC.

Julious, S.A. and S.J. Walters. In press. Estimating effect sizes for health related quality of life outcomes. *Statistical Methods in Medical Research*. Published online 19 February 2013. E-pub ahead of print. DOI: 10.1177/0962280213476379.

Kazis, L.E., Anderson, J.J., and R.F. Meenan. 1989. Effect sizes for interpreting changes in health status. *Medical Care* 27:S178–S189.

Kendall, P.C., Marrs-Garcia, A., Nath, S.R., and R.C. Sheldrick. 1999. Normative comparisons for the evaluation of clinical significance. *Journal of Consulting and Clinical Psychology* 7:285–299.

King, M.T. 2011. A point of minimal important difference (MID): A critique of terminology and methods. *Expert Reviews in Pharmacoeconomics & Outcomes Research* 11:171–184.

Kleinbaum, D. and M. Klein. 2010. *Logistic Regression*, 3rd edition. New York, NY: Springer.

Kunz, M. 2011. On responder analyses when a continuous variable is dichotomized and measurement error is present. *Biometrical Journal* 53:137–155.

Lachin, J.M. 1999. Worst-rank score analysis with informatively missing observations in clinical trials. *Controlled Clinical Trials* 20:408–422.

Lall, R., Campbell, M.J., Walters, S.J., and K. Morgan. 2002. A review of ordinal regression models applied on health-related quality of life assessments. *Statistical Methods in Medical Research* 11:49–67.

Lewis, J.A. 2004. In defence of the dichotomy. *Pharmaceutical Statistics* 3:77–79.

Lipsey, M.W. and D.B. Wilson. 2001. *Practical Meta-Analysis*. Thousand Oaks, CA: Sage Publications.

Liu, J.-P. 2003. Equivalence trials. In Chow, S.-C. (editor). *Encyclopedia of Biopharmaceutical Statistics*, 2nd edition, revised and expanded. New York, NY: Marcel Dekker, pp. 327–332.

Luo, X., Cappelleri, J.C., Cella, D., Li, J.Z., Charbonneau, C., Kim, S.T., Chen, I., and R.J. Motzer. 2009. Using the Rasch model to validate and enhance the interpretation of the Functional Assessment of Cancer Therapy-Kidney Symptom Index-Disease Related Symptoms. *Value in Health* 12:580–586.

Lydick, E. and R.S. Epstein. 1993. Interpretation of quality of life changes. *Quality of Life Research* 2:221–226.

Marquis, P., Chassany, O., and L. Abetz. 2004. A comprehensive strategy for the interpretation of quality-of-life data based on existing methods. *Value in Health* 7:93–104.

Massof, R.W. In press. A general theoretical framework of interpreting patient-reported outcomes estimated from ordinally scaled item responses. *Statistical Methods in Medical Research*. Published online 19 February 2013. E-pub ahead of print. DOI: 10.1177/0962280213476380.

McLeod, L.D., Coon, C.D., Martin, S.A., Fehnel, S.E., and R.D. Hays. 2011. Interpreting patient-reported outcome results: US FDA guidance and emerging methods. *Expert Reviews of Pharmacoeconomics & Outcomes Research* 11:163–169.

O'Connell, A.A. 2005. *Logistic Regression Models for Ordinal Response Variables*. Thousand Oaks, CA: Sage Publications.

O'Leary, M.P., Althof, S.E., Cappelleri, J.C., Crowley, A., Sherman, N., and S. Duttagupta on behalf of the US SEAR Study Group. 2006. Self-esteem, confidence, and relationship satisfaction in men with erectile dysfunction treated with sildenafil citrate: A multicenter, randomized, parallel-group, double-blind, placebo-controlled study in the United States. *Journal of Urology* 175:1058–1062.

Revicki, D., Erickson, P.A., Sloan, J.A., Dueck, A., Guess, H., Santanello, N.C., and the Mayo/FDA Patient-Reported Outcomes Consensus Meeting Group. 2007. Interpreting and reporting results based on patient-reported outcomes. *Value in Health* 10:S116–S124.

Rogers, J., Howard, K.I., and J.T. Vessey. 1993. Using significance tests to evaluate equivalence between two experimental groups. *Psychological Bulletin* 113:553–565.

SAS Institute Inc. 2011. *SAS/STAT® 9.3 User's Guide*, 2nd edition. Cary, NC: SAS Institute Inc.

Schünemann, H.J., Akl, E.A., and G.H. Guyatt. 2006. Interpreting the results of patient reported outcomes in clinical trials: The clinician's perspective. *Health and Quality of Life Outcomes* 4:62.

Sechrest, L., McKnight, P., and K. McKnight. 1996. Calibration of measures for psychotherapy outcome studies. *American Psychologist* 51:1065–1071.

Senn, S. 2003. Disappointing dichotomies. *Pharmaceutical Statistics* 2:239–240.

Snapinn, S.M. and Q. Jiang. 2007. Responder analysis and the assessment of a clinically relevant treatment effect. *Trials* 8:31.

Steiger, J.H. 2004. Beyond the F test: Effect size confidence intervals and tests of close fit in the analysis of variance and contrast analysis. *Psychological Methods* 9:164–182.

Testa, M.A. and D.C. Simonson. 1996. Assessment of quality-of-life outcomes. *New England Journal of Medicine* 334:835–840.

Thompson, J.R., Cappelleri, J.C., Getter, C., Pleil, A., Reichel, M., and S. Wolf. 2007. Enhanced interpretation of instrument scales using the Rasch model. *Drug Information Journal* 41:541–550.

Ware, J.E., Kosinski, M., and S.D. Keller. 1994. *SF-36 Physical and Mental Health Summary Scales: A User's Manual*. Boston, MA: The Health Institute, New England Medical Center.

Ware, J.E., Snow, K.K., and M. Kosinski. 2000. *SF-36 Health Survey: Manual and Interpretation Guide*. Lincoln, RI: QualityMetric Incorporated.

Westlake, W.J. 1981. Bioequivalence testing—Response. *Biometrics* 37:591–593.

Index